Health Promotion

Global Principles and Practice

Health Promotion

Global Principles and Practice

Rachael Dixey

And co-authors:

Ruth Cross

Sally Foster

Diane Lowcock

Ivy O'Neil

Jane South

Louise Warwick-Booth

Judy White

James Woodall

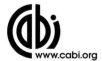
www.cabi.org

CABI is a trading name of CAB International

CABI	CABI
Nosworthy Way	38 Chauncey Street
Wallingford	Suite 1002
Oxfordshire OX10 8DE	Boston, MA 02111
UK	USA

Tel: +44 (0)1491 832111	Tel: +1 800 552 3083 (toll free)
Fax: +44 (0)1491 833508	Tel: +1 (0)617 395 4051
E-mail: info@cabi.org	E-mail: cabi-nao@cabi.org
Website: www.cabi.org	

A catalogue record for this book is available from the British Library, London, UK.

Library of Congress Cataloging-in-Publication Data

Health promotion : global principles and practice / Rachael Dixey ... [et al.].
   p. ; cm.
 Includes bibliographical references and index.
 ISBN 978-1-84593-972-4 (alk. paper)
 I. Dixey, Rachael. II. C.A.B. International.
 [DNLM: 1. Health Promotion. 2. Community Health Planning. 3. Health Communication. 4. Health Policy. 5. Socioeconomic Factors. 6. World Health. WA 530.1]

 613--dc23

2012013388

ISBN: 978 1 84593 972 4

Commissioning editor: Rachel Cutts
Editorial assistant: Alexandra Lainsbury
Production editor: Tracy Head

Typeset by SPi, Pondicherry, India.
Printed and bound by Gutenberg Press Ltd, Tarxien, Malta.

Contents

The Authors   vii

Introduction   ix
Rachael Dixey

1   The Foundations of Health Promotion   1
Rachael Dixey, Ruth Cross, Sally Foster and James Woodall

2   Healthy Communities   30
Louise Warwick-Booth, Sally Foster and Judy White

3   Healthy Public Policy   54
Louise Warwick-Booth, Rachael Dixey and Jane South

4   Communicating Health   78
Ruth Cross, Ivy O'Neil and Rachael Dixey

5   Practising Health Promotion   107
Rachael Dixey, James Woodall and Diane Lowcock

6   Towards the Future of Health Promotion   143
Rachael Dixey

References   183

Index   221

The Authors

Rachael Dixey

Rachael is Professor of Health Promotion at Leeds Metropolitan University. She has a lifelong interest in the politics of health, and in Africa, having lived or worked in a number of African countries. She has a background in development and education. More recently, she has worked on childhood obesity and currently has an interest in health in prisons. She is also involved in developing the public health workforce internationally. Until 2011, she led the Health Promotion group at Leeds Met but is now concentrating more on writing, and developing the Institute of Health and Wellbeing at Leeds Met. She has a long experience in teaching at postgraduate level and in supervising PhD students. She wrote most of Chapters 1, 5 and 6, and contributed to Chapters 3 and 4. She also edited the book.

Ruth Cross

Ruth is Senior Lecturer in Public Health – Health Promotion. She has wide experience in health, health care services and health promotion both in the UK and in sub-Saharan Africa. Ruth contributes to the MSc Public Health – Health Promotion at Leeds Metropolitan University and the two transnational Master's programmes taught in West and sub-Saharan Africa facilitating learning around the foundations of health promotion, health communication, health behaviour and research methods. Ruth wrote half of Chapter 4, and has contributed to Chapters 1, 5 and 6.

Sally Foster

Sally is a Senior Lecturer at Leeds Metropolitan University and a sociologist by background. She has a lifetime's experience of working in higher education, and has a keen understanding of the needs of students for thought-provoking literature. She has recently been involved in researching solid waste management in Tanzania and Zambia, and has interests in women's health, the politics of health and development. She contributed to Chapter 2, and provided material on lay perspectives throughout the book.

Diane Lowcock

Diane is a Senior Lecturer in Health Promotion and has taught research methods and epidemiology at Leeds Metropolitan University since 2005. In her previous role as a public health specialist, she worked with primary care teams in developing a wider health promotion agenda and became interested in the nature of evidence and how it is used in practice to make decisions. She has worked on several research projects within the Centre for Health Promotion Research at Leeds Met, including evaluations of health trainers and self-care in primary care. She contributed the material on evidence-based practice and evaluation in Chapter 5.

Ivy O'Neil

Ivy is a Principal Lecturer and the Course Leader for MSc Public Health – Health Promotion. Her background is in nursing. She is also a Registered Midwife, a Registered Sick Children's Nurse and a Health Visitor. Her MSc is in Research, undertaking primary research into health needs assessment of the health needs of ethnic minority families. She has over 20 years' clinical and 12 years' academic experience. She currently teaches health promotion on a range of health-related under/post-graduate courses within the Faculty.

Her research interests are in health needs assessment, promoting child, young person and family health. She also has an interest in education within the higher education sector and is currently doing an Education Doctorate degree looking into the public health workforce development and the education of public health practitioners. She wrote half of Chapter 4.

Jane South

Jane is Professor of Healthy Communities and Director of the Centre for Health Promotion Research, Leeds Metropolitan University. She has wide experience of research on community-based health promotion, and co-authored a textbook on evaluation for public health practice published by the Open University Press in 2006. Her research interests are focused on community involvement in health and she was the lead investigator on the People in Public Health study that aimed to build understanding of approaches involving volunteers and lay health workers in delivering health programmes. Jane started her professional life as a nurse but moved into health promotion research in 1997 after gaining a Masters in Policy Studies. She worked at the University of Bradford on the evaluation of the Health Action Zone before returning to Leeds Met in 2002. Since then she has built up a portfolio of community research projects and publications, along with developing innovative tools for practice including evaluation and planning frameworks. Jane has jointly authored Chapter 3 as well as contributing the Hamara case study in Chapter 6.

Louise Warwick-Booth

Louise is Principal Lecturer in Health Promotion and a sociologist with specific interests in health policy and social policy. She is the course leader for BSc (Hons) Public Health – Health Studies, and teaches across a range of undergraduate and postgraduate courses delivering modules including sociology, health policy and research methods. Her current research interests are focused around healthy communities and her PhD was concerned with regeneration. Louise wrote parts of Chapter 2 as well as most of Chapter 3.

Judy White

Judy worked for 10 years in the voluntary and community sector and then for 22 years in health promotion in Bradford before coming to work for Leeds Metropolitan University in 2008. She is currently a senior lecturer involved in teaching, evaluation and research primarily in relation to healthy communities, health trainers and community health champions. Judy was responsible for writing the sections in Chapter 2 on community development.

James Woodall

James is a Senior Lecturer in Health Promotion at Leeds Metropolitan University and teaches primarily on their MSc Public Health – Health Promotion degree. His PhD explored the health-promoting prison and how values central to health promotion are applied in the context of imprisonment. James has published in a number of areas related to prison and offender health, including prisoners' lay views on health, the mental health of prisoners and young offenders, the role of prison visitors' centres in reducing health inequalities and the health needs of prison staff. James has also published more broadly on empowerment in health promotion and the contribution that lay people can make to the public health agenda. He contributed most of the section on empowerment in Chapter 1, and the section on settings in Chapter 5.

Introduction

RACHAEL DIXEY

This book is not a guide to 'how to do health promotion'. There are plenty of good books already published that can help with that (Naidoo and Wills, 2000, 2005; Ewles and Simnett, 2003; Hubley and Copeman, 2008), whilst the Health Promotion Glossary provides an explanation of key terms (Nutbeam, 1998b; Smith *et al.*, 2006). Others develop in some detail how to plan, implement and evaluate health promotion (Tones and Tilford, 2001; Green and Tones, 2010). These books are useful further reading in terms of the practice of health promotion. There are a number of books that, although written some time ago, still provide useful chapters debating important aspects of health promotion, such as Sidell *et al.* (1997). Our book aims to set out some of the key principles and ideas or, in more academic terms, to explore the discourse surrounding health promotion in the 21st century. It attempts not only to explore what health promotion is, but also to ask some uncomfortable questions about health promotion – in short, to be critical of it. Being critical, according to some, is what defines our age (Jencks, 2007) – being sceptical and asking questions. This is also the state of mind that postgraduate study encourages, and this book is aimed at the postgraduate reader. As such, then, this book *does* aim to be a guide to 'how to think about health promotion'. It also shows how ideas drawn from social science can aid health promotion theory and practice, and ends by attempting to bring together some of the ideas that might be helpful for the next decades. However, it cannot hope to be comprehensive, and there will be authors and ideas that others might feel should have been included.

It is ambitious to write a book with global relevance, but we believe that wherever health promotion is practised, whether in the rich countries of the global North, middle-income countries or the poorest of the global South, this book will have some use. Although it is written by authors based in the global North, we do teach in the global South; we teach students from all over the globe, and we have used the book to raise issues for practice all over the world.

The book aims to ask some challenging questions, some of which concern a series of implementation gaps – gaps between the rhetoric and the reality in terms of closing inequalities in health, for instance. Why do such glaring inequalities exist between the health of those in the richest and poorest countries, and between groups within the same societies, and has the development of the modern health promotion movement done anything to tackle those inequalities? Another 'gap' is that between the ideology of 'empowerment', 'involvement' or 'participation', and whether any of these concepts have materialized on the ground. Have any of the power structures that shape the determinants of health been changed by the efforts of health promoters and are people any more 'empowered' to take control of the social determinants of their health? A further implementation gap is the failure of many countries to take on the principles of health promotion as in the Ottawa Charter, and instead have approaches to health that are dominated by the medical model and that are not concerned with tackling the social determinants of health. These themes will be returned to later.

The book emerges at a time of changing global governance of health; health, as a 'global public good' (Kickbusch 2005, p. xiii) in a 'borderless world' means that 'a new conceptualisation of health as a new form of global politics' has emerged.

> In health promotion terms this gives a totally new meaning to what we define as healthy public policy. Health is now part of foreign policy, security policy, trade and economic policy and geopolitics. Increasingly therefore in macro terms health is being seen as being 'at the core of human development'.
>
> (Kickbusch, 2005, pp. xiii–xiv)

With the blurring of the boundaries between the public and the private sectors, the relative decline of the power of the WHO and the emergence of new and powerful players (such as the Bill & Melinda Gates Foundation), there are concerns about who sets the direction of global health priorities.

The book thus aims not only to understand global health and global health promotion, but also to ask whether the foundation stones of modern health promotion, principally in the Ottawa Charter of 1986, provide a sound enough foundation in a new century, in which globalization has accelerated and the world has altered in key ways, resulting in new health challenges.

A further aim of the book is to introduce key thinkers in health promotion such as Ilona Kickbusch, whom we have just mentioned and who would qualify as one of the main shapers of the modern health promotion movement, but, of course, there are many others. In this sense, the book describes the 'epistemic community' that makes up health promotion. Peter Haas (1989, p. 378) first used the phrase 'epistemic community' to mean a network of professionals who not only have recognized expertise and competence but who also 'have 1) a shared set of normative and principled beliefs ... 2) shared causal beliefs which are derived from their analysis ... 3) a shared notion of validity and 4) a common policy enterprise'. Or, according to Antoniades (2003, p. 26), epistemic communities are conceptualized as 'socially recognized knowledge-based networks, the members of which share a common understanding of a particular problem/issue or a common worldview and seek to translate their beliefs into dominant social discourse and social practice'. We are not suggesting that everyone involved in what can be called 'health promotion' agrees conclusively on the aims, methods and principles of health promotion – it would be strange if there were no disagreements among a professional community comprising several thousand practitioners and academics operating across the globe – but we are attempting to give a sense of that community and also to articulate our own particular standpoint or 'take' on health promotion.

It is relevant in a book such as this to introduce some of the main writers and practitioners who make up this epistemic community, and to explore exactly what their 'worldview' is. What *is* their 'shared set of normative and principled beliefs', and is there a set of values and principles that forms a consensual platform, which can be called 'health promotion'? And if there is not, what are the key points of divergence? It also raises (but probably does not answer) the critical question of whether this worldview and set of principles has been translated into social discourse and social practice, i.e. whether policy makers have drawn upon this community in order to create a better, more socially just and thus healthier world. One of our concerns in the book is to consider who and what shapes the orthodoxy of health promotion and we point out where health promotion is Eurocentric. The epistemic health promotion community has a place to make its voice heard through the VHPO (Views of Health Promotion Online), which is hosted by the International Union for Health Promotion and Education (Mittlemark, 2009). The latter also has its journal, *Global Health Promotion* (Mittlemark, 2010).

What qualifies us to write this book? Leeds Metropolitan University has played a leading role in academic health promotion since 1972. At that point, three English universities were asked to provide postgraduate training for what were then called health education specialists, and later health promotion specialists. Leeds Met therefore took an early lead, and remains a foremost academic health promotion department. It has contributed a large number of key texts (Hubley, 1993; Tones and Tilford, 2001; Tones and Green, 2004; Cattan and Tilford, 2006; Green and South, 2006; Hubley and Copeman, 2008; Green and Tones, 2010; Warwick-Booth *et al.*, 2012) and has had a tradition of appointing professors of health promotion (Keith Tones, Sylvia Tilford, Jackie Green, Rachael Dixey, Jane South – the latter two are still in post) in a situation where, as an under-recognized discipline, the number of current professors of health promotion in England can be counted on one hand. The view presented in the book is from a Leeds perspective – that is where we are located – and whilst many of us have worked elsewhere and currently work overseas too, principally in Africa, it must be recognized that our view is from where we are – a country of the 'North'. The book aims to be useful for a global audience and we do, of course, include ideas from those countries that have developed academic health promotion. The book *does* present a particular perspective – it is the culmination of our teaching and thinking about health promotion – and as such the reader needs to be critical and to ask whether there are other perspectives, whether our views are partial and whether we have left out important ideas. Inevitably, we cannot cover here all there is to know about health promotion. There are many books currently available about health promotion, and anyone wanting to further their knowledge needs to sample a range.

In terms of defining health promotion, there is an apparent conundrum: on the one hand, for many (including us), health promotion is 'social movement', akin to other social movements fuelled by a concern with social justice and with injustice, such as the feminist movement or the human rights movement. Our concern is with justice in health, and this could be seen as 'big picture' health promotion. On the other hand, health promotion is often seen as synonymous with relatively small-scale activities that are labelled 'health promotion', such as handing out leaflets about healthier eating, running a cardiac rehabilitation group, developing policy for schools on sexual health for young people, delivering insecticide-treated nets to remote villages, and so on. This activity, 'small picture' health promotion is relatively 'downstream' activity (upstream and downstream will be explained later). Thus health promotion is *both* a broad social movement concerned with tackling the determinants of health and also seems to encompass the whole range of activities designed to improve health of populations and (hopefully) to address inequalities in health too. Some of those working in health promotion might not especially be aware of the bigger picture, but simply be motivated by, for example, realizing that there are educational needs of communities affected by diabetes or schistosomiasis and who want to work in more preventive ways. A look through the journals shows the wide range of issues seen as coming under the umbrella of 'health promotion', from all-embracing discussions of social determinants or global governance, to the minutiae of the delivery of the technical elements of a particular campaign or activity.

'Academic health promotion' – i.e. the writings and conference papers about health promotion and public health from academic departments within universities and other higher education institutions and also from practitioners working within major inter-state organizations, government departments and the like – might demonstrate a further 'gap'. It might be that whereas the discourse is predominantly about empowerment, community development, participation and healthy public policy, the majority of (small picture) health promotion on the ground is top-down, non-inclusive, behaviour-change approaches. Thus, students on postgraduate courses might find that what they are being asked to think about and implement is far removed from their day-to-day practice. In our experience, students are often motivated to undertake a course of study precisely because they *do* want to change their practice; very often, they are frustrated by working in predominantly curative roles. Alternatively, they might be working in 'upstream' modes within communities, and want to increase their expertise and confidence in tackling health issues. The key aim of postgraduate courses in health promotion is to provide the theoretical basis for practice; this book aims to provide that, together with critical questioning of that base. This questioning can apply equally to those currently undertaking a course of study, or those who might not be, but who simply want to inform their practice and to increase their reflection on that practice.

A further aim of the book is to comment on the state of 'academic health promotion', a theme taken up in Chapter 6. We need to ask whether the disciplinary base is adequate or relevant in the 21st century. The disciplinary base reflects the development of health promotion itself, which has evolved from health education, and from a concern with how lifestyles impact on health – in effect, with changing the knowledge, attitudes and behaviour of *individuals*. Health education sprang from the realization that modern medicine did not hold solutions to the 'lifestyle' diseases of developed nations, and was essentially an arm of the medical enterprise. It is not surprising that the primary discipline is often seen as psychology. Whilst 'psychology' *can* offer insights, there are three important points: first, 'psychology' is not one undifferentiated discipline, and there are major tensions between its various branches (and perhaps more sympathy among health promoters with critical psychology and community psychology rather than with behaviourism, for example); secondly, psychology developed as a discipline within the wealthier countries of the North, and displays a peculiarly 'Western' and individualistic view; thirdly, and most obviously, there are many disciplines that health promotion *can* draw upon, which more faithfully add value to the contemporary nature of health promotion, based as it is on healthy public policy, supportive environments and the range of activities promoted by the Ottawa Charter.

The second of these points has been made by Airhihenbuwa and Obregon (2000), that not only do Western ideas of 'psychology' fail to capture the realities of societies in which the community and family are the primary reference point for identity, but also any attempts to measure constructs developed outside of those communities can be disrespectful and lead to untrustworthy depictions of those communities. The third point, concerning the variety of disciplines available to inform health promotion thought and practice, will be expanded later in the book, with an exploration of feeder-disciplines and subject areas that health promotion can draw upon.

Our view of health promotion is that it is a social movement with the central aim of tackling the social determinants of health and so bringing about greater social justice in terms of health. Throughout, we assert that the way societies are organized has consequences for health: fairer societies lead to healthier lives. As so many aspects of the way societies are organized impact upon health, this gives us a mandate to consider a very wide range of issues – from spending on armaments, to migration, multiculturalism, climate change, women's rights, crime rates, the 'banking crisis', freedom of speech, tourism, land rights and many more. In short, health promoters do not start with blank sheets – we have to start with the messy, true-life realities of our complex world. We present a view of health promotion that has as its central aim the empowerment of communities and we emphasize the importance of working with people, not 'on' them or through them. We thus implicitly criticize top-down, behaviour-change and lifestyle approaches that attempt to manipulate people into healthier behaviours; not that we do not believe that (some) behaviours need to change – the point is the process by which these are made, and the political processes that underpin them. Health promoters often talk of 'interventions', whereas we prefer the idea of 'implementation with people'. The role of lay people will be explored later in the book.

The Structure of the Book

The organizing principle for the book is based on the postgraduate courses provided by Leeds Met. It generally follows the modules that comprise those courses, taught in Leeds, and also in Zambia and The Gambia. However, the book is very appropriate for, and applies generally to, other postgraduate courses in health promotion, as it covers areas that can be expected to be found on such courses. We start with a chapter that attempts to outline key principles and approaches, exploring the value base of health promotion and trying to define health and health promotion, and to consider how health promotion relates to 'public health'. It introduces 'threshold concepts' and those ideas and documents that are essential to know about, such as the Ottawa Charter and the Commission on the Determinants of Health.

Three chapters follow the introductory one; the second chapter explores the idea of healthy communities and why working with communities is so important. The third chapter takes up the idea of healthy public policy and explores why there is so much stress on this as an essential part of the health promotion endeavour. The fourth chapter considers communication for health, picking up the role of health education and of how people learn about health so that they can make changes as appropriate.

The fifth chapter attempts to provide ways forward in terms of implementing change, and thereby realizing the vision that health promoters espouse. It considers key aspects of practice, explaining and exploring central ideas such as evidence-based practice, evaluation, ethics, settings for health and innovative ways of providing leadership for organizational change. It introduces the attempts, such as the Galway Consensus, to outline the competencies required of health promotion practitioners.

The final chapter considers the role of the academic health promotion community and questions where health promotion is going, and its potential as a social movement to effect global health and to bring about a fairer, more just world in which everyone has good health and can achieve their potential.

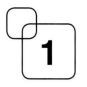

1 The Foundations of Health Promotion

RACHAEL DIXEY, RUTH CROSS, SALLY FOSTER
AND JAMES WOODALL

This chapter aims to:

- explore concepts of 'health' held by lay people and health promoters;
- introduce recent work on the social determinants of health;
- introduce certain threshold concepts including salutogenesis, social models of health and upstream thinking;
- establish the value base of health promotion;
- outline in more detail 'empowerment' as a key value in health promotion; and
- describe the key WHO conferences, which provide the milestones in the development of health promotion.

The aim of this chapter is to provide an orientation to current thinking in health promotion and offers some of the material that would be covered in an introductory module, laying the foundations for a course of study. It is essential to understand that health promotion is a political and ethical activity, with a sound value base providing the platform for practice and setting its direction.

The introductory chapter above stated that our view of health promotion is that it is a social movement with the central aim of tackling the social determinants of health and so bringing about greater social and health justice. By the 'social determinants of health' we mean those factors that enable people to live healthy and productive lives – these factors include the obvious ones of decent housing, access to education, employment opportunities, nourishing food, well-functioning and accessible health care, cohesive communities, good systems of government and peaceful, safe nation-states. Social justice is harder to define, and is often used interchangeably with related concepts such as 'fairness', 'equality' and 'equity'. Aristotle's *Ethics* suggest that equity is where like but different individuals are both regarded and treated justly because they are equally valued. Thus, regardless of ability/disability, gender, sexual orientation, ethnicity, age or any other variable that differentiates people, *all* individuals have equal value. Treating individuals with equal value is *just* and therefore contributes to

social justice. Logically, following from this is the idea that 'social goods' such as health should be distributed fairly. Harvey (1973, p. 98) in his attempt to outline the 'skeleton concept' of social justice, says that it starts with a 'just distribution justly arrived at'. We can argue that where access to a good, decent and productive life is not available to some, where some live in abject poverty and others in excessive wealth, then there is clearly not 'a just distribution'. This raises the question of whether people have the *right* to good health, and we would assert that people do indeed have the right to those determinants that produce good health. This is enshrined in the Universal Declaration of Human Rights: that people have the right to the conditions necessary to achieve the highest possible standard of health (United Nations, 1948; Marks, 2004). Health promotion has, at its heart, the drive to eliminate health inequities, if inequity means the failure to regard and treat 'like but different' individuals and groups justly because they are not equally valued.

Individual readers might pause at this point and think that they do indeed see all individuals as having equal worth. However, an extra-terrestrial being from another planet, making a visit to Earth, would plainly see that at a global scale we do not treat individuals as having equal worth – otherwise children would not be dying in the 'developing' world due to preventable diseases such as diarrhoea, respiratory infections or measles, whilst others live in unimaginable luxury. There would not be the less dramatic differences between individuals within the same country, such as in England, with children growing up in situations described as below the poverty line (for a 'developed' country) and those living in very comfortable wealth.

This central concern with health equity has been present since the Ottawa Charter, and was present in the WHO from 1946. According to Whitehead and Dahlgren (2007, p. 5), health equity

> ... implies that ideally everyone could attain their full health potential and that no one should be disadvantaged from achieving this potential because of their social position or other socially determined circumstance. This refers to everyone and not just to a particularly disadvantaged segment of the population. Efforts to promote social equity in health are therefore aimed at creating opportunities and removing barriers to achieving the health potential of all people. It involves the fair distribution of resources needed for health, fair access to the opportunities available, and fairness in the support offered to people when ill.

> The outcome of these efforts would be a gradual reduction of all systematic differences in health between different socioeconomic groups. The ultimate vision is the elimination of such inequities, by levelling up to the health of the most advantaged.

The concern with health inequities recently culminated in the global health promotion community cohering behind the work of the Commission on Social Determinants of Health (CSDH). The Commission was established by the World Health Organization (WHO) in 2005 and chaired by Sir Michael Marmot. It was essentially an independent enquiry into the social and environmental issues affecting health and planned to investigate actions with the potential to promote greater health equity. The CSDH reported in August 2008 and concluded that social injustice is killing people on a grand scale. Publication was followed by a conference in London in November 2008, which constituted the first major international event to attempt to develop a global agenda to address the issues. The conference had the ambitious title of 'Closing the Gap in a Generation' and the optimistic task of turning the CSDH framework into practical action.

A paper written by Friel and other writers (2009), including Marmot, to explain the purpose of the London conference is worth considering here (and worth reading in full too). With regard to whether closing the gap in a generation is possible,

they point out that under-5 mortality in Egypt fell from 235 to 35 per 1000 live births in 40 years (to 2005). They start by asserting that 'money matters' – whereas the UK found US$900 billion and the USA US$700 billion to save the banks in the current credit crisis, the CSDH estimated that upgrading the slums where globally one billion people live, could be achieved for US$100 billion. Between US$11 and 17 billion is needed to enable every child to attain free schooling. The point they are making is that the money can be found if the political will to do so is in place. They call for social solidarity in terms of public sector leadership – to enable redistributive justice such as in tackling poverty through fairer redistribution of taxes for example – and social solidarity in terms of the power of communities. Social groups and communities could be empowered to engage in decision making and agenda setting, and to form the grassroots organizations that would lead to the 'nutcracker effect' described by Baum (2007), who was one of the CSDH commissioners. She has called for 'combining top down political commitment and

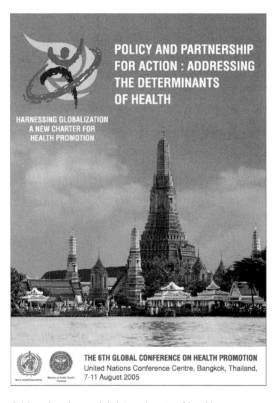

Addressing the social determinants of health.

policy action with bottom up action from communities and civil society groups' (Baum, 2007, p. 192). To turn the dream of health equity into reality, Friel *et al.* (2009) list the challenges. First is rebalancing the distribution of power and tackling the 'entrenched structural inequities' along the lines of class, education, gender, age, ethnicity, disability and geography. The CSDH calls for: the strengthening of political and legal systems to protect human rights, especially those of marginalized groups, and particularly indigenous groups; empowerment of social groups through greater representation in policy making and in grassroots action; and a fundamental shift in the balance of power. Secondly they call for engagement from political leadership at the highest levels, to commit to global health equity as a goal. Thirdly, they call for market regulation and implicitly, a reining in of the unfettered neo-liberal agenda. More will be said on this later, but basically, it calls for a return to a more welfarist and humane approach to global politics. Fourthly, they call for greater accountability so that governments can be measured on how their policies affect health inequities. This requires the development of measuring and monitoring tools so that quality of life and health status can be accurately assessed.

Fran Baum (2009, p. 72) takes up the theme of how the gap can be closed in a generation and asserts that

> ... the 21st century will be dominated by two questions: How can we learn to live within our ecological means? How can we do this in a way that is democratic and equitable? These answers will be crucial in building the global community's response to the very real threats to our collective health, especially those from global warming and persistent inequity.

She too questions the assumption that economic growth can bring about improvements to the lives of the poor and she calls for a challenge to the 'basic tenets of neo-liberalism'. (This will be returned to in Chapter 6.) Outlining a vision for 2040, she quotes the Charter of the People's Health Movement:

> Equity, ecologically-sustainable development and peace are at the heart of our vision of a better world – a world in which a healthy life for all is a reality; a world that respects, appreciates and celebrates all life and diversity; a world that enables the flowering of people's talents and abilities to enrich each other; a world in which people's voices guide the decisions that shape our lives.
>
> (Baum, 2009, p. 73)

This captures part of what health promotion is all about – that is, the wish to envision what kind of world we want to create – for ourselves and for future generations. Envisioning the future has been a central activity of health promotion since its inception at the Ottawa conference in 1986. The Ottawa Charter, coming up to its 25th anniversary, remains a central document for anyone studying health promotion. It is the cornerstone of the modern health promotion movement. Its value lies in its outline of strategies and activities to achieve health for all. Whereas 'Health for All by the Year 2000' was a call to mobilize governments, the Ottawa Charter is more of a guide to how to go about putting the vision into practice.

The central concern with the social determinants of health is what distinguishes health promotion from public health. Health promotion takes a different approach from 'mainstream' public health, and we suggest that health promotion is more a form of politics than a part of the medical enterprise – that it is more allied to social policy than it is a profession allied to medicine. The politicized nature of health promotion is captured nicely by Larsen and Manderson (2009) when they write that health promotion is about:

> ... representing marginalized populations, advocating equity, giving voice to the powerless and educating people in civic rights, democracy and politics, that is, in citizenship. In this respect, health promotion represents a humanist discourse aimed at creating a more equal and just society.
>
> (Larsen and Manderson, 2009, p. 608)

More will be said on citizenship in subsequent chapters.

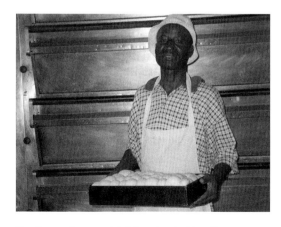

Employment – a social determinant of health.

That we do not live in an equal and just society is easy to demonstrate. Data on inequalities in health abound, whether this is within rich countries such as the UK, between richer countries, such as the USA and Japan, or in poorer countries of the global South. The reasons for the existence of these inequalities are more contentious. Wilkinson and Pickett (2009) claim to have produced an undeniable argument that inequalities in health within countries are explained by inequalities in wealth, not by the absolute wealth of that country, and that the more unequal a society, the more inequalities in health there are in that society. As epidemiologists who have worked on health inequalities, they show the socially corrosive impacts of inequality, and how 'almost everything – from life expectancy to mental illness, violence to illiteracy – is affected not by how healthy a society is, but how equal it is' (2009, back cover). Their work, *The Spirit Level*, has received a great deal of attention and also criticism. The Black Report of 1980 was the first major report in the UK to highlight how health is systematically related to social class, and it put forward a number of reasons for this. Later work has refined analysis of health inequalities, and most notably the Marmot review of the social determinants of health highlights the role of psychosocial factors in explaining the fine gradients in health between social groups.

Whilst this body of work shows that inequalities in health *do* exist, why should we be concerned? Could we not simply agree that some people will 'naturally' experience better health, and also that it is inevitable that the better off, whether in 'developed' or 'developing' countries, in 'good' jobs and living in nicer neighbourhoods, with no major stresses, will be healthier? If we accept that inequality is an inevitable feature of capitalist societies, then surely so are inequalities in health? This *is* the position adopted by many, and can be seen in the discourse that describes 'differences in health' rather than inequalities. Although there may be disagreements on this point among all those working in public health and health promotion, we would argue that these inequalities are *not* inevitable, thus providing a political justification for action. Whitehead (1992) has argued that a health difference becomes a health inequity when it is avoidable, unnecessary and unjust. If these three criteria are met, she argues that a response is needed, in the cause of social justice.

Ethical justification for intervention to tackle inequalities, or to improve *anyone's* health, needs to be mentioned here too. It would not, at first sight, appear to be contentious that we ought to 'help' those less fortunate than ourselves, whether this is in terms of richer countries giving foreign aid, directing resources to poorer areas and communities within rich countries, or aiding individuals living in deprived circumstances. The parable of the good Samaritan is a powerful motif in Western cultures, Islam and other cultures and religions, i.e. of providing charity to the less fortunate; it informs our moral codes whilst appealing to a human sense of 'natural justice'. Thomas Pogge (2007; Jaggar, 2010) is perhaps the most outspoken of those arguing the moral case for intervention. He suggests that citizens commit a monumental crime against humanity when they collude with their governments in wealthy countries in maintaining the injustices of the world order.

We are entering a series of debates, however, which could turn into a minefield. It is also possible to stray into condescension, paternalism and unwanted interference. The Zambian economist, Dambisa Moyo (2009), in her critique of overseas aid to Africa, argues that aid is part of the problem, not part of the solution. Her thesis is that the aid-based development model currently in place will not generate sustained economic growth in Africa and that it can lead to corruption. Riddell (2008) similarly provides an in-depth analysis of the failures of aid to promote development, and although he tentatively suggests that aid *is* necessary, he makes persuasive arguments for radical changes in the way that aid is administered. The entry of wealthy philanthropists such as Bill Gates, in the form of the Bill & Melinda Gates Foundation, provides huge quantities of money for health projects, but there is also the danger of distorting priorities (as these are seen through a particular lens of the benefactors), and secondly, those funds can be withdrawn at any time, which is the weakness of a 'charitable' as opposed to a rights-based approach.

Cuba provides an example of a country that has managed to improve its health statistics such as infant mortality and life expectancy whilst being effectively cut off from aid for more than half a century. Other regions – the most often cited is Kerala in India, but also Sri Lanka, Costa Rica and Brazil (Carr, 2004) – have also improved a whole range of indices, from women's literacy to maternal

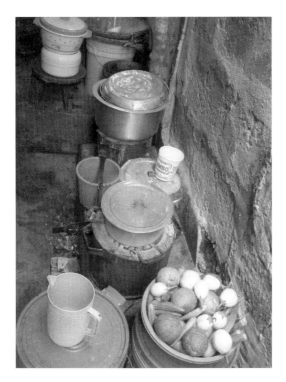

Nutrition – a social determinant of health; a kitchen in Tanzania.

mortality, by the way they have organized their societies rather than being recipients of aid. *They have not seen the 'interventions' regarded by the international agencies as essential to improving public health.*

David Sanders (Sanders with Carver, 1985), who was one of the most influential practitioners to highlight the 'struggle for health' in much of the developing world, and particularly in Africa, writes that the 'concerned health worker' will have to think carefully about their role, given that 'health in the underdeveloped world can only come by the actions of the people themselves – it will not come from outside' (Sanders with Carver, 1985, p. 218). He continues,

> The concerned health worker may arrive in a village, overflowing with brilliant, progressive ideas for preventive or promotive schemes, only to discover that the inhabitants are obstinately uninterested in them ... And the visiting health worker must accept that more often than not, the villagers are right.
>
> (Sanders with Carver, 1985, p. 218)

Sanders' views have since become mainstreamed and so may seem less radical than they were in the 1980s, the so-called lost decade of development. This questioning of how communities can be 'helped' continues to be a vexed one, even in situations of dire emergency, such as after a tsunami or earthquake, where help from 'outside' may not always be welcome or may not actually help. The idea that health can only be achieved by people taking action for themselves will be returned to later, particularly in discussing empowerment.

At the level of the individual or of communities, what right do we have to intervene in order to improve health and at what point do we have the right to constrain people's behaviour if it is felt that it is damaging to health? It is possible to see health promotion being hijacked by governments who wish to propagandize and manipulate, to even force people to live in 'healthier ways'. Thus Larsen and Manderson (2009, p. 608) suggest that

> another way of seeing health promotion is as an 'extended arm' of the neo-liberal discourse ... health promotion is one way of 'governing the masses' and health education is explicit in this task: people are directed to eat healthy foods, not to smoke cigarettes or use drugs, consume alcohol moderately, exercise regularly, participate in community life, and be responsible for their own life.

At best, this can be seen as part of the 'nanny state' and at worse, could be seen as a form of 'health fascism'. However, if governments do not take responsibility for ensuring the health rights of their populations, they could be accused of negligence. It is not a 'nanny state' that provides decent housing, employment opportunities, and good education and health systems, though it might be a 'nanny state' if it forbids people to smoke. A key question therefore is: what is the proper role of the state in ensuring that citizens enjoy the best possible health and what are the responsibilities of individuals for their own health? This debate is a key one in health promotion and it returns to the whole question of the determinants of health – to what extent is my health determined by factors external to me, such as the country I live in, the levels of pollution, level of development, the opportunities in my neighbourhood for good schooling, a satisfying job, good parenting ... and so on, and to what extent is my health determined by those factors under my control – by the choices I freely make, my lifestyle and so on? Of course in reality these two – the external and internal – are intertwined.

The focus on lifestyles and the need to adopt healthier behaviours is a recurring theme in public policy and is propagated in the mass media. A recent example from the UK (as of December 2011) is the reporting of findings from the Cancer Research Report UK, which proposed that more than 100,000 cancers per year in the UK are caused by four lifestyle factors – smoking, unhealthy diets, alcohol and obesity. The report estimated that up to 40% of cancers in women and 45% in men are preventable through lifestyle changes – the most significant factor in this appears to be cigarette smoking. The report was based on research carried out by Parkin *et al.* (2011), which examined 14 lifestyle and environmental risk factors in an attempt to estimate what proportion of cancers were avoidable. Interestingly only two of the 14 factors could really be labelled 'environmental' (exposure to radiation and occupational exposure to carcinogens). Attention was not paid to the wider socio-environmental factors, which we, in health promotion, would pay heed to. We need to be critical of information that solely focuses on poor health outcomes as being down to issues of behaviour and personal choice. For example, childbearing is statistically linked to a lower risk of breast cancer (Peto, 2011), yet few people would advocate that women should be forced to have children to reduce their risk of developing breast cancer.

The focus on lifestyle factors and individual behaviours is not peculiar to industrialized countries now that we are witnessing the rise of non-communicable diseases (NCDs) within less wealthy countries. In 2008, the WHO estimated that a total of 58 million deaths occurred around the world; of these 35 million were due to NCDs; of these 35 million, 28 million deaths were in developing countries and of these 28 million, 14 million were estimated to have been preventable (WHO, 2009b). NCDs were cited as being *the* major challenge to development in the 21st century. The modifiable risk factors were identified as being tobacco use, unhealthy diets, physical activity and harmful use of alcohol. This global focus in health policy at the individual level was also reflected in the High-level Meeting on Non-Communicable Diseases, which took place at the General Assembly of the United Nations (UN) in New York in September 2011. The Secretary General's report published in advance of the meeting in May 2011 clearly outlined the evidenced-based link between individual behavioural risk factors and wider socio-environmental determinants such as poverty, lack of education and levels of economic development (UN, 2011). At the meeting in September 2011, however, the focus on the wider determinants was lost.

So far, we have established that health promotion is both a political and ethical activity. Broader ethical questions are taken up again in Chapter 5. Health promotion is both political and ethical because it asks the question: what sort of society do we want to live in? This implicitly asks questions about who has power and who does not, and about how societies can be re-organized so that they are fairer.

Before offering a short history of the development of health promotion, noting the key milestones in its development, we suggest that there are a number of concepts that require understanding. In our teaching, we have found it useful to think in terms of threshold concepts, where, as the name suggests, the learner steps over into another realm of understanding. The point about a threshold is that once it is crossed, there is no going back. In educational terms, they are important, as they are concepts that have to be understood before being able to proceed to the next idea. They have proved useful for example in mathematics education, where one block of knowledge has to be mastered before being able to progress. Meyer and Land (2005) suggest that crossing a threshold can transform a person's worldview and additionally cause fundamental shifts in that person's sense of identity and reconstruction of who they are (Meyer and Land, 2005; Meyer *et al.*, 2010). Thus crossing a threshold can lead to fundamental questioning of, for example, one's career to date. We introduce three threshold concepts early on in our courses – 'upstream thinking', salutogenesis and the social model of health.

Threshold Concepts

Upstream thinking

Zola (1970, in McKinlay, 1979) is credited with developing the river analogy, which has become such a potent image within health promotion (Box 1.1). It refers to the medical enterprise of rescuing people once they have got into difficulties. Whilst this is essential for those who have become ill or contracted a disease, it would be better to have stopped them becoming so in the first place.

Whilst we would assert that health promotion is the profession that walks up the river bank to find out what is pushing all the people into the river (i.e. health promotion is *the* profession dedicated to tackling the determinants of health), it remains the case that many who work within health promotion are actually working downstream. This is perhaps one of the gaps identified above – that although much of the international, epistemic health promotion community talks about upstream working, many or even most, frontline workers in health promotion are not in positions where they *can* affect change upstream. Furthermore, they may be located in arenas that are strictly *not* political organizations, such as the UK's NHS. Many health promoters are civil servants with explicit contracts not to engage in political activity, and, as we saw above, health promotion is inherently political – hence a contradiction! The move in the UK by the current coalition government to locate health promotion and public health within local authorities (which are political organizations) and not in the NHS is thus to be welcomed.

A further issue is that the further upstream one looks, the harder it is to be sure of the chain of causality. A death downstream will have a series of causes: a child who dies of diarrhoea in a poor country will most likely also have an infection, be malnourished and live in a poor household. Whilst intervention that is most close to the diarrhoea and infection would be effective, those conditions are likely to reoccur; a health worker could treat those conditions but malnutrition is not likely to be within their remit or expertise. Tackling under-nutrition and food security would require a strategic intervention, as would tackling the causes of poverty, and would require politicians and policy makers both nationally and globally to take action. Similarly, in England, a common cause of death for primary school-aged children is through a pedestrian accident. Creating a 'problem tree' of causes, one could trace this to children playing out on the street, cars driving too fast, lack of adequate play spaces, lack of adequate traffic planning, which separates vulnerable road users from vehicles, lack of resources to upgrade lower class neighbourhoods, lack of government investment, and so on. Others of different ideological persuasions might simply say that child pedestrian accidents are caused by lax parental control. Thus the causal pathways have both technical and political dimensions, and the further up the chain, the less likely are those with 'health' in their job title able to tackle the issue.

Medical and social models of health

Health promotion holds a 'social' model of health. The central ideas about the social model of health are that understandings of health are broad and complex. The social model of health encompasses 'lay' perspectives about health, taking into account subjective experience and understandings. Crucially it also takes into account the wider determinants of health (Dahlgren and Whitehead, 1991, 2006, 2007; Commission on the Social Determinants of Health, 2008; Marmot, 2010) regarding health as holistic and multidimensional and emphasizing *social* responsibility for health. These ideas are in direct contrast to more biomedical perspectives, which view health rather more narrowly, focusing on disease and disability at the individual level, elevating objective, scientific and expert ideas and emphasizing *personal* responsibility for health.

An analogy that might be useful is of attempting to understand the game of football. It might not be useful to start by dissecting the ball. This would give clues to a problem with the football – if it was not bouncing properly, for example. But it would not tell us much about football in its entirety, as a game that has captivated the world. To understand modern football, it would be necessary to know something about economics, politics, psychology, sociology, culture, ritual and sport. Transferring this to health, the medical profession does often start by dissecting the body – modern medicine is highly reductionist, and capable of understanding bodies at the cellular level. This is very helpful and has saved lives! But it doesn't help very much in understanding health in its modern context, or the conditions that create health in its entirety.

A social model of health views the 'health service' as a sickness service, essential when people become ill and are in need of medical help, but not the key player in terms of *creating* health, except where services are preventive, such as in immunization and screening. A social model tends to see the health service as treating symptoms and not causes – the causes of ill health are rooted in society, in poor housing, food insecurity, lack of employment, lack of money, poor education and so on. In short, the causes are 'upstream' and the medical model 'saves' people in a downstream fashion. Whereas the medical model sees ill health as caused by disease, the social model sees ill health as caused by social conditions (Table 1.1).

A social model of health naturally begins to question the 'illness', negative view of health, and moves towards asking what a positive view of health would look like. If we are not measuring health in terms of mortality, morbidity, years of life lost, or years of life compromised by poor health, how should we measure health? We can begin to realize that most of our measures or indices of 'health' are actually measures of ill health. It is clearly important to have these facts about negative health – (life expectancy *is* a matter of life and death!) – but we also need to develop positive concepts of health and the means to measure this. Several writers are attempting to do this, based on Antonovsky's idea of salutogenesis.

Salutogenesis

Salutogenesis will be discussed below in some depth as part of an attempt to define health. It is mentioned here as a threshold concept, as it represents a

Table 1.1. Comparing and contrasting the medical and social models of health (adapted from: Lyons and Chamberlain, 2006; Earle, 2007; Warwick-Booth *et al.*, 2012).

Negative view of health	Positive view of health
Narrow or simplistic understanding of health	Broad or complex understanding of health
Explanations of disease and illness are rooted in biological science	Explanations for ill health are rooted in a range of social factors. Ill health is caused by structural factors such as poverty and inequalities
Medically biased definitions focusing on the absence of disease or disability; the focus on pathology emphasizes individual risk factors	More holistic definition of health taking a wide range of factors into account such as mental and social dimensions of health
Wider influences on health not taken into account (outside of the physical body)	Takes into account wider influences on health such as the impact of the environment and inequalities
Health is located within the individual body; the physical body is seen as separate to social and/or psychological processes	Health is socially constructed and subjectively experienced
Influenced by scientific and expert knowledge, a high value is put on this and it is privileged over other types of knowledge	Takes into account lay knowledge and understandings
Emphasizes personal, individual responsibility for health	Emphasizes collective, social responsibility for health
Quantitative scientific evidence and the positivist paradigm is more highly valued	Qualitative scientific evidence and the interpretative paradigm is more highly valued
Forms the basis of 'Western' health care systems	Forms the basis of traditional and 'alternative' health care systems
Reductionist	Inclusive
Ill health requires expert intervention	Ill health requires collective intervention

real attempt to move towards seeing health differently. Often when we talk of 'health', we are actually talking about 'ill health', and it is easier to describe what illness and sickness, or sanity, are, compared with health, well-being, wellness or sanity. It can be very difficult to re-conceptualize health away from illness and the negative, towards a positive notion of health – from the pathogenic to the salutogenic. Salutogenesis has a major following in the epistemic health promotion community (Bengel *et al.*, 1999), most notably in the Scandinavian countries (Lindstrom and Eriksson, 2006; Eriksson and Lindstrom, 2008). Antonovsky (1996) attempted to show how the model can be used to guide health promotion, and more recently, Lindstrom and Eriksson (2009) have used the theory to guide healthy public policy making: 'This paper is probably the first ever describing a salutogenic approach to the making of a healthy public policy on a national level' (Lindstrom and Eriksson, 2009, p. 26). More will be said in this chapter about salutogenesis when we start to discuss in detail what we mean by 'health'.

A Short History of the Development of Health Promotion

A history of health promotion usually starts in 1974 with the publication of the Lalonde Report in Canada, and then proceeds to the Ottawa Charter in 1986, which was followed by a series of conferences that further explicated the WHO agenda for health promotion. The Ottawa conference was aimed at 'industrialized countries', and from a global perspective, the Alma-Ata conference on primary health care in 1978 is an equally, if not more, important milestone.

A useful WHO publication provides a synopsis of the key points from each of the health promotion conferences from Ottawa, Adelaide, Sundsvall, Jakarta, Mexico and Bangkok. It also includes notes on the 1984 Copenhagen discussion document on the concept and principles of health promotion (WHO, 2009a).

The Lalonde report (1974) was the first attempt by a western democracy to assert that the approach to health was misguided, and it called for a radically new approach to tackling the issues of 'lifestyle' in a rich country. It started the trend to thinking that health was not merely the responsibility of the health service, but needed a broader approach, first to stem human misery caused by illness, but also to reduce the runaway costs of health care. It focused more attention than hitherto on the role of the environment and on lifestyle, thus calling for a shift towards prevention. Much of this thinking subsequently found its way into the Ottawa Charter, and Canada has remained a power house for health promotion ideas ever since (Pederson *et al.*, 2005).

The Ottawa Charter provided a definition of health promotion: 'Health promotion is the process of enabling people to increase control over, and to improve, their health' (WHO, 1986a, p. 1).

The Charter provided a list of the prerequisites for health (Box 1.2).

It suggested three processes through which to work: Advocate, Enable and Mediate (Box 1.3).

And it proposed five areas of action:

- Build healthy public policy.
- Create supportive environments.
- Strengthen community actions.
- Develop personal skills.
- Reorient health services.

Box 1.2. Prerequisites for health.

The fundamental conditions and resources for health are:

- peace;
- shelter;
- education;
- food;

- income;
- a stable eco-system;
- sustainable resources; and
- social justice and equity.

Improvement in health requires a secure foundation in these basic prerequisites.

(WHO, 2009a, p. 1)

These five areas should be seen as having equal worth, not as being ranked. The Charter made the powerful statement, 'health promotion goes beyond health care', to assert the fact that health care is but a minor part in creating health. It called for all policy makers to consider the health consequences of their decisions and made the point that many government sectors contain the key to health creation – especially employment, trade and industry, education, transport, housing and so on – 'It is coordinated action that leads to health ...' (WHO, 2009a, p. 3). Thus healthy public policy requires joint action and is a foundation for tackling the social determinants of health.

Creating supportive environments explicitly recognizes the importance of the natural environment and sustainability of ecosystems, calling for a socio-ecological approach to health. That people live their lives inextricably bound up with the environments in which they live is obvious, but tends to be overlooked by a medical model of health. Health promotion 'generates living and working conditions that are safe, stimulating, satisfying and enjoyable' (p. 3) – and clearly not everyone enjoys this in the world today.

Strong communities are the third central plank of the infrastructure for health promotion:

> Health promotion works through concrete and effective community action in setting priorities, making decisions, planning strategies, and implementing them to achieve better health. At the heart of this process is the empowerment of communities, their ownerships and control of their own destinies (p. 3).

As Farrant (1997, p. 223) points out:

> Endorsement of this principle implies at the very least:

- acknowledging inequalities in power, ownership and control, and vested interests in maintaining inequalities;
- challenging professional control of health promotion; and
- validating and supporting community health initiatives that are seeking to transform the distribution of power, ownership and control.

The fourth area concerns helping people to develop personal skills, and is centred on the need to support personal development, provide information and education for health, and to enhance life skills. If people really are to take control of the factors influencing their health, they need to be equipped to learn throughout their lives, but action is also required by educational institutions, workplaces and the voluntary sector to enable and provide such learning opportunities.

Finally, health services need to be reoriented, 'embrace an expanded mandate' and move beyond their curative focus, but must also be more sensitive to the needs of individuals and communities and respect diverse cultural needs.

Two subsequent conferences, in Adelaide and Sundsvall, took up the first two action areas, expanding on what these might mean in practice. The Adelaide conference took up the theme of building healthy public policy, reasserting that 'inequalities in health are rooted in inequities in society' (WHO, 2009a, p. 7). Healthy public policy explicitly places at the forefront the importance of health and equity in all areas of policy and requires all policies to consider their health impacts. In terms of immediate action, the Adelaide conference suggested four areas:

- Supporting the health of women: ensuring that countries develop healthy public policy around equal sharing of caring work, birthing practice based on women's preferences, and supportive mechanisms for the caring that women do in terms of childcare and other caring. It emphasized the rights of all women 'especially those from ethnic, indigenous and minority groups, have the right to self-determination of their health and should be full partners in the formation of healthy public policy to ensure its cultural relevance'.
- Food and nutrition: the elimination of hunger and malnutrition must be a fundamental objective, incorporating agricultural, economic and environmental policy. Taxations and subsidies should be used to enable better access to healthier diets.
- Tobacco and alcohol: these are 'two major health hazards that deserve immediate action'. It was noted that tobacco, not only as a direct cause of ill health and premature death, but as a cash crop in impoverished countries, has serious ecological consequences and can be linked to crises in food production and distribution. It called upon all governments to reduce tobacco growing and alcohol production, marketing and consumption.

- Creating supportive environments: as so many people live and work in hazardous environments, coordinated inter-sectoral efforts are needed to protect health across national borders. It argues: 'Policies promoting health can only be achieved in an environment that conserves resources through global, regional, and ecological strategies' (WHO, 2009a, pp. 8–9).

The Sundsvall conference took up the theme of supportive environments, suggesting that they comprise four aspects:

- The social dimension, including the way that norms, customs and social processes affect health; changes to traditional ways of life are not always health-enhancing.
- The political dimension, requiring governments to guarantee democratic participation in decision making and decentralization of responsibilities and resources, and to make a commitment to peace, human rights and a shift of resources away from armaments.
- The economic dimension, requiring a re-channelling of resources to achieve better health.
- A gender dimension, whereby women's skills and knowledge are recognized in all sectors, including policy making and the economy in order to develop a more positive infrastructure for supportive environments (WHO, 2009a, p. 14).

It could have been expected that subsequent conferences might have taken up the other key planks of health promotion, after the Adelaide and Sundsvall tackled the first two. However, Jakarta took a different tack, and although it built very much on Ottawa, it was the first to be held in a so-called 'developing country' (the Ottawa conference was aimed at 'industrialized countries'), and was the first to include what it called the 'private sector'. It wished to reflect on what had been learnt about effective health promotion and to re-examine the social determinants of health. It asserted that there were new challenges, including greater integration of the global economy, financial markets and trade, changed access to the media and communications technology, greater environmental degradation, new and re-emerging infectious diseases. Demographic trends such as increases in older people, greater urbanization, more sedentary behaviour and a host of other emerging issues led the conference to call for new responses, greater investment in health, more capacity in health promotion by

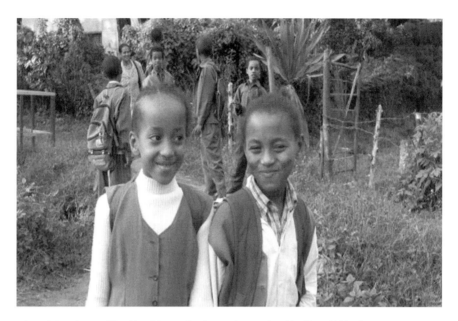

Education – a key determinant of health: girls coming home from school in Jima, Ethiopia.

developing its infrastructure and maximizing its impact. It called for emphasis on 'settings for health' (taken up in Chapter 5 of this book). It also called for new kinds of partnerships and a more robust documentation of experiences in health promotion so as to develop the evidence base.

Mexico, in 2000, took up the last point, asserting that there was 'ample evidence that good health promotion strategies of promoting health are effective' (WHO, 2009a, p. 22). The Mexico conference had the subtitle of 'Bridging the Equity Gap', and in the spirit of 'From Ideas to Action', 88 countries signed up to support country-wide plans of action for promoting health, to take a lead role in ensuring the active participation of all sectors and civil society, to expand partnerships for health and to support national and international networks to promote health.

The Bangkok conference (2005) reiterated many of the key aspects of the previous conferences and noted that action had not always followed the signing of the resolutions by national governments. It therefore offered a series of actions and called for four commitments, to make the promotion of health:

- central to the global development agenda;
- a core responsibility for all of government;

- a key focus of communities and civil society; and
- a requirement for good corporate practice (WHO, 2009a, p. 26).

The Nairobi conference was the first to be held in Africa, in 2009. It wished to mainstream health promotion into priority programmes such as HIV/AIDS, malaria, tuberculosis, mental health, maternal and child health, violence and injury, neglected tropical diseases, and NCDs such as diabetes (WHO, 2009a). The Nairobi Call to Action put great emphasis on countries to strengthen leadership and workforces, empower communities and individuals, enhance participatory processes, and apply knowledge for the effective implementation of health promotion. According to the call to action, countries are to build capacity in health promotion, to strengthen health systems, to ensure community empowerment, to develop partnerships and intersectoral actions relevant to addressing the determinants of health, and to help improve health literacy and healthy lifestyles (Petersen and Kwan, 2010).

It can be seen that whereas Ottawa, Adelaide and Sundsvall explored and expanded on key principles of health promotion, the subsequent conferences aimed at developing high-level political commitment for health promotion. They thus involved ministers and others in powerful governmental roles in signing up to the actions necessary to tackle health inequalities. Whilst this is necessary, it did mean that the two action areas – building healthy public policy and creating supportive environments – were more fully developed compared with the other three. The whole ethos of the Ottawa Charter was, to a large extent, a reaction against the individualistic approach of health education where individuals were exhorted to adopt new behaviours in the face of personal risks to their health. Building healthy public policy was seen by some as a panacea and an alternative paradigm. At the same time, activities in many countries are called 'health promotion' but do not appear to be touched by the Ottawa vision. Rather, health promotion is seen as health education, behaviour change approaches and lifestyle advice. The entire political point of the need for structural change is missed, and these activities persist in what some would regard as 'victim-blaming'.

Of course, health promotion has a history that is wider than this series of conferences, but they do provide a backbone for our movement. A number of writers consider whether the radical intention of Ottawa has been diluted in subsequent years (Baum and Sanders 1995; Potter, 1997) providing commentaries on what has happened in the intervening years, and these are covered in Chapter 6, where we discuss where health promotion is going to next. An excellent series of discussion papers was published in December 2011 in a supplement of the journal *Health Promotion International*, which draws together the reflections of key thinkers in health promotion on the 25th anniversary of the Ottawa Charter.

An overview of the key conferences is presented in Table 1.2.

What are the Inequalities that Health Promotion is Attempting to Address?

We could start this section by copying Venkatapuram's (2011, p. 1) approach, when he starts his book *Health Justice* by saying,

> I am going to skip the usual graphic story describing the wretched life of some poor girl or woman in some poor country. I am also going to skip over the mind-boggling statistics on the millions of avoidable deaths and causes of serious disease and disability occurring every year. Nor will I dwell on their conspicuous social distribution patterns across every country and across countries.

Kaufmann (2009) argues that figures don't mean very much – the fact that 15 million people die as a result of infectious diseases every year is impossible for most of us to grasp. It is harder still to comprehend the loss of life-years due to sickness, disability and early death.

However, we do want to point out some of these statistics, to show the scale of the task of tackling inequalities. The world's richest country, the USA, has lower life expectancy (77.0) than countries with less income (such as Sweden 79.7 and Japan 80.7). There are also middle-income countries that have higher life expectancy than might be expected. Sri Lanka is one such example, with average life expectancy of 73.1 (World Bank, 2002; UNDP, 2003). Sri Lanka and Cuba are both examples of high health-achieving countries as a result of national-level policies that created access to basic social services (Mehrotra, 2000).

The WHO has stated that extreme poverty is the most serious cause of disease, with 70% of deaths in developing countries attributable to five causes that can be easily and cheaply combated – pneumonia, diarrhoea, malaria, measles and malnutrition (WHO, 1995). In 2001, the deaths of two million people could have been prevented simply if they had been given access to uncontaminated food and clean drinking water (Kindhauser, 2003). Those in weak social, economic and political positions, such as women, are much more at risk of certain conditions such as malnutrition, violence, sexually transmitted infections and respiratory conditions. Women and children bear the main burden of global health inequalities. In 2007, women made up 61% of HIV infections in sub-Saharan Africa (UNAIDs, 2007). In addition there are many deaths from maternal mortality (Hill *et al.*, 2007). Put simply, within all societies death rates are typically highest amongst the poorest and marginalized. In Australia for example,

> There are many statistics that document the vast difference in health status between Indigenous and non-Indigenous Australians, but perhaps one of the most telling is that while 70% of Indigenous peoples die before they are 65, only 21% of non-Indigenous Australians do so.
>
> (Baum and Simpson, 2006, p. 178)

Data on many sources of inequalities go uncollected – information on the health of refugees, asylum seekers, prisoners, indigenous peoples, uncontacted

Table 1.2. Summary of the key global conferences on health promotion.

Meeting of the World Health Organization at the 30th World Health Assembly (1977)	• 'Health for All by the year 2000' launched
Alma-Ata Declaration (1978) – seen as the means to achieve 'Health for All'	• Focus on primary health care Key issues: • Social justice • Addressing inequalities • Government responsibility
First International Conference on Health Promotion in Ottawa, Canada (1986), resulted in the **Ottawa Charter**	Five key areas: • Building healthy public policy • Creating supportive environments • Strengthening community action • Developing personal skills • Reorienting health services To be achieved through: • Advocacy • Enabling • Mediation
Second International Conference on Health Promotion in **Adelaide**, Australia (1988)	• Focus on healthy public policy • Alliances for health
Third International Conference on Health Promotion in Sundsvall, Sweden (1991), resulted in the **Sundsvall Statement on Supportive Environments for Health**	• Focus on supportive environments for health

Fourth International Conference on Health Promotion in Jakarta, Indonesia (1997), resulted in the **Jakarta Declaration on Leading Health Promotion into the 21st Century**	• Reinforced health as a basic human right
	• Identified *settings* as key to promoting health
	• Set out the following priorities:
	  ○ Promote social responsibility for health
	  ○ Increase investments for health development
	  ○ Consolidate and expand partnerships for health
	  ○ Increase community capacity and empower the individual
	  ○ Secure an infrastructure for health promotion

Fifth International Conference on Health Promotion in Mexico City, Mexico (2000)	• Highlighted the need to invest in health • Create an infrastructure for health promotion • Reduce inequity
Sixth International Conference on Health Promotion in Bangkok, Thailand (2005), resulted in the **Bangkok Charter for Health Promotion in a Globalized World**	• Emphasized policy and partnership • The need to address determinants of health
Seventh International Conference on Health Promotion in Nairobi, Kenya (2009), resulted in **The Nairobi Call to Action**	Five sub-themes: • Build capacity for health promotion • Strengthen health systems, partnerships and inter-sectoral action • Community empowerment • Health literacy • Health behaviours

tribes, Romanies and gypsies, the homeless, and a range of other marginalized groups is not available, often for obvious reasons. Data are often aggregated too, disguising inequalities within regions and groups. Infant mortality is often used as a rough guide to the scale of inequalities (Box 1.4).

What is Health?

Thus far, we have seen health as a common-sense concept and assumed that we have a working definition of it. We need to consider in some detail what we really *do* mean by health – if we are trying to promote it, we need at least to be clear that

Box 1.4. Infant mortality as an indicator of health inequalities.

Using the example of infant mortality as a crude indicator of health we can map clear health inequalities at local, regional and global levels. If we start with Leeds, which is where we are based at Leeds Metropolitan University, we can see differences within the city itself:

- The Annual Report of the Director of Public Health 2011 for Leeds stated that, despite a steady decrease in infant mortality over the last few years, the rate is higher in the more deprived areas of the city (5.6 deaths per 1000 live births for Leeds as a whole from 2000–2004 *but* 8.2 deaths per 1000 live births for the most deprived areas of the city).

Moving to the regional level, we can see differences between Yorkshire and Humber (the region where Leeds is located) and the rest of England:

- In 2006, the average infant mortality rate for the whole of England was 5.0 deaths per 1000 live births and 5.6 deaths per 1000 for Yorkshire and Humber. Within the Yorkshire and Humber region, there were variations from 3.8 (East Riding) to 7.2 (City of Bradford) (Yorkshire and Humber Public Health Observatory, 2008).

There are differences between England and the rest of Europe:

- In 2005, the average infant mortality rate was 5 in England per 1000 live births compared with, for example, Turkey at 24 per 1000 live births and Luxembourg at 3 per 1000 live births (UNICEF, 2009).

There are differences between Europe and the rest of the world:

- In 2006, the average infant mortality rate in the countries comprising Latin America and the Caribbean was 27 per 1000 live births compared with the average infant mortality rate in the countries of Europe, which was 6 per 1000 live births. There is a clear difference here between 'developed' and 'developing' countries (UN, 2009).

There are also differences within continents:

- Within the continent of Asia for example, in the year 2000, the infant mortality rate was over 150 per 1000 live births in Afghanistan, compared with fewer than 10 per 1000 live births in Japan in the same year (CIESIN, 2005).

health is a complex, multifaceted and contested concept, a consensual definition of which is virtually impossible. The examples given above of inequalities in health are from literature, which is disease orientated. Health is usually measured in disease terms – mortality, morbidity, life expectancy are the key features. These are not to be minimized, but they only give a partial picture. When asked what makes them well and happy, people will usually produce a list (assuming that they have had their basic needs satisfied, such as for shelter, food, clothing and so on and are living free from terror, war or violence) that includes all or some of the following: feeling loved and wanted, being close to family and friends; doing something useful and with purpose, such as paid or unpaid work; being part of a community; having leisure time, being able to relax and rest, sleeping well, feeling alive, being in touch with nature, enjoying a cultural life; being free from violence, feeling safe, being able to access health care when needed; having hope for the future ... This list could continue, but what is clear

is that the items on it do not feature on indices of 'health'. We do not know how many people in the world, for example, feel safe most of the time, how many feel loved or how many enjoy reasonable leisure time. In other words, we know little about those things that most cause us to be at ease, happy and healthy, in terms of official statistics. There are international attempts to develop 'happiness' indices, but these remain to be inserted into the debates about how to address the social determinants of health. These issues will be taken up in Chapter 6.

The professional view

The health promotion community necessarily puts a high value on health – as something worth trying to promote. Duncan (2007) offers a critical discussion about the nature of health, emphasizing the importance of examining what 'health' is in order to determine how we might create or improve it. He concludes that continuous dialogue is needed 'as part of a strategy for examining and understanding perspectives on health' (2007, p. 214) as well as the constant awareness that alternative (and perhaps equally valid) positions exist. Different discourses on health hold different views about ideas such as where health is located (whether it is at the individual, community, societal or even global level), how health is defined, how health is experienced and how health is valued. If people do not hold health in high regard then there is little impetus to try to promote it.

The nature of health and how it is defined have been extensively discussed and debated in the wider literature. In summary, health is conceptualized in many ways – as abstract (Earle, 2007), as contested, as subjective, as difficult to define (Chronin de Chavez *et al.*, 2005) and as dichotomous (Green and Tones, 2010). Differing theoretical, ideological and philosophical perspectives influence the way in which health is viewed (Warwick-Booth *et al.*, 2012). In addition, we know that concepts of health are influenced by a range of different factors including our culture (Aidoo and Harpham, 2001; Burns and Gavey, 2004), our socio-economic position (Blaxter, 2004; Duncan, 2007), our individual experiences across the lifespan (Brannen and Storey, 1996; Chapman *et al.*, 2000; Lawton, 2003) and our gender (Emslie and Hunt, 2008). Calnan (1987), Blaxter (1990, 2004), Seedhouse (2001b), Stainton-Rogers (1991) and Murray *et al.* (2003), among others, have examined lay perspectives on health and offer interesting accounts and understandings. Lay perspectives are discussed in detail later in this chapter.

Salutogenesis

One of the key critiques of research that has claimed to have investigated perspectives on health is that relatively few of them have actually examined concepts of *health* and instead have focused on aspects of illness (Hughner and Klein, 2004). Clearly, health *can* be viewed in negative or positive ways, and the classic WHO definition of 1946 (cited in WHO, 1986b) highlights how health should be seen as much more than the absence of illness, disease and disability. But if it is not simply the absence of these things, what *is* health? It is rather easier to frame health in negative rather than positive ways, and easier to talk about those things that create ill health rather than those that create health – just as more has been written about what causes war rather than what causes peace. Biomedical accounts of health remain the most

influential within Western contexts (Sidell, 2010) but salutogenic ways of thinking about health are more positive and focus on what creates health and well-being rather than on what causes ill health (Antonovsky, 1996). Logically, health promotion should align itself with more salutogenic ways of understanding and conceptualizing health.

'Salutogenesis' is one attempt to capture a positive view of health and its causes and challenge negative ways of conceptualizing health. It is the opposite of pathogenesis, which is the attempt to understand disease. Antonovsky (1996) coined the term 'salutogenesis' and challenges the 'pathogenic' nature of the medical model of health by arguing that we should be focusing on wellness not illness. Rather than emphasizing the biomedical dichotomy of health versus illness and disease, Antonosky argues that we are all on a continuum that he calls the 'health-ease-dis-ease' continuum and that we move up and down this continuum all of the time – no-one ever really achieving 'full' health. He argues that this is impossible, given that we are all biological beings subject to the pathogenic forces of disease and decay. He also called for a move away from focus on the unwell and those deemed 'at risk' (a key tenet of public health approaches; Green and Tones, 2010).

Antonovsky further developed his ideas of what health is composed of with what he calls a Sense of Coherence. This encompasses three key elements – comprehensibility, meaningfulness and manageability. These relate, in turn, to our understanding of our world and making sense of our experiences, how we feel about these and to what extent we can cope with the demands that we face (Sidell, 2010). This idea becomes crucial in terms of understanding and accounting for our 'place' on the 'health-ease-dis-ease continuum' – those with a stronger Sense of Coherence, Antonovsky argues, are more likely to be able to move towards the 'health' end of the continuum. Given this perspective then, the question for health promotion is: how do we enable people to develop a Sense of Coherence?

Health as happiness

Intuitively, it makes sense that happiness is fundamentally related to health. A recent focus on the links between happiness and subjective experiences of health is evident in the UK government plans, from April 2011, to introduce measures of well-being and quality of life in order to determine people's experience and obtain indicators of 'progress' above and beyond economic ones. Exactly how this will be done, however, remains to be seen. Measuring 'happiness' and 'well-being' is not an exact science, although there does appear to be a direct and positive correlation between health and happiness (Gerdtham and Johannesson, 2001). Well-being is another term that is well used yet not well defined. Grant *et al.* (2007) offer a useful way of conceptualizing 'well-being'. They draw on the WHO's 'holistic' definition of health as a starting point for discussion then go on to bring together ideas about well-being from the wider literature, drawing on psychological, philosophical and sociological definitions. Their summary is presented in Box 1.5.

Another useful model of health is offered by Labonte, in Fig. 1.1.

This places well-being in the centre, which is the point of reference for many people when thinking about their health. (In the UK for example, a common greeting is 'Are you well?' We do not say 'Are you healthy?')

The model also centralizes the notion of 'control', a notion that is central to definitions of health promotion. Kobasa *et al.* (1979) assert that *control*, the idea that an individual is able to influence the course of events, is one of three common factors in salutogenesis. The other two factors are *commitment* – having a sense of curiosity for life and a sense of meaningfulness in life – and *challenge* – the expectation that life will change and that change is beneficial. Helping people to make appropriate changes, as individuals, families, communities and organizations, is a key task of health promotion.

The model captures the importance of meaningfulness and a sense of purpose – to be meaningfully occupied is almost a definition of health (Dixey, 2010).

The material presented so far is from the viewpoint of professionals – thinkers, academics, health workers – and not from lay people's perspective. We use the term 'lay' to mean the ideas of those who are not professionally trained in health – people in communities and in cultures who have developed their own ideas about health. It is important that we explore these beliefs in some detail, as, in keeping with our philosophical standpoint, we start with where people are, regarding their views on health and illness as a form of knowledge that needs to be recognized and respected.

Lay health beliefs

What do we know of lay people's ideas about health, and how these relate to their health-related behaviours? Anthropology, in its attempt to 'make the strange comprehensible' (Lambert and McKevitt, 2002, p. 212), has long studied lay ideas about health in non-Western cultures. Sociology and psychology have come more recently to the study of lay beliefs, often engaging in research motivated by health professionals' concerns to explain what was seen as problematic patient behaviour, for instance not consulting doctors appropriately or not complying with their advice.

However, the growing interest in health that has come with an emphasis on the prevention of illness and health promotion has led to a growth of research, especially since the 1970s, on ideas about health and health-relevant behaviours. However, as Hughner and Kleine (2004) point out, in their comprehensive review of the literature on views of health in the lay sector, much of this research has focused on particular conditions and people's behaviours in relation to the prevention of these,

---

Box 1.5. Capturing 'well-being' – core elements.

Grant *et al.* (2007) identify three dimensions of 'well-being': the psychological dimension, the physical dimension and the social dimension. Each dimension contains several core elements as follows:

- *Psychological*: includes agency, satisfaction, self-respect and capabilities.

- *Physical*: includes nourishment, shelter, health care, clothing and mobility.
- *Social*: includes participating in community, being accepted in public and helping others.

(Adapted from Grant *et al.*, 2007, p. 52)

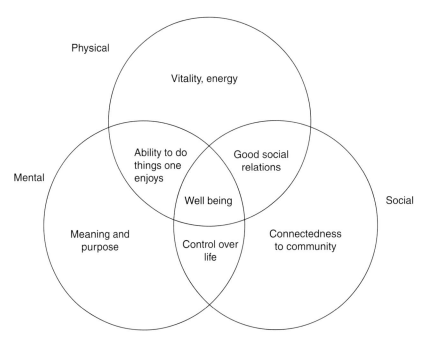

Fig. 1.1. Labonte's model (1998, cited in Orme *et al.*, 2003, p. 287).

rather than their views on health as such. Therefore the research evidence on health beliefs is relatively small, but what follows is an account of some of the main findings, followed by a discussion of the ways in which lay people feel that health can be promoted, or illness prevented. Important to this discussion is recognition of the importance of culture, ethnicity, social class, gender and age in relation to ideas about health.

As in the biomedical model, a common lay conception of health is as the absence of disease; indeed Kleinman (1980) points out that professional, folk and popular ideas about health co-exist, and are not distinct. In the Health and Lifestyle study in the UK reported on by Blaxter (1990), 'absence of illness' was one of the main definitions of health. However, she also noted that illness and health were not always conceived as dichotomous states, and that respondents talked about being healthy *in spite of illness*. A much more recent study by Abbott *et al.* (2006) of post-soviet citizens in Russia and the Ukraine also found that the 'most frequently cited indicator of health included in people's accounts was absence of illness (or in some cases serious illness), mentioned by nearly half our informants' (p. 231). However, in a study of Polynesian ideas about

health, Capstick *et al.* (2009) point out that 'for Samoans, it is inaccurate to conceptualize health as absence of illness and illness as absence of health – instead illness is seen as an inevitable though potent disruption to life and social systems' (p. 1342). They also say that the Polynesian languages have no equivalent to the biomedical constructs of 'health' and 'disease' (p. 1342).

'Health as instrumental' is another conception of health, which is outlined in Blaxter's (1990) study, where she describes responses that linked health with ability to function. In Abbott *et al.*'s postsoviet study, they note that a quarter of their informants talked about health as a resource: 'A healthy man should be able to easily walk 20 km and be able to lift with one hand a 50 kg sack of potatoes' (2006, p. 231). This quote also suggests elements of 'health as fitness', another category in Blaxter's typology (1990), and Williams (1983) also found concepts of health as fitness in his study of elderly Aberdonians, although this was less to do with strength and more to do with absence of disease; by contrast, in French studies, functional fitness is dependent on strength as well as on freedom from disabling disease (Williams, 1983). Abbott *et al.* (2006) report that a third of their respondents mentioned physical appearance as part of a definition of health, with sporty appearance also mentioned. Physical appearance and fitness relate to more positive concepts of health, but in such positive concepts social and psychological well-being feature the most. Abbott *et al.* (2006) found that many of their respondents saw healthy people as happy and positive about life. Similarly Blaxter (1990) found that health was described as well-being. Abbott *et al.* (2006, p. 231) quoted one respondent who said: 'if a person is psychologically healthy he will be physically healthier'.

Underpinning many of these ideas about health are also important notions of balance or equilibrium. In the classic study by Herzlich (1973), 'health as equilibrium' was one of three main conceptualizations of health. Interestingly, according to Stacey (1986, cited Pierret, 1993, p. 17), 'this positive conception of health as an equilibrium is more frequently found in French than British studies'. Harmony was also a feature of Polynesian ideas about health (Capstick *et al.*, 2009), as were notions of balance and harmony in Kwok and Sullivan's (2007) study of Chinese Australians; this same study highlighted the emphasis on 'everything in moderation' in Chinese culture. And what needs to be kept in equilibrium? For Polynesians, health is about harmony with the environment and the family (Capstick *et al.*, 2009). Omonzejele (2008) in his study of concepts of health in Nigeria also concludes that health is about more than individual stability: 'Good health for the African consists of mental, physical, spiritual, and emotional stability for oneself, family members, and community' (p. 120).

Whilst the different concepts of health have been presented here as discrete, people often express health as combining many elements. For instance, in Abbot *et al.*'s study of post-Soviet citizens' health world views, one respondent noted: 'A healthy person is rarely ill, does not have any chronic diseases – is always in a good mood, has a healthy complexion, good hair and shinning [*sic*] eyes and allocates time for work and rest' (Abbott *et al.*, 2006, p. 232).

There are other themes that emerge from the studies, which relate more to how much health can be maintained, and where responsibility for this lies. For instance, some studies explore the degree to which people feel health is under their control. Pill and Stott (1982), in an early study of lay health beliefs in Wales, suggested that their respondents' ideas about health and illness could be grouped into those ideas that were 'fatalistic', where health

and illness were regarded as states that were not preventable, and those that emphasized 'lifestyles' where, in contrast, it was felt that an individual's behaviours could affect health and the occurrence of illness. However, in a later paper, Pill and Stott (1987) cautioned against categorizing *people* as 'fatalists' or 'lifestylists', and observed that rather than seeing these as opposing views, respondents tended to combine elements of each view. Similarly, Davison *et al.* (1992) argued that 'fatalism' is not a contrast to a lifestyle-orientated viewpoint, but rather tends to arise from people's observations of the limitations of a purely lifestyle-focused discourse; in other words, people are well aware of messages that particular behaviours are linked to health maintenance or to the causes of illness, but if their own experiences do not support this view, they may become more fatalistic. Exploring the relationship between people's ideas and the messages they receive about health is clearly important, as so much of current health promotion discourse focuses on health lifestyles. However Abbott *et al.* (2006) found that amongst post-soviet citizens few explicitly mentioned health lifestyles in their definition of health, and the authors attributed this to a lack of understanding of 'healthy lifestyles' as promoted in the West.

Conceiving of health as something that can be controlled also raises questions about how that control can be achieved. On the theme of control and responsibility, Mullen (1994) gives an account of male Glaswegians' concepts of health in which both activist and fatalist dimensions can be found. He points out however that:

… activist thinking was seen to have three strands: personal activism, social activism, and religious activism. Further, fatalistic thinking was not about passive submission but rather the belief that control lay outwith the person in the realm of the social, natural or supernatural worlds.

(Mullen, 1994, p. 414)

From her findings, Pierret (1993) suggested that whilst one conception of health was as 'health-product', as an objective to be reached, yet in this conception there were also tensions, and the need for balance, as health was seen as a product of controlled risk on the one hand, and pleasure on the other. This theme of tension is also pursued in Crawford's (1984) work in the USA, where he discussed health as 'release' and health as 'self-control'.

So how much do people accept that they are responsible for their own health? In Abbot *et al.*'s

(2006) study, virtually all their respondents felt that individuals were responsible for their own health, and this is a theme in many studies. For instance, the issue of health as an achieved rather than an ascribed status is evident in the work of Backett (1992). This study of middle-class Scottish respondents also revealed that 'healthiness was defined on moralistic grounds' (p. 261). Crawford (1984) also highlighted the moral dimensions of health, pointing out that as health comes increasingly to be seen as a state to be achieved by effort and self-control, health becomes an issue of morality.

Another conception of health highlighted by Pierret is that of 'health-institution', where health is seen as a matter of public policy and institutions; Pierret comments on the peculiarly French nature of this construct, which might be a product of French social policy (Pierret, 1993, p. 19). Certainly in Abbot et al.'s (2006) study, few respondents felt the post-soviet state was responsible for their health.

Throughout this overview of findings about lay concepts of health, there has been evidence of cultural differences in such concepts. This reminds us of the importance of the social context of such ideas, or worldviews. There is also evidence of the importance of social location in terms of social class, gender and age. A number of studies have compared and contrasted concepts of health among middle- and working-class respondents. For instance, in d'Houtard and Field's study (1984) of 4000 French respondents, when socio-economic status was taken into account, clear differences emerged, with those in the higher and middle groups associating health with hedonism, equilibrium, vitality and the body, whereas those in the lower socio-economic groups were more likely to see health as the absence of sickness, and link it with hygiene and psychological well-being. d'Houtard and Field conclude that the more personalized representation of health in the higher groups contrasts with a more socialized conception of health in the lower groups, where health is instrumental and about performing one's social duties and these differences reflect 'corresponding roles of mastery on the one hand and the execution of social tasks on the other' (p. 47). These findings are echoed in the Welsh study by Pill and Stott (1982), who also found that functional definitions of health were more common among working class women. However, Calnan (1987) cautions against overemphasizing social class differences in defining health, suggesting that seeming differences may relate more to the way people respond in interviews, and also to whether respondents are referring to their own health or that of others.

Another dimension that has received increasing attention in recent years is the role of gender in ideas about health. Blaxter (1990) found women more expansive in their ideas about health than men; she also found that younger women saw health as being about vitality, energy and functioning, whereas younger men were more likely to see health as being about physical fitness. Many of the early studies were purely on women (e.g. Herzlich, 1973; Pill and Stott, 1982); however, recent studies have focused on men and their definitions of health. For instance, Robertson (2006) found that direct questions about defining health were problematic for his male respondents, and he attributed this to cultural notions of masculinity, which made it harder for men to express concern about health: 'It's [health] important to women, innit? But blokes don't really bother about it' (Robertson, 2006, p. 178). He goes on to describe echoes of Crawford's description of health as an outcome of control and release, as shown in this quote from a respondent (p. 179):

> I do keep fit. Um, don't drink too much, don't smoke too much, well I probably do at times [laughs]. Watching what I eat to a certain extent, eating fruit and vegetables. Um, so keeping fit, eating healthily and not living life in too much of an excess.

However, Macintyre et al. (2006) concluded from their Scottish study of both men and women that there were no significant sex differences. They comment: 'This suggests the need for caution in interpreting single sex studies from which implicit comparisons might be drawn with the opposite sex on the assumption that there are always gender differences' (p. 737). Age is also a factor in concepts of health. Blaxter (1990) found definitions of health varied through the life course, with negative concepts and views of health as ability to function perhaps unsurprisingly more common among older people. Jolanki (2004), in a study of Finnish older people aged 90 and above, noted that the responses suggested people's concerns to challenge the discourse of old age as decline.

Much of the research on concepts of health and maintenance of health also contains evidence about lay people's ideas about the causes of illness. For instance, if health is seen as a product of harmony and social relationships, then disruption to this balance and problems with relationships might be assumed to be the causes of ill health. However, it is important to realize that causes of health and causes of illness may not be conceptualized as opposites. For instance, in Herzlich's (1973) work, health was seen as something that could be enhanced by individual actions, but illness was seen as a something that was beyond control. Broadly, however, lay ideas about the causes of illness have been categorized as internal or external, as under control or beyond control. An example of a focus on external factors is the following: 'Illness in the Pacific may be perceived as coming about through conflicts with family members, or because of otherwise unbalanced or unsettled social relations' (Capstick *et al.*, 2009, p. 1343). Similarly, Swami *et al.* (2009) conclude that among their Malaysian respondents, the social world was seen as an important source of both health and illness. In Nigeria, Omonzejele (2008) stresses ideas about disequilibrium with ancestors, or evil spirits as the cause of disease.

The research on lay health beliefs outlined here has revealed rich and complex ideas, despite their differing methodologies. As the studies show, people offer many accounts for health and illness, and it would be wrong to assume that an understanding of such accounts might allow us simplistically to predict behaviours; if people are in 'two minds', they will have more than one way of making sense of health and illness and acting on it (Stainton Rogers, 1991). How health promotion both needs to take account of, and might work with, lay knowledge will become a theme of the book. We now turn to another key theme – empowerment.

Empowerment

From what has been said so far, it is becoming apparent that our view of health promotion will favour an approach that puts people at the centre, is empowering and that challenges the social structure. Sen (1993) articulated the idea of capability, meaning all those aspects that enable people to live lives with meaning and value to themselves; capability also contains aspects that constrain individual agency – the ability to act freely. As health promotion is defined as the ability to take control of the determinants of health, it follows that people need a certain amount of power in order for them to do so. Empowerment is essential in terms

of becoming the author of one's own life (Baxter Magolda, 2001).

We are thus clear in our view that empowerment is the key to promoting health. This view has been consistent from Leeds Met from the work of its first professor of health promotion, Keith Tones, who asserted that 'empowerment is central to the philosophy and practice of health promotion' (Tones, 1997, p. 39), through to our current work trying to assess the effectiveness of empowerment approaches (Woodall *et al.*, 2010). Empowerment is mentioned in all the key conference documents from Ottawa to Nairobi. Empowerment fits with humanistic approaches, where we assume that people are competent and capable of making changes in their own lives; that competence is gained through life experiences and not from being told what to do; and that empowerment cannot be 'given', it can only be worked on collaboratively in a process where workers or 'professionals' aim to decrease the powerlessness felt by individuals and communities. It is also clear that power and thus empowerment, like capability, are distributed in massively unfair ways.

Despite the central importance of empowerment, there have been difficulties in articulating exactly what it means. Victoria Grace (1991), for example, highlighted the inconsistencies and contradictions of 'empowerment' within health promotion and our recent review reiterated the ambiguity and confusion surrounding the term, suggesting that 'empowerment' was being deployed somewhat 'casually' in the health promotion literature (Woodall *et al.*, 2010). Raeburn and Rootman (1998) have been two prominent authors highly disparaging of empowerment and its status as a 'buzz word' in the health promotion discourse. They, like Rissel (1994), argue that the absence of a clear definition leads to misuse of the term. Its use has thus become problematic (Minkler, 2000; Labonté and Laverack, 2008).

Describing a vicious theory-practice circle, Catteneo and Chapman (2010, p. 646) argue that '... one might argue that the lack of precise definition has made it amenable to diffuse applications, which have then exacerbated the lack of precision in its definition.'

Somewhat compounding this issue is that the discourse of empowerment within health promotion has not evolved consistently throughout the world, so it is little wonder that the term has been misrepresented so frequently within health promotion. For example, empowerment has been viewed by some as a 'Eurocentric phenomenon' (MacDonald, 1998, p. 40), perhaps because it was a central tenet in the original WHO European Healthy Cities programme in the late 1980s (Heritage and Dooris, 2009) and because of the burgeoning amount of academic writing on the issue from European authors. However, in Africa, community development and empowerment approaches have been a key strategy for some time (Nyamwaya, 2003), but very little academic commentary has been provided by authors from the continent. In contrast, Anme and McCall (2011) argue that empowerment is a reasonably new concept in Asian countries. These semantic difficulties should not divert attention from the overwhelming importance of empowerment. A working definition has been suggested by the Altogether Better programme in the UK (Woodall *et al.*, 2010).

Power and powerlessness

The concept of power is at the heart of empowerment – empowerment can only occur when communities take power (Rappaport, 1985). The radical roots of empowerment can be traced to the Brazilian humanitarian and educator, Paulo Freire (1921–1997), whose key text, the *Pedagogy of the Oppressed* (1972) introduced key ideas such as critical awareness or 'conscientization', which have entered the health promotion discourse. Freire necessarily brings in the issue of oppression, necessitating a working definition of this term too, but as Dalyrymple and Burke (2001) argue, oppression is a complex and emotive term and to explain it simply would be to deny this complexity. Empowerment approaches should inevitably be anti-oppressive approaches, and we would assert that health promotion needs to develop anti-oppressive practice. 'Anti-oppressive practice … means recognizing power imbalances and working towards the promotion of change to redress the balance of power' (Dalyrymple and Burke, 2001, p. 15). This requires reflection on the power imbalances between professional health promoters and communities, and challenging oppression wherever it is encountered, a task taken up again in Chapter 6.

Within health promotion, empowerment is generally regarded as a process enabling people who lack power to become more powerful and gain some degree of control over their lives and health (Green and Tones, 2010). Empowerment is associated with re-addressing causes of powerlessness and addressing the causes of disempowerment. In its widest and most radical sense, empowerment concerns combating oppression and injustice and is a process by which people work together to increase the control they have over events that influence their lives and health (Laverack, 2006). This suggests that empowerment approaches must operate at various levels, from the individual through to organizations and communities. Real empowerment only happens when a person makes the links between their personal position and structural inequalities, i.e. when they not only feel a sense of personal power but when they begin to question their position in society. An example of this awakening is this:

> During the depression years of the 1930s, cookery classes were organised for women in poor communities in an attempt to help them to provide nutritious meals for their families despite low incomes. One particular evening a group of women were being taught how to make cod's head soup – a cheap and nourishing dish. At the end of the lesson the women were asked if they had any questions. 'Just one', said a member of the group, 'whilst we're eating the cod's head soup, who's eating the cod?'
> (Quoted in Popay and Dhooge, 1989; a cod is a fish commonly eaten in Europe)

Powerlessness, in Solomon's view, comes from three potential sources: first there are systems that systematically deny powerless groups opportunities to take action; secondly there are the negative images that oppressed people have of themselves, a form of self-oppression; and thirdly there are the negative experiences that oppressed people undergo in their everyday interactions with systems, institutions or the media (Solomon, 1976).

Experiencing powerlessness means that people feel further excluded, rejected, treated as inferior and in a downward spiral, then feel that they are inadequate, unworthy and deserving of the role of 'second-class citizen'. Those experiencing powerlessness could occupy a stigmatized role, such as a 'traveller', Gypsy, 'ethnic minority', 'gay', 'asylum seeker', 'ex-convict', 'mentally ill', and/or could be facing insecurity in terms of joblessness, income, housing, education, literacy. Dalyrymple and Burke (2001, p. 15) comment:

> If we consider that people's relations are structured by power then we are less likely to stereotype, make assumptions or misinterpret other people's actions. It is when we do stereotype, make assumptions and misinterpret other people's actions that we start to oppress.

Individual and community empowerment

Empowerment is a necessary stage in the process of transformation. As Freire (1972, p. 34) said:

> In order for the oppressed to be able to wage the struggle for their liberation, they must perceive the reality of oppression, not as a closed world from which there is no exit, but as a limited situation which they can transform.

Empowerment resonates with the important sociological concept of agency: 'agency' suggests that people have 'internal powers and capacities which, through their exercise, make her an active entity constantly intervening in the course of events going on around her' (Barnes, 2000, p. 25). It means that people have the will, power and capacities to act. Agency, however, also requires an understanding of how one stands in relation to others – an appreciation of one's identity and standing in relation to the rest of the community in which one is located. This moves us into considering individual empowerment and its relationship with community empowerment. These two concepts are often presented as being separate but, of course, they are connected, as summed up in the basic tenet of the feminist movement, that 'the personal *is* political'.

A prominent theme within health promotion discourse has been that of fostering individual forms of empowerment. Individual empowerment (also referred to as psychological or self-empowerment) can occur without participation in collective action or political activity and is concerned with developing attributes that are needed for people's personal capacity to be realized – it is associated with people having the genuine potential for making choices (Tones and Tilford, 2001). Choice is an embedded term in the empowerment process, as empowered people often have better health because they are more capable of making informed decisions about their life (Rodwell, 1996; Linhorst *et al.*, 2002; Larsen and Manderson, 2009). Staples (1990) suggests that individual empowerment concerns the way people think about themselves and also the knowledge, capacities, skills and mastery they actually possess. At the individual level, individuals who become more empowered feel better about themselves (Staples, 1990). Indeed, there is good evidence showing that empowerment interventions focusing on the individual increase participants' psychological well-being, including self-efficacy, confidence and self-esteem (Gibbon, 2000; M.L. Crossley, 2001; Jacobs, 2006; Laverack, 2006; Wallerstein, 2006; Aday and

Kehoe, 2008; Fisher and Gosselink, 2008). Two comprehensive reviews, for example, both showed how participation in various groups and programmes had led to increases in these particular health related outcomes (Laverack, 2006; Wallerstein, 2006). Whereas powerlessness can lead to depression and immobilization, increasing empowerment can enable a shift in the individual's perspective, away from self-blame and towards feeling that change is possible. Greater individual empowerment is not at the expense of others and is thus a non-zero-sum form of power. This type of power is infinite – an increase in one person's individual empowerment is not at the expense of anyone else's – it is a 'win-win situation' (Rissel, 1994, p. 40).

Individual empowerment, however, may not consider or challenge the social determinants of people's health (Wallerstein, 2006) and in our view does not constitute full empowerment in the sense of transforming the relations of power. Individual empowerment alone has a limited impact on addressing health inequalities and may be illusory in that it does not lead to an increase in actual power or resources. In reality, empowerment simply at the individual level does little to influence social change:

> Individual empowerment is not now, and never will be, the salvation of powerless groups. To attain social equality, power relations between 'haves,' 'have-a-littles,' and 'have-nots' must be transformed. This requires a change in the structure of power.
>
> (Staples, 1990, p. 36)

This is not to say that individual empowerment is unimportant, but if it remains at this level, it overlooks change in the political and social context in which people live (Riger, 2002).

Individual and community empowerment should be seen as linked (South and Woodall, 2010). Community empowerment (Box 1.6) is a 'synergistic interaction' between the individual and broader social and political action (Laverack, 2007, p. 14). It refers to processes by which individuals join together to make changes to their situation and is tied to principles of social justice. Tones and Green (2004) suggest that if empowerment consists of facilitating voluntaristic decision making and 'free choice', then it should not only target the individual but also the community and environment. This is encapsulated by Wallerstein (1992, p. 198) who defines community empowerment as:

> … a social-action process that promotes the participation of people, organizations and communities towards the

goals of increased individual and community control, political efficacy, improved quality of life and social justice.

Community empowerment (Boxes 1.7 and 1.8) has a political orientation in which members are made conscious of their powerlessness and actively participate in redistributing resources to challenge social injustice and oppression (Ward and Mullender, 1991; Rissel, 1994). Wise (1995) believes that the underlying philosophy involves enabling the oppressed to understand how structural processes (e.g. gender inequality, social inequalities etc.) impact upon them as individuals and concerns mobilizing people to take community action (Baum, 2003). Community empowerment in this respect is a zero-sum relationship – power in essence is finite.

For example, resources being directed at some people can cause the displacement of power (disempowerment) from others due to competition for the same resources (Riger, 2002; Heritage and Dooris, 2009). Consequently, Gutierrez (1991) suggests that this form of empowerment is based on a conflict model.

'Outcome' or a 'process'

Whether community empowerment is an 'outcome' or a 'process' has been a debated issue. An empowerment outcome could, for instance, be the redistribution of resources to redress health inequalities or a change of policy in favour of community groups that have come together to create change. Laverack

---

Box 1.6. Similarities and differences.

According to Laverack and Wallerstein (2001), community empowerment has been superseded by a plethora of other terms, such as community capacity, community competence, community cohesiveness and social capital.

Community empowerment has similarities with, but is still different from, terms like community capacity and social capital. In summary, community empowerment concerns power relations and intervention strategies which ultimately focus on challenging social injustice through political and social processes (Wallerstein, 2006). The overall aim is to allow people to take control of the decisions that influence their lives and health.

Box 1.7. Yuannan women's reproductive health and development programme.

Participation in the Yuannan women's reproductive health and development programme involved women documenting their life conditions using 'photovoice', a participatory strategy that uses photographs for creating discussion between people. The women were given cameras to capture their lives as they saw them. The images collected were then used to promote dialogue, critical thinking and to identify causes of powerlessness. The images allowed the women to better advocate for change and resulted in an improvement in the reported levels of self-esteem and confidence. Photos produced as part of the programme led to the establishment of day-care centres, midwifery programmes and scholarships for rural girls.

(Laverack, 2006)

Box 1.8. New Zealand Prostitutes Collective (NZPC).

Laverack and Whipple (2010) report how a group of sex workers in New Zealand were able to bring about reform in the legislation regulating sex work. Through a process of community empowerment the women achieved social justice and equity for all sex workers in New Zealand. Although it took 15 years to reform the legislation, started only by a small group of sex workers, NZPC were eventually able to influence public policy and safeguard the human rights of sex workers through building partnerships and alliances with agencies.

(2004) has developed a continuum of community empowerment, which outlines the process of community empowerment. As illustrated in Fig. 1.2, Laverack has proposed a series of actions that progressively contribute to more organized community and social action. Starting with an individual's concerns about a given issue, the process of community empowerment starts with the development of small mutual groups, then community organizations, partnerships and ultimately to groups of people taking political and social action to create social change through the redistribution of resources and power (Wallerstein, 2002; Laverack, 2006). The continuum is useful from a theoretical perspective, as it allows practitioners to identify how they can be involved in empowerment approaches in their everyday work. However, in reality, the process of community empowerment is dynamic, iterative and complex as opposed to linear (Laverack, 2010).

Participation is an important feature of Laverack's continuum. Individuals have a better chance of achieving their health goals if they can share these matters with other people who are faced with similar problems. Through participation, individuals are likely to experience some degree of control as they are better able to define and analyse their concerns and together they are capable of finding joint solutions to act on their issues (Laverack, 2005). Figure 1.3 demonstrates the assumed relationship between levels of participation and degrees of empowerment.

While participation forms 'the backbone of empowering strategies' (Wallerstein, 2006, p. 9), participation alone does not guarantee empowerment, as it can often be manipulative and passive, rather than truly engaging and empowering. It is perhaps also naive to consider empowerment a panacea for improving people's health and well-being (Hyung Hur, 2006), as Baistow (1994, p. 40) argues that 'problems' are often complex and interconnected, and a simple 'dose of empowerment' is unlikely to provide the full solution. Notwithstanding this criticism, it is imperative that the relationship between the professional and the community is equal in order to facilitate empowerment-based

approaches (Jacobs, 2006). Empowerment cannot be given to people, but comes from individuals and communities empowering themselves. The health promoter may create a situation where empowerment may be more likely, through facilitation and support, but only when groups of people gain their own momentum, acquire skills and advocate for their own change will empowerment have been fully realized (Rissel, 1994; Wallerstein, 2006). Yet this does raise some interesting issues, such as how do we know if our intentions and practices to empower really are empowering and can we and should we attempt to facilitate the empowerment all people? According to Allah Nikkhah and Redzuan (2009), if power cannot change, i.e. if it is inherent in social structures, then empowerment is not possible. The question as to whether health promoters should work toward empowerment with all people returns to our view of health promotion as a moral activity. Riger (2002) argues that there are some groups who should become less empowered, rather than more powerful, but who should decide which groups? Our work on health in prisons presents interesting contradictions between the central tenet of empowerment and the stripping away of power that the prison experience engenders.

Prisons arguably represent an environment where empowerment cannot be fostered. It is a setting where little choice can be sanctioned, where autonomy and personal agency are frowned upon and where prisoners are under surveillance, controlled and forced into subservience and obedience (Maeve, 1999; Smith, 2000; de Viggiani, 2006). The 'power over' individuals can be particularly damaging to health and contribute to a loss of control and disempowerment (Woodall, 2010). The empowerment of people in prison is a potentially contentious area, but the WHO (1995) claim that prisons should be concerned with empowerment. This has been reiterated more recently by the UK government in their delivery plan for health and criminal justice (DOH, 2009), where the strategy alluded to the increased participation and empowerment of offenders. The rationale for empowering prisoners

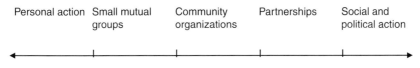

| Personal action | Small mutual groups | Community organizations | Partnerships | Social and political action |

Fig. 1.2. Community empowerment as a continuum (Laverack, 2004, p. 48).

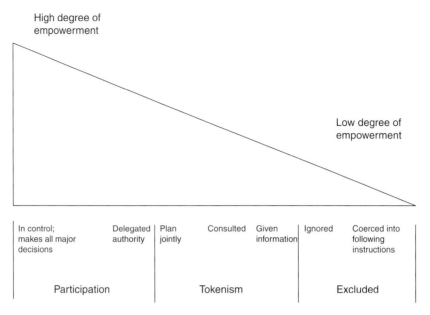

Fig. 1.3. Participation and empowerment gradient (from Green and Tones, 2010, p. 46).

is justifiable, given the fact that most people serve short prison sentences and return back to the community. However, there are some writers who feel that the empowerment of prisoners is 'morally questionable and politically dangerous' (The Aldridge Foundation and Johnson, 2008, p. 2)

The Altogether Better initiative (Woodall *et al.*, 2010) has attempted to provide a working definition and model of empowerment, captured in Fig. 1.4.

The Value Base of Health Promotion

So far, this chapter has explicated a number of key values held by health promotion, including the importance of listening to lay views, empowerment and participation. We will end this chapter by further outlining the value base, by presenting the views of a number of thinkers writing recently. Seedhouse (1997) has usefully summarized the debate about whether health promotion is, and should, be driven by values or by evidence. Wills and Woodhead (2004, p. 12) argue that a 'technical-rational model' of public health with its focus on 'applying expert knowledge objectively to analyse problems and provide the solutions' gives 'little attention to value based questions about what outcomes are desirable, how situations are framed

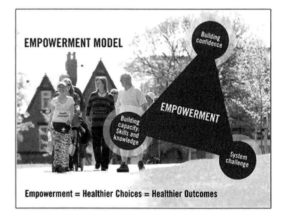

Fig. 1.4. The Altogether Better Empowerment Model (Woodall *et al.*, 2010).

as problems, and what constitutes valid professional knowledge'.

We would assert that not only is health promotion driven by values, but also that some sets of values *are* better than others: justice, peace and democracy are all values, and we would say that they are better than their opposites. We (the authors) are thus not value-neutral. Furthermore, we believe that health promotion should be underpinned by a set of values and principles that guide practice. If health promotion is values-driven, it raises the question of how the evidence base for health promotion should be used, as evidence-based practice not only is part of current professional life, but it also ethical to work in ways that we believe will work (however 'working' is defined). Evidence-based practice is taken up in Chapter 5, with the obvious caveat that not everything that counts can be counted, and with a scepticism towards the current obsession with not doing anything that cannot be 'evaluated'. A values-based approach should not be seen in opposition to an evidence-based approach – it is not necessarily an 'either/or'. Incorporating evidence-based practice is an ethical value, and should be one of the principles of practice *within* a values-based approach. Some attempts at delineating sets of values for health promotion work will be discussed here.

The WHO in 1986 developed a set of concepts in its Copenhagen discussion paper mentioned above (WHO, 2009a). These principles are covered in Box 1.9.

Health promotion focuses on the population as a whole in their everyday life, not just those seen to be 'at risk' of particular disease conditions; it is directed towards action on the determinants or causes of health; it combines diverse but complementary methods and approaches; it aims to obtain effective public participation; it requires professionals to play an enabling role.

In an attempt to detail what a 'people-centred' health promotion might look like, Raeburn and Rootman (1998) wrote a book with that title, which provided a set of principles. Health promotion should be concerned with real, living people and focus on positive, life-enhancing factors and not on social problems or disease symptoms; it should focus on people's strengths rather than their weaknesses; it should focus on health outcomes rather than more general (but equally important) outcomes such as social justice or social equality; empowerment, justice, equity, cultural appropriateness and spirituality are central values to health promotion; health promotion takes time and should not be judged on 'quick results'; health promotion must be efficient, well-organized and systematic.

Those countries – Australia, Canada, the USA and New Zealand – with a large indigenous population that was subsequently overwhelmed by the invading Europeans have attempted to develop ways to make health promotion meaningful for those native populations. Durie (2004), for example, has argued that for health promotion to be useful to indigenous peoples it must be consistent with their values, attitudes and aspirations. (The same could be said of all communities, of course.) An Indigenous model of health promotion has been developed in New Zealand that combines

---

Box 1.9. Health Promotion Principles.

1. Health promotion involves the population as a whole in the context of their everyday life, rather than focusing on people at risk for specific diseases. It enables people to take control over, and responsibility for, their health as an important component of everyday life – both as spontaneous and organized action for health. This requires full and continuing access to information about health and how it might be sought for by all the population, using, therefore, all dissemination methods available.

2. Health promotion is directed towards action on the determinants or causes of health. Health promotion, therefore, requires a close cooperation of sectors beyond health services, reflecting the diversity of conditions that influence health. Government, at both local and national levels, has a unique responsibility to act appropriately and in a timely way to ensure that the 'total' environment, which is beyond the control of individuals and groups, is conductive to health.

3. Health promotion combines diverse, but complementary, methods or approaches, including communication, education, legislation, fiscal measures, organizational change, community development and spontaneous local activities against health hazards.

4. Health promotion aims particularly at effective and concrete public participation. This focus requires the further development of problem-defining and decision-making life skills both individually and collectively.

5. While health promotion is basically an activity in the health and social fields, and not a medical service, health professionals – particularly in primary health care – have an important role in nurturing and enabling health promotion. Health professionals should work towards developing their special contributions in education and health advocacy.

(WHO, 2009a, pp. 29–30)

Maori world views and health perspectives. Given the importance of the symbolism of the Southern Cross constellation (Te Pae Mahutonga), the model adopts an Indigenous icon to increase understanding and to make health promotion relevant. The model proposes four key areas for health ('ora'), each representing one of the central Southern Cross stars.

> Waiora refers to the natural environment and environmental protection; Mauri Ora is about cultural identity and access to the Maori world; Toiora includes wellbeing and healthy lifestyles; and Whaiora encompasses full participation in the wider society. The two pointer stars symbolize capacities that are needed to make progress: effective leadership (Nga Manukura) and autonomy (Mana Whakahaere).
>
> (Durie, 2004, p. 181)

Another excellent guide to health promotion using an 'aboriginal lens' is provided by the Mungabareena Aboriginal Corporation and Women's Health Goulburn North East (2008), in a guide that is useful to everyone working in health promotion, wherever they practise, as it presents ideas on how to work in culturally appropriate, participative ways. It considers each stage of a health promotion work cycle through an 'aboriginal lens':

> There are 10 components within the framework. Each section describes a health promotion concept, and then presents it through an Aboriginal lens. Following this are examples of practice and useful resources. The 10 components of the framework are:
>
> 1. Identifying guiding values and principles
> 2. Identifying theoretical underpinnings and frameworks
> 3. Analyzing health promotion practice environments
> 4. Evidence gathering and needs analysis
> 5. Identifying settings and sectors for health promotion
> 6. Determining and implementing health promotion strategies and approaches
> 7. Evaluation design and delivery
> 8. Partnerships, leadership and management
> 9. Workforce capacity building for the Aboriginal community and generalist (non-Aboriginal) health and community sector.
> 10. Infrastructure and resources for sustainability.
>
> (Mungabareena Aboriginal Corporation and Women's Health Goulburn North East, 2008, p. 3)

Health promotion has been influenced by the principles of community development, such as described by Ife (2000), and we would assert that these principles would provide a suitable basis for health promotion too:

- social justice principles, which address structural disadvantage, power differentials, institutionalized prejudice;
- local principles, valuing local knowledge, cultures, skills, ways of working, assets;
- process principles, working ethically and with integrity, processes which have appropriate timing and pace, are inclusive and lead to community building, engender cooperation, consensus, peace, non-violence, conflict resolution, and enable vision and outcomes to be realized;
- ecological principles, which consider sustainability, diversity, holism, and the environment;
- global principles, which link the global and local (thinking globally, acting locally), makes connections, using anti-colonial practice.

The principles of working with communities are the focus of the next chapter.

The detailed discussion of the concept of health shows that it is not a simple one, is seen differently by different people, and changes over time; discussion of the social determinants of health show that health is the product of complex processes. Thus promoting 'health' is not a straightforward matter. Health promotion has attempted to distance itself from the reductionist, narrow approaches adopted by the medical and psycho-behavioural models, and ways of working that shows a gap between the rhetoric of health promotion and the reality in practice:

> ... a significant proportion of present health promotion practice is underpinned by a conventional biomedical model of health that is concerned primarily with the physical body and its diseases ... many health promoters find themselves focusing primarily or exclusively on the conventional immediate or proximal behavioural risk factors for specific disease conditions, without the opportunity to address the distal or social determinants of health.
>
> (Gregg and O'Hara, 2007a, p. 10)

To address this gap, Gregg and O'Hara (2007b) propose a new model that is explored more fully in Chapter 6, when we offer some ways of thinking suitable for the 21st century. Whether the values and principles are adequate for providing a reliable foundation and whether this foundation is translatable into action remains a moot point, and some of this discussion is taken up again at the very end of the book. For now, distilling the key points from this discussion, we propose (in no particular order), that health promotion therefore should:

1. Resist biomedical models of health and advocate for the broader social model of health to be adopted at policy making levels.
2. Place empowerment and the redistribution of power at the centre, so as to bring transformation to individuals, communities, organizations and societies with the aim of producing greater health.
3. Involve collaborative working and strong partnerships.
4. Take a salutogenic approach and promote the importance of 'good health'.
5. Take an assets perspective (rather than a deficits one), with a stress on capability.
6. Prioritize the most vulnerable and disadvantaged communities, thus tackling areas facing the worst inequities.
7. Start with where people are, use 'constructionist epistemologies', respect and value local knowledge and lay epidemiologies.
8. Use ethical change processes.
9. Have capable, skilled health promotion workers working alongside communities as allies.
10. Adopt anti-oppressive practices, challenge racism, sexism, disablism and any other practices and institutions that oppress people.
11. Adopt ecological principles, sustainability and a concern for the environment.
12. Invest in the capabilities of the health promotion workforce (both professional and lay), paying attention to life-long learning.
13. Use evidence-based practice, 'real world' evaluation methods.
14. Produce 'big picture' change at the societal level and also 'small picture' change, working with communities and individuals.

Summary

This chapter has provided a foundation upon which to base further study; it has presented the key values and principles of health promotion; emphasized the need to tackle the social determinants of health; presented a history of health promotion's development through the WHO-led conferences; introduced some threshold concepts; outlined professional and lay concepts of health; and suggested that empowerment approaches are the essence of health promotion. The next three chapters provide detail on three central aspects of health promotion, which follow logically from what we have outlined thus far: working with communities, developing healthy public policy and communicating about health. These three areas also, logically, form modules of study on many postgraduate courses.

Further Reading

Commission on Social Determinants of Health (2008) Closing the Gap in a Generation: Health Equity through Action on the Social Determinants of Health. Final Report of the Commission on Social Determinants of Health. WHO, Geneva.

Douglas, J., Earle, S., Handsley, S., Lloyd, C. and Spurr, S. (2007) *A Reader in Promoting Public Health: Challenge and Controversy*. Sage, London.

Global Health Watch (2011) *Global Health Watch 3: An Alternative World Health Report*. Zed Books, London.

Health Promotion International (2011) Volume 26, supplement 2, December – all papers.

Minujin, A. and Nandy, S. (2012) *Global Child Poverty and Well-being: Measurement, Concepts, Policy and Action*. The Policy Press, London.

Myers, J.C. (2010) *The Politics of Equality*. Zed Books, London.

Venkatapuram, S. (2011) *Health Justice*. Polity Press, Cambridge, UK.

2 Healthy Communities

LOUISE WARWICK-BOOTH, SALLY FOSTER AND JUDY WHITE

This chapter aims to:

- explore 'the community' as a vital context for health promotion;
- explore different meanings of community participation, community involvement and community development;
- discuss the importance of social capital;
- explore the role of lay involvement in health promotion; and
- suggest that working *with* communities and not merely *in* communities is essential.

Introduction

In the previous chapter, a view of health promotion was developed which emphasized a focus on the social determinants of health, social justice, and empowering and participatory approaches. This chapter addresses the central importance of community in such a view of health promotion, and of people as active producers of health and agents of change. In it, we argue that there is a need to see the world through the community's eyes, to appreciate the contribution that people and communities can make to improve their health. We start by exploring both the term 'community' and the centrality of community involvement to health promotion; we then move to a consideration of the health-enabling community, through networks and social capital, before moving on to explore the growing recognition of the importance of lay people's health knowledge and the contribution they can make in terms of health care and health promotion. There are many ways of involving and working with communities and we explore various models, especially the community development approach, before concluding with a consideration of other ways in which people may address health issues through social action.

Communities as a Context for Health Promotion Practice

Although the community is the central focus for health promotion practice, the term community itself, however, is used to mean different things and

there is debate about who the community is (Laverack and Wallerstein, 2001). The notion of community is frequently linked to place – thus a community can be understood to be a setting; however, it is too simplistic to say that community is just neighbourhood (Green and Tones, 2010). Communities are also formed upon the basis of collective identity, sense of belonging, shared values and network membership (Piper, 2009). Advances in technology mean that virtual communities exist and are perceived as real communities to those who are members (De Leeuw, 2000). The Standing Conference for Community Development (2001, p. 4) defines community as 'the web of personal relationships, groups, networks, traditions and patterns of behaviour that exist amongst those who share physical neighbourhoods, socio-economic conditions or common understandings and interests'. Despite the existence of such definitions, the notion of community remains a fuzzy concept. Mayo (1994, p. 48) says 'It is not just that the term has been used ambiguously. It has been contested, fought over and appropriated for different uses and interests to justify different politics, policies and practices.' The term can be used at both descriptive and evaluative levels and is defined as much by community members as by academics (Shaw, 2004); therefore, the notion of community continues to be contested. Despite these issues with understanding communities, health promoters will continue to work in communities as part of their work in

---

addressing the broader social determinants of health (Kinder *et al.*, 2000) because communities are fundamentally linked to both health and health inequalities.

However, debates about the nature of such work in communities are central to health promotion practice. Many professionals have the word community in their title: community suggesting the location of their work, for instance community nurses and police community support officers, to name but two. But to say one works *in* the community is not necessarily to say one works *with* the community. McKnight (2003), for instance, talks about the relationship many professionals have with their clients, and points out that the word client is derived from the Greek, and means 'one who is controlled', whereas he argues strongly for a model of practice that frees people from medical clienthood to act as 'citizens', meaning those who hold power. Indeed, McKnight argues that health is a political communal issue and that to 'convert a medical problem into a political issue is central to health improvement' (1978, p. 39), and we will return to this claim, and McKnight's work, later in the chapter.

This focus on community health action is reflected in various global initiatives and statements from the WHO, such as the Alma-Ata Declaration: '… people have a right and a duty to participate individually and collectively in the planning and implementation of their health care' (WHO, 1978, p. 1). Similarly, the WHO Regional Office for Europe argued: 'it is a basic tenet of the health for all philosophy that … health developments in communities are made not only for, but with and by people' (WHO, 1985, p. 4). Finally, the Ottawa Charter states:

> Health promotion works through effective community action in setting priorities, making decisions, planning strategies and implementing them to achieve better health. At the heart of this process is the empowerment of communities, and the ownership and control of their endeavours and destiny.
>
> (WHO, 1986b, c)

In order to help facilitate the development of healthy communities, the WHO (1986b, c) launched the global healthy cities programme in which a network of places has been created that attempts to get health on the social, economic and political agenda of local government as well as demonstrating the influence of all sectors upon health and well-being. This programme is focused upon community as a geographical location in its present format, links the local to the global and outlines key components described as producing a healthy city (Box 2.1).

Developing healthy communities and healthy cities is seen as an important tool to tackle inequalities, in which community development is used within the context of health promotion practice. This is spelled out clearly in a report on evidence from the New Deal for Communities Programme in England, which was initiated by the then Labour Government to address inequalities in health. In the report, Pearson *et al.* (2010) stress that community development is a vital contributor to improved health outcomes. The reason why community is so central is because this is the level of social experience where the possibilities of action and the constraints of structures meet (Popple and Shaw, 1997); in communities, we see the interface, where the social, economic and environmental determinants of health and individuals' lives and experiences meet, and they are thus the potential site of struggle. Indeed, in relation to health inequalities, Baum (2007) talks about the 'nutcracker effect' and makes a case for

---

Box 2.1. The concept of a healthy city.

- A healthy city is defined by a process, not an outcome.
- A healthy city is conscious of health and is trying to improve it, so any city can be a healthy city.
- The requirements of being a healthy city are simply a commitment to health and a process and structure to achieve it.

- A healthy city is one that continually creates and improves its physical and social environments and expands the community resources that enable people mutually to support each other in performing all the functions of life and developing to their maximum potential.

(Adapted from WHO, 2011)

---

an approach to tackling such inequalities, which has not only top-down actions involving policies, but also bottom-up involvement from civil society. Thus communities have become a central focus of health promotion and Syme (2004) suggests that the work of health promotion is to help build people's sense of control and to embrace the community as an empowered partner. The rest of this chapter explores key issues in such control, and debates about participation, community development and empowerment. In addressing issues of control and participation, we stress throughout the vital importance of the lay perspective, of seeing the world through people's eyes, and acknowledging and valuing people's contribution.

However, our starting point is communities themselves, and evidence about what makes a health-enabling community (Campbell, 2001). Ecological studies suggest that social capital is a collective resource and an important determinant of health at the collective level (Poortinga, 2006). Whilst debates abound within the literature about social capital,

> A construction of social capital which explicitly endorses the importance of transformative social engagement, whilst at the same time recognizing the potential negative consequences of social capital development, could help community organizers build communities in ways that truly promote health.
>
> (Wakefield and Poland, 2005, p. 2829)

Thus, the concept of social capital has become central to health promotion, and so we start by looking at debates about social capital, communities and health.

Communities are People Working Together: Social Capital and Health

Social capital has been given much attention within academic literature and policy circles in recent years. Wakefield and Poland (2005) stress the importance of social connections in relation to health promotion indicating the importance of community ties and relationships for health. Much attention has been afforded to the concept in relation to how it affects health and communities via social support mechanisms.

All definitions of the concept suggest that it has positive consequences for members of communities (Box 2.2), achieved through shared norms, networks and trust. As different theorists highlight a variety of interpretations of the concept, these will be considered now with particular attention being paid to how health relates to these varying conceptualizations.

Communities are Connections and Social Obligations

Bourdieu describes social capital as a potential resource linked to networks and relationships of mutual acquaintance and recognition, giving members collectively owned capital (Schuller *et al.*, 2000). More recently, Bourdieu (1999) identified the superimposition of social and physical space, and the associated disadvantages that are bestowed upon less powerful social groups by their residence in poorer communities.

Bourdieu emphasizes the structural constraints on individuals and the unequal access that people have to resources based on class, gender and race (Everingham, 2003). For Bourdieu (1999), access to resources and issues of power within society

---

Box 2.2. Social capital, social support and health.

There is a large amount of evidence showing social capital as an important determinant of health (Szreter and Woolcock, 2002).

Social capital has been empirically linked to:

- increased mental health (Kawachi and Berkman 2001);
- improved child development (Keating, 2000);
- reduced mortality (Kawachi *et al.*, 1997);

- lower susceptibility to binge drinking (Weitzman and Kawachi, 2000);
- sustained participation in anti-smoking programmes (Lindstrom *et al.*, 2000);
- self-related health (Kawachi and Kennedy, 1999; Rose, 2000a); and
- less inequality – income inequality leads to poorer health outcomes via disinvestment in social capital (Kawachi *et al.*, 1997).

---

are the key to social capital (Harper, 2001). Social capital effectively viewed as connections and social obligations in Bourdieu's (1986) understanding can be converted under certain conditions into economic capital. This notion has greatly appealed to policy makers as it appears a quick-fix solution but this fails to focus upon the complexity of the 'conditions' under which such a process actually happens (Leonard, 2004). There is, however, growing consensus that area effects do exist. Reviews of American research (Jencks and Mayer, 1990; Brooks-Gun et al., 1993; Ellen and Turner, 1997) all conclude that there are causal connections between poorer neighbourhoods and other social problems, as well as poorer health outcomes. Atkinson and Kintrea (2004) argue that individuals living within deprived communities are held back because of where they live rather than by their individual characteristics. Hence, what is important from this perspective is the way in which individual networks operate to enhance or constrain health outcomes. For example, in Russia after the collapse of communism, life expectancy decreased. Men reporting high levels of mistrust in local government had higher rates of total mortality (Kennedy et al., 1998), demonstrating that in communities with lower levels of social capital, health outcomes are poorer. Furthermore, where communities are unequal, health outcomes are poorer (Marmot and Wilkinson, 2001). Indeed, democratic societies tend to have fewer health inequalities and better population health (Wilkinson and Pickett, 2010). The importance of social capital levels within communities in relation to health is illustrated through the example of Roseto (Box 2.3).

The Roseto example highlights the importance of the function of social capital in relation to health within a community context. Coleman (1998) defines social capital by its function. Here social capital is similarly conceived of as a resource to be drawn upon and is more positively conceptualized in the sense that social relations constitute useful capital resources for actors through processes such as obligations, expectations, trust, information channels and setting norms. Coleman (1998) sees these resources as less exclusionary than Bourdieu (1999). According to Coleman (1990), social capital takes three forms:

- first, the obligations and expectations, which depend upon the trustworthiness of the social environment;
- secondly, the capacity of information to flow through the social structure in order to provide a basis for action; and
- finally, it is the presence of norms accompanied by effective sanctions.

Social capital differs from other forms of capital in that it does not necessarily bring benefits just to the individual; rather, it brings benefits to all of those who are part of the social structure such as community members.

Despite this recognition of the wider benefits of the concept, Coleman's theorizing primarily focuses upon individuals and the family. Coleman also argues that social capital creation is a largely unintentional process (Schuller et al., 2000). Hence, if social capital production is unintentional, how can it be encouraged or developed within the context of communities for health promotion? Furthermore,

---

Box 2.3. The Roseto effect.

- From 1955–1965, Roseto, an Italian American community in Eastern Pennsylvania, displayed a high level of social capital through ethnic and social similarities, close family networks and good community cohesion (Stout et al., 1964).
- Roseto community members had a very low rate of myocardial infarction (heart attacks) in comparison with nearby communities (Bruhn and Wolf, 1979).
- It was suggested that the stable and supportive structure of the community and strong family

cohesion may have led to a protective effect against heart attacks (Bruhn and Wolf, 1979).
- As the community evolved and changed during the 1960s and 1970s, family and community ties became less important. Greater rates of heart attacks were seen as well as higher mortality rates. This shows the importance of social networks and community ties in relation to health because there were no significantly different risk factors for Roseto and its neighbouring communities (Egolf et al., 1992).

Coleman's concept, if applied in practice, would lead researchers to focus upon social capital as inherently good (Everingham, 2003). Critics say that this approach overstates the importance of closure and dense ties within the social structure and treats social capital in an unproblematic manner (Schuller *et al.*, 2000). Despite critique, Coleman's view of social capital highlights the community benefits of the concept. If social capital benefits the community as a whole and can be developed through effective social policy, it can consequently serve as a useful tool in health promotion practice. However, the uncritical stance taken by Coleman requires caution. Even if human capital can be increased, this does not necessarily ensure better community-level prospects because structural factors also need to be considered. For example, social capital levels within communities relate to economic and political contexts as well as material resources (Wakefield and Poland, 2005).

Communities are Networks of People

Putnam's work on social capital popularized the concept enabling it to find its way into mainstream political discourse (Schuller *et al.*, 2000). According to Putnam (2000), social capital refers to the connections among individuals, social networks and other forms of reciprocity and trust, which arise from them. Networks, norms and trust dominate his definition of the concept whilst activity is situated at the heart of civic life and therefore is a crucial aspect of his conceptualization

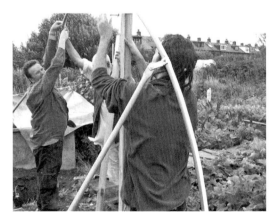

An allotment project – growing your food in your own community, Bradford, England.

(Schuller *et al.*, 2000). Putnam (1993a, b) suggests that the more people work together, the more that social capital is produced. This relates to the notion that communities that work together are indeed healthier. Putnam's work imbues community with highly positive connotations portraying an image of helpful, friendly interactions between individuals based upon personal knowledge and face-to-face contact. This ignores the downside of community life (Leonard, 2004), in which negative relationships may be detrimental to both physical and mental health.

Central to Putman's (2000) conceptualization of social capital is his description of different types of networks, all of which operate within communities to produce differential health effects.

1. Bonding networks – bonding social capital is essentially related to a common identity with group members having some factors in common (Jochum, 2003). The literature highlights the potential negative impact of excessive bonding social capital because it can serve to create exclusivity (Taylor, 2000a, b).
2. Bridging networks – these are the weak connections between people such as business associates and acquaintances. Bridging social capital is likely to be greater in communities and organizations that have a collaborative approach (Jochum, 2003). Narayan (1999) pays particular attention to the potential for less powerful and more socially excluded groups to benefit from bridging ties. Narayan (1999) argues that effective bonding and bridging ties are required to avoid social exclusion, suggesting that social capital can be a helpful resource in community development approaches.
3. Linking networks – these are the connections made to those in positions of power by those less powerful (Putnam, 2000). Linking social capital is useful in terms of enlisting and engaging support from key agencies and key players within community contexts.

These different types of social capital are also said to interact with each other. However, there is some debate about whether this interaction occurs automatically and recent empirical findings suggest that moving from bonding to bridging social capital is beset with contradictions. In order to set in motion the framework for bridging social capital to develop, the conditions that lead to the emergence of bonding social capital may need to be undermined

(Leonard, 2004). Thus, the interaction between the different types of social capital requires further exploration and is not as simple as some suggest. Despite complexities, evidence does show that network membership and related social support are important in relation to health, as Box 2.4 demonstrates.

There is some contradictory evidence here in the sense that network membership can detrimentally affect health. For example, network phenomena are relevant to obesity because obesity appears to spread through social ties (Christakis and Fowler, 2007). Furthermore, the mechanism of action between social support activities, membership of networks and health outcomes is not very well understood. The relationship between social capital and health outcomes at the community level is largely hypothesized (Halpern, 2005).

Communities are People that Trust Each Other

Fukuyama primarily presents social capital as trust by defining the concept as 'a set of informal values or norms shared amongst members of a group that permits co-operation between them' (1999, p. 16). Most social capital definitions pay attention to trust and give equal weight to trust and networks, but some prioritize one over the other (Berman and Phillips, 2003). For Fukuyama (1999), trust leads to cooperation, which makes both groups and networks operate smoothly. Central to this conceptualization is the radius of trust, where it is argued that the further trust expands outside of the family then the more likely it is to be based upon moral resources and ethical behaviours (Fukuyama, 2001). Where groups have a narrow radius of trust, their in-group solidarity reduces their ability to cooperate with outsiders. It is arguably difficult for people to trust those outside of narrow circles especially in the absence of weak ties. This argument about in-group trust reflects parallels to Putnam's emphasis on close, tight-knit networks not always being beneficial. Communities with broader networks of trust are more likely to care about individual members; therefore, they are more predisposed to provide political mandates for the redistribution of wealth via taxation (Halpern, 2005), which will ultimately benefit health. Furthermore, in communities with higher levels of trust, wider interactions between people are likely to be more cooperative and less stressful. Family, neighbours and friends are likely to provide more social support as a result of higher levels of trust (Halpern, 2005), and social support has already been shown to be beneficial for health.

However, Fukuyama's (1999) approach has again been criticized because of his monoculturalist standpoint in which he asserts that societies need to share the same language, norms and moral values in order to avoid disintegration. Other commentators such as Kymlicka (1995a, b) offer a more multiculturalist perspective.

Social Capital and Health Promotion within a Community Context

These definitions of social capital all highlight elements such as trust and associational linkages, although they give different weight to their importance. The different definitions also emerge from a

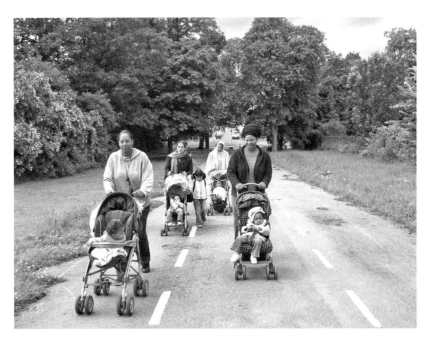

Changing lifestyles – getting out and being more active with others in the community, England.

variety of theoretical traditions. Bourdieu draws upon Marxism, Coleman is concerned with function, Putnam politically locates his interpretation and Fukuyama's discussion is inherently conservative. Despite these different traditions, all of these interpretations suggest that the concept is useful for understanding communities and in achieving positive health outcomes. The benefits of social capital in relation to health can seemingly be conferred upon individuals and communities via several different pathways (Kawachi and Berkman, 2001). Clearly, if social capital can provide community-level benefits then it is important for health promotion practice (Box 2.5).

However, a cautious approach is required when examining the links between health promotion and social capital. There are complex and subtle ways in which inequality manifests itself within community relationships, which on the surface seem to be based upon trust and reciprocity (Leonard, 2004). For example, inclusion and exclusion occurs based upon gender, ethnicity, age and religious affiliation. The key lesson to be drawn from the empirical evidence for health promoters is that although social capital can have positive health outcomes, it is not a thing that can be promoted via public health interventions and simply given to people. Health promoters

need to get to grips with the concept because 'understanding social capital is part of understanding the operations of power in daily life and how social structure as practiced in daily life creates and perpetuates inequalities' (Stevens, 2008, p. 1182). Understanding the concept involves examining its complexities, including the problems and criticisms highlighted within the literature.

Problems with the Concept of Social Capital

There are a number of criticisms of the concept, which is still in its infancy. Several theorists argue that social capital as a concept is nothing new and that it is simply being exported wholesale from America to the UK, which ignores the cultural context of its conceptualization within research studies (Harper, 2001). Davies (2002) suggests that the concept is gender blind and ethnocentric, whilst other theorists recognize that it is narrow in its focus (Walker and Wigfield, 2003). These are just some of the broader criticisms of social capital. Other general criticisms focus upon definitional diversity (Portes and Landolt, 1996; Schuller *et al.*, 2000; Everingham, 2003), lack of precision (Flora, 1998; Wall *et al.*, 1998; Everingham, 2003) and

Box 2.5. Social capital and health promotion practice.

- Social capital is important for community development, which is central for health promotion practice (Wakefield and Poland, 2005). A social action approach to community development is the most useful approach, as it is concerned with social justice in social activity (Rose, 2000b).
- Involvement and empowerment are central to health promotion practice; similarly, associating together and engaging in community affairs are crucial to social capital development for Coleman (1998).
- Social capital is a resource that may have positive use in relation to health promotion initiatives.
- Putnam (2000) marshals evidence to demonstrate that in high social capital areas, public spaces are cleaner, people are friendlier and the streets are safer. Certainly, in some communities, more positive levels of health are achieved when social capital is developed to a higher level.
- At the level of the individual, social capital has been argued to improve quality of life via psychological and biological processes. Individuals rich in social capital with high levels of social,

economic, cultural and collective resources cope better with traumas and fight illness more effectively (Putnam, 2000).
- Social capital can act as a buffer against economic disadvantage by reducing the effects of a lack of economic resources (Campbell, 1999).
- Putnam (2000) also discusses participation and reciprocity. The concept may be useful in explaining collective action in terms of mutual involvement and the creation of alliances to achieve group and community goals including those related to health improvement.
- Social capital indicators can be used to assist in evaluating and measuring health-enabling communities, as well as acting as an intermediary stage between health promotion approaches at the micro-level (such as individual behaviour change) and the macro-level (empowerment approaches). Furthermore, understanding social capital can help health promoters to develop both policies and interventions that promote health-enhancing social and community contexts (Campbell, 2001).

measurement difficulties (Portes and Landolt, 1996; G. Green *et al.*, 2000; Walker and Wigfield, 2003). Given that there is no agreed consensus about the definition of the concept, the operationalization of a shared definition for measurement is simply not achievable (Harper and Kelly, 2003). Furthermore, there are ongoing debates about the concept in relation to its theoretical underpinnings and epistemological foundations (Portes and Landolt, 1996; Gamarnikow and Green, 1999; Hooge and Stolle, 2003). With specific reference to health contexts, the way in which policy makers view social capital can involve victim blaming, because poor people may be viewed as unhealthy as a result of not participating enough in community activities (Muntaner and Lynch, 1999). Attention therefore needs to be paid to attempts to build social capital via health promotion initiatives delivered within communities. Box 2.6 outlines some of the complexity of building social capital in the community.

Thus, social capital creation in the context of healthy communities needs both a considered and critical approach. Social capital development is

certainly not a magic bullet for health promoters nor is it a cheap option, because the quality of relationships is important within networks. Policy makers have become engaged with social capital development because its implications within policy appear cheaper than attempting to reduce health inequalities (Campbell, 2001). Indeed, 'taking social capital seriously in the context of health promotion in rich or poor countries is therefore not in any sense a cheap option; it is an additional dimension – and one necessarily requiring additional costs – which has been too neglected in the past' (Szreter and Woolcock, 2002, p. 26). All of this ultimately begs the question of how social capital relates to the concept of a healthy community.

Healthy Communities and Social Capital

There is no simple answer to what a healthy community will look like when measured against the concept of social capital because there are many complexities here. This is demonstrated in the lack of clarification of healthy community indicators within the wider literature. The key lessons for

Box 2.6. Issues with attempts to build social capital at a community level.

1. Trust within any neighbourhood is not guaranteed. The impact of historical divisions within areas, contemporary housing policies, intense deprivation and the sudden presence of streams of money can all act to undermine levels of trust between individuals and groups within neighbourhoods (Hibbitt *et al.*, 2001).

2. Secondly, building social capital may not be a suitable goal for all community contexts or purposes. Social capital is highly context dependent (Jochum, 2003), different factors in different places create success (Groves *et al.*, 2003) and as a result, consideration must be paid to the socio-economic situation and the institutional environment within any community (Jochum, 2003).

3. Some individuals are better placed within a community to lead others forward in developing social capital. Despite this suggestion, the literature on social capital has largely ignored the importance of leadership. Purdue (2001) suggests that community leaders play a crucial role in accumulating internal social capital through their work at the grassroots level and are at the forefront of developing external social capital through partnerships with outside elite groups.

4. Social capital is only valuable to the extent that community members recognize and sustain its value. It may be the case that the use of social capital terminology brings out a negative reaction from people working within community settings (Begum, 2003), including health promotion practitioners.

health promoters in relation to social capital as part of healthy communities are outlined here.

- Healthy communities are not necessarily those with more social capital.
  - Cattell's (2001) study of working class communities in East London demonstrates that social networks are crucial in helping individuals survive and negotiate disadvantage. Thus an absence of social capital per se is not automatically linked to an unhealthy community.
  - Cohesive communities can also be characterized by distrust, fear and racism as well as exclusion of outsiders (Baum, 1999). Therefore, health promoters should carefully examine the types of social capital present when engaged with community work.
- Healthy communities are more likely to have the right kind of social capital in which network access serves to link to resources that help improve situations (Gibson, 2010).
  - Building bridging social capital will not necessarily lead to healthier communities because only particular individuals are likely to participate and so this becomes exclusionary (Wakefield and Poland, 2005). In communities divided along many lines such as race, class and gender, developing shared norms and networks is difficult (Gibson, 2006).

- Healthy communities have health-promoting social relations such as good local governance; they are effective communities with strong participation, inter-sectoral collaboration and political and managerial accountability (Campbell, 2001). Again, this requires the examination of the types of social capital present within any given community.
- Healthy communities are happy communities.
  - There are links between happiness and health with subjective well-being strongly influencing health and all-cause mortality (Deiner and Chan, 2011). Holistic definitions of health examine the interaction and relationship between the self, the community and the environment. Thus, being part of happy communities is important for individual mental health.
  - There are many determinants of happiness but whether a person is happy depends upon whether others in that person's individual networks are also happy, suggesting that happiness is related to groups and levels of social capital (Fowler and Christakis, 2008). Interventions to enhance subjective well-being are therefore useful tools for public health practitioners (Deiner and Chan, 2011).
- Healthy communities are salutogenic.
  - Antonovsky (1996) raised the question of what is the origin of health, asking health

promoters to explore this rather than focusing upon the causes of disease. He argues that an individual sense of coherence, the way in which people view their lives, has a positive influence upon health. This definition of health is at the individual, group or societal level; therefore, communities that enable people to build sense of coherence are salutogenic and healthier. Salutogenic communities can be measured according to social capital levels and network support.

- Healthy communities have assets (assets model).
  - Communities have numerous assets – individual and community resources that they can draw upon, which are useful in protecting against negative health outcomes. Community-level resources include social capital such as networks, solidarity and community cohesion. These are health promoting irrespective of the level of inequality and disadvantage within the community (Morgan and Ziglio, 2007). Health promoters therefore should work in ways to develop assets rather than simply examining community deficits.

Despite the debates about the evidence base for social capital and the various theoretical interpretations of the concept, it has made its way into contemporary health promotion practice as part of the notions of healthy communities and the importance of working with communities. We now turn to the issue of working with communities as a central component of health promotion practice, by exploring lay knowledge and the lay contribution, and various models of community participation.

Communities are People Working Together: the Lay Contribution

Lay health knowledge

Much of the preceding discussion has indicated that a focus on healthy communities requires an approach that goes beyond seeing people as passive recipients of professional action to regarding them as an essential resource in enhancing the health of the community. For instance, when communicating about health in the traditional biomedical model, health knowledge is the domain of health professionals who transmit this knowledge to patients and the public. However, the problems of this

approach are well illustrated in a classic paper by Nichter (1985), which describes a health promotion message about safe water in Sri Lanka that failed because it did not recognize people's ideas about health. The paper describes how diarrhoeal diseases continued to be a major cause of morbidity and mortality in spite of preventive interventions emphasizing the importance of drinking boiled water. The assumption was that people had misunderstood the message about boiling water, but Nichter began to understand that water use needed to be set in a cultural context. Only sick people were seen to need water that has had its properties mitigated by boiling it; moreover, such people were also not to be subjected to shock, so even though they were offered boiled water, this water may need cooling with unboiled water. By contrast, healthy people were not seen to need boiled water, as this is no longer fresh and 'full of life' (p. 668). His paper illustrates clearly that for health messages to be communicated effectively, recognition of lay beliefs and cultural systems is vital. Box 2.7 offers a contrasting example of an approach to behaviour change rooted in an acknowledgement and valuing of people's ideas about health, and a participatory approach.

From 'Expert Patients' to Lay Health Work

The importance attached to lay knowledge by so many writers, and the recognition of the need to understand and involve people in efforts to improve their health means the public are now no longer seen as 'passive recipients of paternalistic professional efforts to improve their health' (Taylor, 2007, p. 98). Indeed, Stacey reminded us in 1976 that a 'patient can be said to be a producer as much as a consumer of that elusive and abstract "good health"' (Stacey, 1976, p. 194), and in recent years there has been increasing recognition of lay expertise in encounters with health professionals. In 1985, Tuckett *et al.* talked about the medical encounter as the meeting of two experts, with not only the professional but also the lay person who had considerable experiential knowledge of their own body, health and illness. Debates about this professional–patient relationship have centred on the term 'compliance' and 'adherence', both of which connote a relationship of inequality and obedience; in recent years the term 'concordance' has been used to signify greater equality and shared decision making in the medical encounter (Britten,

Box 2.7. Grandmothers in Senegal.

Aubel *et al.* (2004) describe a community intervention in Senegal that involved grandmothers and older women. The authors are critical of what they call the dominant transmission–persuasion paradigm in health education and communication, where top-down, one-way messages are aimed at changing people's behaviours. They point to the failure of this paradigm in maternal and child health nutrition practices, and the findings of a review in Senegal, which outlines the following factors as limiting health and nutrition education:

- the use of directive methods;
- failure to involve influential household and community members;
- failure to include discussion of existing socio-cultural values and beliefs in discussions of recommended practices (p. 945).

As a result of a study, which highlighted the significant role played by grandmothers and older women in the community in relation to maternal and child health, a 'grandmother strategy' was developed. Working in communities that were very traditional in their ideas and practices in relation to health, the strategy:

- aimed to develop existing human resources in the community and enhance social networks;

(Aubel *et al.*, 2004)

- focused on encouraging 'learners' to actively and critically analyse both their own experience and alternative solutions and construct their own strategies to deal with everyday problems (p. 950).

This approach was participatory and empowering, with activities such as songs and problem-posing 'stories-without-an-ending', which encouraged 'discussion of problematic nutrition-related situations and possible solutions' (p. 951). After initial scepticism, the grandmothers were won round by the respect shown for their roles, ideas and experiences, and they participated enthusiastically. Both quantitative and qualitative findings suggested the strategy had been successful, with not only improved nutritional practices but strengthened family and community ties. Whilst there are various factors in this success, a key one was the acknowledgement of the lay perspective, and the integration of this.
The grandmothers themselves said:

- 'Grandmothers are human beings like everyone else';
- 'We can learn and change our ways';
- 'We feel much stronger now because not only do we have our traditional knowledge'; but, in addition,
- 'We have acquired the knowledge of the doctors' (p. 954).

2003; Bissell *et al.*, 2004) and, more recently, shared decision making, mutuality and 'co-production' (Boyle *et al.*, 2010) have been terms used to reflect the changed nature of the relationship. In addition, the term 'lay expert' has entered the vocabulary of health care, particularly with the initiatives associated with 'expert patients' in chronic disease management (DOH, 2001a). Such initiatives are partially rooted in the growing literature, outlined in Chapter 1, about lay health knowledge and behaviour, but they are also rooted in the rising consumerism in welfare services, and in critiques of medical power (e.g. Illich, 1976; Doyal with Pennell, 1979).

We also have considerable evidence of the role of people in self-care and care of others, covering activities as disparate as diagnosing and treating one's own cold, to spending 50 or more hours a week engaged in the care of someone with a chronic illness or disability. (The ONS, 2003, reported that the 2001 census showed that there were 5.2 million unpaid carers, that is 1 in 10 of the population of England and Wales.) Recognition of the enormous contribution of such unpaid care for health and social care policy is clearly important, but the lay contribution is wider even than this and covers lay roles in the services themselves, as volunteers and lay health workers, and it is to these roles we now turn.

As noted above, people engage in health care work all the time, in looking after their own health, or that of family and neighbours. Indeed, historically and globally deprived communities have often had no access to other forms of care; women, for example, have assisted in childbirth, often combining what Kleinman calls the 'popular' and 'folk' sectors. However, the development of programmes for lay or community health workers (CHWs) has its origins in the shift to primary health care (PHC) from the late 1970s onwards, and the community health movements of the 1970s.

The PHC movement that arose post-Alma-Ata grew out of critiques of the nature of urban hospital-focused health care systems (e.g. Morley's 'three quarters rule', in Sanders with Carver, 1985), and the alternatives being developed in post-colonial and socialist countries such as Tanzania and China, with a focus on poor communities and the use, for example, of barefoot doctors. Thus PHC was seen to address two agendas: one was that of creating an alternative to the high-cost urban health systems with highly trained health professionals; the other was the 'transformative agenda, which saw ill-health as rooted in the poverty and inequality in people's lives' (Standing *et al.*, 2008, p. 2097). Community mobilization and the training of local people to provide basic services was seen as central to PHC, and as a result, CHW programmes proliferated, although Standing *et al.* (2008) point to their decline from the late 1980s onwards. Whilst CHWs go by many names, and, as we shall see, are surrounded by many issues, the WHO defines them thus:

Community health workers should be members of the communities where they work, should be selected by the communities, should be answerable to the communities for their activities, should be supported by the health

system but not necessarily a part of its organization, and have shorter training than professional workers.
(WHO, 1989, as cited by Lehman and Sanders 2007, p. 3)

This definition suggests that CHWs are more than cheap alternatives in a health care system; rather, they are seen as embedded in communities, as well as performing an important linking role between health care systems and their communities (Lehman and Sanders, 2007). The issues that surround them are many; two recent reviews (Lehman and Sanders, 2007; Standing *et al.*, 2008) have explored these and a summary can be seen in Box 2.8.

Much of the research on CHWs has been carried out in countries of the global South. However, in the global North, the use of lay health workers is also advocated and has been well researched in the USA, although often in relation to very different agendas. There are two key questions – is the main motivation for the use of lay health workers that they are able to stand in for health professionals and thus 'create breathing room for physicians and other health professionals, allowing them to make best use of their limited time' (Canadian Health Service Research Foundation, 2007, p. 1) or is there a positive value to the use of their knowledge and skills 'that allows lay health workers to serve as change agents to others within their community' (Canadian Health Service Research Foundation, 2007, p. 2)?

Box 2.8. CHWs.

1. Who volunteers and who selects? The issues here relate to power in the community as well as the possible use of patronage to select particular members for training.
2. Should they be paid, and if so, by whom? The general evidence is that volunteering does not sustain most CHW schemes, as by definition, they are often in poor communities. Thus most CHWs are remunerated, and more usually by the state rather than the local community.
3. What training do they receive? Again, by definition, training is short, but without ongoing training and support, CHWs may be put in situations where they cannot meet the expectations of the communities in which they work. This may be particularly true where the CHWs have specialist roles in relation to, for example, TB, or maternal and child care. There is

also the issue of how much CHWs are trained as community mediators, rather than as health care practitioners.
4. To whom are they accountable? On the one hand, CHWs may become embedded in the government services of which they are a part, and struggle then to obtain status and recognition within this service (this may lead them, for example, to seek further training and remuneration to enhance their professional status). On the other hand, if CHWs see themselves as embedded in the community, their roles and actions may bring them into conflict with the very government services that pay them.
5. How sustainable are CHW programmes? The evidence suggests that without the support of both established services and the communities themselves, the failure rate of CHW programmes is high.

(Lehman and Sanders, 2007; Standing *et al.*, 2008)

The first of these questions is primarily functional in terms of service delivery but the second one is more relevant to health promotion and recognizes the particular advantages of the use of CHWs in reaching communities; this has meant that the use of CHWs in the global North is very much associated with reaching 'hard-to-reach' groups. In North America for instance, CHWs have been used to encourage underserved groups to access preventive services; for instance encouraging Vietnamese-American women to attend for cancer screening (Mock *et al.*, 2007). A more radical approach is that of Poder es Salud/Power for Health in Oregon, USA, where a project worked with CHWs from local African American and Latino communities to address the root causes of health disparities (Farquhar *et al.*, 2008). Farquhar *et al.* (2008) explore in their paper the experiences of the CHWs themselves, rather than the communities, and they describe the multiple roles of the CHWs, their work as community organizers and their experiences as members of the Steering Committee for the project. What comes through vividly in their account is the activist roles of the CHWs and the importance of an increasing sense of power; not only do the participating families and neighbours 'have a greater sense of community … and now because of that they know they have the power to change things' (Farquhar *et al.*, 2008, p. 4), but the CHWs themselves felt empowered by the project.

In 2004, a role similar to a CHW, the health trainer, was introduced in England (DOH, 2004) and health trainer programmes now exist in most parts of the country, albeit on a small scale. Health trainers are recruited to work with communities with the poorest health, and the majority are drawn from those communities. They do outreach work in order to engage with communities that professionals have found 'hard to reach', offer one-to-one support for people who want to make a change to improve their health, and connect them to activities in their local area. As Attree *et al.* (2011) point out, health trainers do not address structural inequalities in health, but they are addressing inequity of access and engaging with many diverse, disadvantaged communities. There can be challenges with combining community engagement with achieving public health targets for behaviour change (Wills and Cook, 2011), but evaluations of local services have consistently shown that the peer-led, person-centred approach health trainers take is hugely popular and is helping people make changes that they want to make to improve their health (South *et al.*, 2006; Kime *et al.*, 2008; White *et al.*, 2010a, b; Kinsella *et al.*, 2011; White *et al.*, 2011).

Also in England, a recent study entitled People in Public Health (South *et al.*, 2010a) explored the many public health roles lay people are taking and the myriad ways they are contributing to improving the health of their communities. It covered many of the issues outlined above and concluded that a particular strength of lay people in health roles is their ability to act as a bridge to communities to connect to groups and communities who are seen as 'hard-to-reach'.

Such approaches allow people who are accepted and trusted in communities to deliver health messages and offer support in appropriate ways to people who might otherwise be disengaged or who face barriers to participation. Findings suggest that lay workers and volunteers add an important dimension and therefore such approaches need to be considered as a way of addressing persistent health inequalities (South *et al.*, 2010a, p. 226). The People in Public Health study formed the basis of a book entitled *People Centred Public Health*, which sets out a radical vision for a different public health system with citizen engagement at its core (South *et al.*, 2012).

South *et al.* (2012) explore the challenges for health professionals working with lay health workers; for a number of years, there have been suggestions that a process of deprofessionalization might be occurring in relation to the medical profession in particular (Cooper *et al.*, 2011). Deprofessionalization has been linked to, among other trends, the changing nature of health professional relationships with their patients, and a more knowledgeable and demanding public. Clearly, having lay people acting in public health or health care roles, together with the shift we saw earlier to recognizing lay ideas about health as a form of knowledge, suggests a possible challenge to the idea of the all-knowing and all-powerful professional. There are also issues about how professionals and lay health workers work together and how much they value each other. In a study of five community partnerships in South Africa, El Ansari *et al.* (2002) outline five key domains of partnership working, which include educational competencies, partnership fostering skills, community involvement expertise, proficiency as change agents, and strategic and management skills. They conclude from their study that whilst community members valued the skills of professionals especially in relation to proficiency as change agents and strategic and management skills, professionals had limited appreciation of community skills in all domains. Whilst this study was not specifically about CHWs, it does suggest potential problems in valuing those without professional training. South *et al.* (2010a) also found that there were concerns about acceptance by health professionals:

> I think some of the professionals boo hoo us. (L25)

> I think they [lay workers] need credibility, I think they need that, I think a lot of … a lot of health care professionals see themselves as the professionals and they know best. (P23)
>
> (South *et al.*, 2010a, p. 193)

The other issue for lay health workers is their own potential professionalization, the possibility of pursuing further training and gaining greater remuneration and the challenges of working within bureaucratic institutions. An example of the ways in which a lay health project goes 'mainstream' is shown by the Fag Ends project (Box 2.9).

The challenge engaging lay people in public health roles can present to professional power has been discussed above. CHW programmes have also been challenged as a diversion from addressing structural inequalities in health and as part of a right wing agenda to 'shrink the state' and replace paid workers with volunteers. South *et al.* (2012) address these challenges and put forward a strong argument in support of engaging lay people as part of a more people-centred public health. Lay engagement is not about saying there can be individual solutions to structural problems and it need not undermine professionals or replace paid jobs. Rather, it is a way of people gaining more control over their health and is supported by a growing evidence base, which demonstrates that lay engagement can make a real difference to health at a community level.

Community Participation

The claim earlier that the public are now no longer seen as 'passive recipients of paternalistic efforts to improve their health (Taylor, 2007, p. 98) is nowhere more evident than in the emphasis on community participation in promoting health. The previous discussion of lay health work is a reflection of this focus, but community participation can also be seen to go further than this by involving communities in processes relating to the identification of health problems and action on these. Central to debates about community participation and health are issues of power and empowerment, and the concepts of community participation and empowerment have become central tenets of health promotion in the years since the 1978 Alma-Ata Declaration.

Box 2.9. Fag Ends Smoking Cessation Service.

The Fag Ends Service had its origins in a community development self-help project, started in Everton in 1994 in a deprived area of Liverpool, in which ex-smokers volunteered to help others give up smoking. Over time, there were changes in the project and by 1999 it had become the main smoking cessation service for Liverpool, with the lay advisers working as employees. Springett *et al.* (2007) provide an account of the way in which the service used local knowledge to provide a successful service, appropriate and responsive to users' needs, whilst also meeting the requirements from national guidance. The critical role of the lay health workers is clear; as the workers themselves said, their clients:

> … want real people, don't they. People they meet every day, on the same level, talking in everyday terms. Sometimes they get frightened of too much medical jargon. Most of our clients don't understand that. (p. 251)

(Springett *et al.*, 2007)

At the heart of the account is the recognition of the tensions between the lay world and the professional world, and the conflicting ideologies of bottom-up and top-down provision:

> What lay beneath the Fag Ends experience … is an issue of conflicting ideologies that still reverberate at the centre of health promotion and public health, situated as it is in the dominant discourse of medical science … many established power relationships including the devaluing of local knowledge by the professional remain undisturbed. (p. 254)

Yet the Fag Ends Service offers a glimpse into how a service can manage to be responsive to its users, recognizing their own knowledge, culture and complex lives, and retaining the ethos of a self-help group.

So what is meant by community participation in health? If people have a 'right and a duty to participate individually and collectively in the planning and implementation of their health care' (WHO, 1978) and if at the heart of health promotion is 'the empowerment of communities, and the ownership and control of their endeavours and destiny' (WHO, 1986b, c), what does this mean in practice? A number of writers have developed models of participation that reflect the degree of actual involvement and power of lay people; perhaps the most used are those of Brager and Specht (1973, as cited by Tilford and Tones, 2001) and Arnstein (1969), who uses a ladder (Fig. 2.1) to demonstrate how participation may move from the lower rungs of manipulation, therapy and informing, to middle rungs of consulting and placating; only the top three rungs of partnership, delegated power and citizen control demonstrate citizen power (Tritter and McCallum, 2006). Similarly, Tones and Green (2004) link degrees of participation to degrees of empowerment, suggesting that often what is called participation is really about involving communities in health promotion initiatives that come from professional agendas and are professionally led. In a similar vein, Rifkin et al. (2000) identified three different approaches to

community participation and health; the medical approach, the health planning approach and the community development approach. In the medical approach, community participation is envisaged as communities responding to professional directives and taking action to improve their health. In the health planning approach, community participation is again professionally led, with the community participating in planning and delivering appropriate health care. In the final approach, that of community development, the focus goes beyond health services to the wider determinants of health and it is the community that identifies and acts on the conditions affecting their health. McKnight (1978) offers an account of such an approach in Chicago (Box 2.10).

The example overleaf of the community development approach to participation and health illustrates the centrality of empowerment to such participation, and the move from a model of *clients* to one of *citizens*, who rather than being controlled, are actually wielding power themselves. It also stresses the importance of *associations* rather than *institutions* in promoting health in communities, and this issue has been explored earlier in this chapter in relation to social capital. Finally, this approach is firmly rooted in a recognition of the social determinants of health that require action beyond the provision of health services, and again, as an approach to community participation it is explored more in a later section.

However, it is clear that this more radical understanding of what is involved in community participation and health is not always reflected in programmes or policies. Whilst participatory approaches in health found favour in the 1970s, when the progressive agenda reflected the greater power of Third World countries and the socialist world (De Vos *et al.*, 2009), the 1980s ushered in a 'lost decade' of debt and structural adjustment programmes, and the health planning and medical approaches to community participation gained popularity, with an emphasis on the 'cultural sensitivity' and appropriateness of health services and initiatives, which could be achieved by involving the community in issues of design and delivery. Such programmes were also often about cost sharing or cost cutting, as illustrated by the Bamako initiative and community control and financing of health centres, making them essentially about 'rural development on the cheap' (Jewkes and Murcott, 1998). The World Bank's enthusiastic support of community participation is seen as further

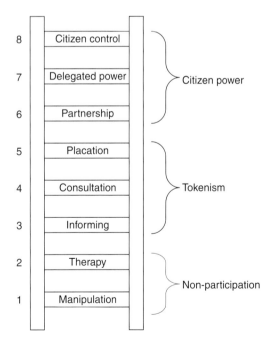

Fig. 2.1. Arnstein's ladder of citizen participation.

Box 2.10. Community action in Chicago.

McKnight's example centres on a community of about 60,000 mainly poor and black people in Chicago. Their initial efforts were focused on 'recapturing' the two hospitals, which had originally serviced the community when it was a predominantly white community, and which were not accessible to the current residents of this poor, black community. Yet after gaining access to these hospitals and changing their policies, there was little evidence of improvements in health, so the community set about getting information about the nature of the problems for which people were being hospitalized. The seven most common (in order of frequency) were:

- automobile accidents;
- interpersonal attacks;
- accidents (non-auto);
- bronchial ailments;
- alcoholism;
- drug-related problems; and
- dog bites.

The community organization was struck by the fact that the problems were mainly social rather than medical ones, and they set about tackling the one they felt they could be most successful addressing, that of dog bites. Drawing on community resources, they set up a scheme to pay 'dog bounties' and over a short period of time, a number of stray dogs were caught, and the cases of dog

(McKnight, 1978, p. 39)

bites decreased. The sense of achievement here led to the next action: dealing with car accidents. By mapping where the accidents had taken place, the community organization identified places where they could take action (e.g. the entrance to the parking area for a local store) and places where the community had less power (e.g. major highways for suburban commuters dissected their community). In the case of the latter, it became clear that communities affected by such through traffic would need to coordinate efforts to convince the city authorities to change policies.

The third issue to be addressed was that of 'bronchial problems' and one factor in these: good nutrition. To address the problem of affordable fruit and vegetables, a greenhouse was erected on the roof of an apartment building where fruit and vegetables could be grown. Not only did this provide a source of income, but an unexpected advantage of this greenhouse was that it conserved heat in the building; it also became a popular place with older people from a local retirement home, who came to help, and began to feel more useful in the community.

McKnight concludes that:

> Health action must lead away from dependence on professional tools and techniques, towards community building and citizen action. Effective health action must convert a professional-technical problem into a political, communal issue.

evidence of this association with cost reduction, and Rifkin (1996) describes such community participation programmes as being products of a 'target oriented framework', rather than an 'empowerment framework', i.e. community participation is seen as a means to improve service delivery, in what is a utilitarian model of community participation (Morgan, 2001), rather than as a form of mobilization that will lead to the 'increased ability of marginalized communities to control key processes that influence their lives' (De Vos *et al.*, 2009, p. 123). In the latter framework, community participation is both a means and an end, and it is inescapably political, involving a paradigm shift to a bottom-up rather than top-down approach to health promotion and placing power relations at the centre. Such an understanding of community participation and empowerment recognizes the potential for conflict with both professionals and their health agenda, as well as with those who have

economic and other resources, and whose power may be challenged.

These conflicts are illustrated well in the account of participatory budgeting in the city of Porto Alegre in Brazil, by Guareschi and Jovchelovitch (2004). Improvements in indicators such as sanitation, housing, health and education in Porto Alegre have been linked to the implementation in the city of participatory budgeting, which allows democratically elected representatives of communities to carry forward their communities' views about allocation of public resources; in addition most city departments have participatory councils where any citizen could discuss issues to do with city services. These processes were not imposed from above, but were the outcome of community participation, and have created a 'new public sphere' and 'a real redistribution of power in the city' (Guareschi and Jovechelovitch, 2004), which has mobilized primarily poor people in the struggle against health inequalities. Yet in the process of participation, difficulties have been encountered in terms of the political culture, the power structures of the city's budget definition, and the resistance of professionals, especially health professionals, to accepting community involvement in what were deemed to be specialist areas. In addition, differences within and between communities also became clear, and those who became very involved in the participatory processes were themselves criticized for becoming too close to those in power (issues about the degree to which community representatives can, or do, actually represent their communities have long been a theme in the literature about community participation, e.g. Jewkes and Murcott, 1998). However, overall Guareschi and Jovechelovitch (2004) conclude that:

> Through participation individuals develop competencies for both themselves and their communities to achieve real gains in all areas deemed essential for health. As individuals become vocal and active, they emerge as conscious actors of their own culture.
>
> The capacity of communities for effective participation generates gains at the personal, community and political levels. It not only empowers individuals and the community, but also poses to the institutional structures of the state the need to incorporate and take into account the insights and demands coming from grassroots movement.
> (Guareschi and Jovechelovitch, 2004, p. 319)

This account focuses on a participatory experience that is widely seen as successful, and indeed Draper *et al.* (2010) point out that whilst approaches to community participation may differ, there are shared assumptions that the 'involvement of communities enhances the delivery and uptake of health interventions to address inequalities' (Draper *et al.*, 2010, pp. 1102–1103). However,

there are many problems in evaluating community participation; as it is both a process and an outcome, involving different degrees of power in different contexts, capturing the complexity of community participation can be difficult in evaluation studies, and the same issues arise when looking at replicating and scaling up strategies. One attempt to capture this complexity can be seen in Rifkin, Muller and Bichman (1988, as cited in Rifkin *et al.*, 2000), where five factors that characterize community participation are identified: needs assessment, leadership, organization, resource mobilization and management. For each of these factors, there is an assessment of the degree of community participation, from narrow (almost exclusively professionally or externally controlled) to wide (community 'ownership') and a diagram is constructed to represent this (Fig. 2.2). In a more recent development of this approach, Draper *et al.* (2010) disaggregate five different components or indicators of community participation, with much more importance attached to community participation in evaluation, and to women's involvement generally (they link the latter to their focus on maternal and child health, but this might be seen as significant for many community health programmes). The five components are:

1. Who leads (community or professionals?).
2. Planning and management (to what extent is there a partnership between professionals and the community?).
3. Women's involvement (seen as critical for maternal and child health, the issue here is the degree of active participation by women).
4. Support for programme development in terms of finance and programme design (to what extent does the community mobilize and control resources?).

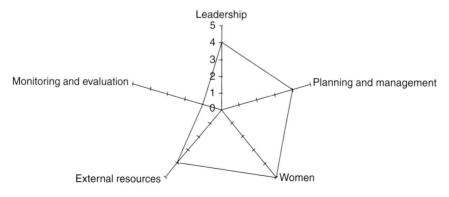

Fig. 2.2. Spidergram of participation.

5. Monitoring and evaluation (to what extent is the community involved in this?).

Using the participation continuum to create process indicators for these five factors, they are then able to create a spidergram, which maps participation for all five factors in a simple, yet powerful way and then links these to outcome measures such as health indicators, uptake of services and sustainability. However, Draper *et al.* (2010) note that whereas, from the case studies offered, there is significant evidence for the critical role of community participation, it is not possible to offer firm prescriptions about the nature of such participation, given the heterogeneity of communities and the impact of local contexts. Indeed Rifkin (2009) suggests that trying to define terms such as 'community' and 'participation', and creating a standard model for community participation in health is unrealistic; all will depend on the context, and especially the political context. She concludes:

> Communities are composed of different people at different times, and depending on the needs and capacities of its members, participation runs along a continuum from merely responding to professional advice to empowerment. It therefore appears that the success of community participation is situational and attempts to replicate it on a massive scale are futile. Leadership, trust, building partnerships and solidarity are critical and are a result of history, culture and tradition.
>
> (Rifkin, 2009, p. 35)

However, one example of the replication and scaling up of a successful initiative is that of the Tostan approach in Senegal (Easton *et al.*, 2003) in Box 2.11.

Box 2.11. The Tostan approach.

Tostan is a rural village empowerment programme (VEP) that originated in Senegal. The word *tostan* means 'breakthrough' or 'coming out of the egg' in Wolof, and the programme, which started in the late 1980s, focused on non-formal education and literacy for rural women, although men were not excluded and some did enrol. The orientation of the education programme was participatory, and the curriculum, which was problem focused, responded to women's expressed interests and needs.

The initial education modules led to follow-up activities and there was demand for more continuing education, so that further modules were added. The most popular were those on human rights and women's health and soon men began to join the modules too, and men's health was included as an issue. It was after these two modules that one community resolved to address the issue of female genital cutting (FGC), a centuries-old practice that had both short- and long-term effects on the health of girls and women, but which was a requisite for marriage. In a very short time, the community publicly renounced the practice, and others showed interest, including a 'cutter', who had seen herself the consequences of FGC. However, the critical turning point came when a locally respected imam became involved. Whilst initially concerned about the threat to tradition, tales from his own female relatives changed his mind, and he supported the women. However, he pointed out that efforts to eradicate such an embedded practice might only divide communities where actually it needed to unite them, as, unless all the intermarrying communities renounced the practice, those who had not experienced FGC would not be marriageable. The decision was made to speak to other communities avoiding explicit and condemnatory language – indeed to invite the communities themselves to go through some of the processes experienced by the initial community. The outcome of this process was that more villages joined the opposition to FGC, and the movement started to spread through Senegal.

At this point, the President of Senegal became involved, and a law was introduced abolishing FGC and punishing violators, but this was counterproductive, leading to resistance and greater difficulties for those attempting to follow Tostan's approach and initiate changes from below. Indeed, key elements of the success of the approach were that it was collectively owned, grounded in the local context and empowering. However, requests for Tostan to develop initiatives in other areas and countries has tended to go along with a more goal-oriented approach to participation, which has led to selecting only elements of the original approach to achieve social change. For instance, where the original focus was on literacy and non-formal education this was replaced with a more limited focus on health and human rights, reflecting the particular focus of the donors behind these new programmes, which was FGC. However, the authors report success in other countries, especially Sudan and Mali, and in the case of the latter Monkman *et al.* (2007) write of the way in which the revised VEP retained key elements that have empowered the communities involved and its 'transformatory potential' for gender relations.

The spread of the Tostan approach allows us to see the central role of participation in the bottom-up approach adopted, and to contrast this with the top-down legislative approach. Monkman *et al.* (2007) also suggest that there is a potential in the process of such programmes to move from *mediated empowerment*, which in this case relates to the key role of the non-governmental organizations (NGOs) involved, to a form of *socio-political empowerment*, with 'the transformation of the community from an object that is acted upon by outside forces, to a subject capable of acting upon and transforming its world' (Rocha, 1997, as cited by Monkman *et al.*, 2007, p. 461). Not only does such action no longer require the aid of intermediaries, its very nature suggests a degree of empowerment, which Laverack (2004) places at the far end of the community empowerment continuum, and we will return to social action and social movements at the end of the chapter. Participation and empowerment are central concepts for health promoters working with communities and fundamental components too of community development approaches.

The Community Development Approach

In this section, community development as an approach to building healthy communities is explored further, including the theory underpinning it. Community development has been defined in a number of different ways (Tones and Tilford, 2001). Here we will use a definition from the National Institute for Health and Clinical Excellence (NICE) in the UK:

> Community development is about building active and sustainable communities based on social justice, mutual respect, participation, equality, learning and co-operation. It involves changing power structures to remove the barriers that prevent people from participating in the issues that affect their lives.
>
> (NICE, 2008, p. 38)

As noted in the previous section, the principles and values underlying this approach to community development distinguish it from other community-based work. Key principles revolve around a belief in and respect for people and of what they are capable, asserting that people have skills as well as needs and have the right to participate in things

A community arts event, Bradford, England.

that affect their lives. These principles underpin the assets-based approach to work in communities, which has gained currency in recent years and which starts with communities' strengths and resources, not their deficits (IDeA, 2010). Community development is founded on values of equity and social justice and the need to address inequalities in order to build a fairer world.

In community development, *process* is very important with empowerment at both individual and community levels being central. According to Green and Tones (2010, p. 35) 'an empowered community has a sense of community, an identification with fellow members, an active commitment to achieve community goals and possesses social capital'. As described earlier, Laverack (2009) describes community empowerment as developing along a continuum from personal action, development of small mutual groups, community organization around key issues, partnership work with other organizations through to social and political action. Community development is a way in which community activists, health promoters, community development workers and others can work with people, either in a geographical/neighbourhood setting, or with a community of interest, to help them progress along this continuum.

The major theorist and activist whose work underpins community development was Paulo Freire. His influence was mentioned in Chapter 1, and his educational ideas will be referred to in Chapter 4, but it is important to mention his work here too as it relates to working with communities. Central to Freire's approach is the concept of 'conscientization', which Ledwith (2005, p. 95) describes as 'the process of becoming critically aware of structural forces of power which shape

people's lives as a precondition for critical action for change'. Freire developed his ideas through years of practice as an educator and an activist. He believed in 'praxis', which is the constant interaction of theory and practice. He was a passionate advocate for poor communities and believed that through a process of critical dialogue people become empowered and that this would in turn lead to them taking collective action to improve their lives. Freire's ideas have been criticized by Marxists for insufficient analysis by class, by feminists for his lack of attention to patriarchy and by those who considered him a dangerous revolutionary, but his ideas have prevailed and are still central to community development thinking and practice.

The case study in Box 2.12 illustrates how a primary school teacher who became a 'community organizer' took a Frierian approach to engaging with people in the community where he was based. This involved moving over a number of months from getting to know the community by doing a lot of listening and networking, through to helping them identify the things that most concerned them and work out what they wanted to do about them. Then, where the community felt sufficiently empowered, moving on to supporting collective action by community members to address the things they had prioritized.

Community development work is highly skilled and national occupational standards and competencies have been developed in the UK to reflect this (Box 2.13). Part of the skill set community development workers employ is in using many and varied methods to engage communities, as the example on the use of storytelling as a way of engaging very marginalized communities in Box 2.14 illustrates.

Box 2.12. Using a community development approach in practice.

This case study centres on the story of a primary school teacher who became a community organizer. His training taught him how to listen and really hear what people are saying and feeling. He worked on a farm but spent as much time as possible getting closely involved in the life of the community. He listened for 'generative themes', topics that people have strong feelings about. He gained the confidence of a number of village people and was soon invited to a number of meetings of women's groups, church meetings, etc. He prepared 'codes'

on the generative themes and presented these in picture form or through story and drama. He engaged the people in dialogue about the possibilities of change. One theme considered particularly important was the lack of money to buy vegetables from wealthy landowners. As a result the group pooled their savings and rented land on which they grew their own vegetables. The best product of the garden, however, was the discovery that they could work together to solve a problem.

(Tones and Tilford, 2001, p. 402)

> **Box 2.13. Key roles for community development workers.**
>
> - Develop working relationships with communities and organizations.
> - Encourage people to work with and learn from each other.
> - Work with people in communities to plan for change and take collective action.
> - Work with people in communities to develop and use frameworks for evaluation.
> - Develop community organizations.
> - Reflect on and develop own practice and role.
>
> (Federation of Community Development Learning, undated)

> **Box 2.14. Storytelling, an example of an effective tool for community development.**
>
> Katrice Horsley uses storytelling to work with many and varied groups of people from Bangladeshi women to young male offenders in the UK. She has also worked in Ghana. Through recounting both traditional and current stories, people can explore a range of feelings within a safe space through drawing parallels between the situation within the story and their experience. Sometimes telling stories can be part of another activity such as sewing and collage making and the narratives can be woven into the textile being made. This helps to build confidence and connections between people. Storytelling can also be a non threatening way to challenge discrimination and prejudice, and to develop self and political awareness.
>
> > Every culture has a story to tell but few people have the confidence or platform to share them. Storytelling projects can promote the telling and sharing of both personal and traditional stories challenging negative stereotypes and assumptions in a positive and non-threatening way. Every culture has a history of storytelling and this shared link makes storytelling powerful as a tool in exploring conflict and diversity.
>
> (Horsley, 2007, p. 4)

Community development inevitably takes an assets-based approach (Fig. 2.3).

Community development can be an effective way of engaging communities and ultimately of improving health and reducing inequalities as the evaluations of many community health projects and other interventions using community development methods illustrate (Tones and Tilford, 2001). In recent years, the UK Department of Health (DOH) has provided limited support to community development, as illustrated by the HELP project in Box 2.15, but in general, public health in the UK and elsewhere has been dominated by the medical model of health. However as outlined in the previous section of this chapter, there has been a revival of interest in the global South in the last few years in training CHWs from disadvantaged communities to help address priority health issues, although it remains to be seen whether the CHW programmes currently being established will adhere to the original empowerment principles.

As noted earlier, community development initiatives in the past have all too often been about governments expecting those in poverty to solve their own problems rather than about addressing the structural inequalities that make them poor in the first place (Tones and Tilford, 2001). Arguably, not much has changed and community development, participation and engagement are paid lip service to by government. For example, the current UK Government has endorsed the report *Fair Society, Healthy Lives* (Marmot, 2010), and claims to support community engagement, whilst pursuing economic and social policies that undermine this approach. Worldwide neo-conservative ideology dominates, reflecting the interests of big business and the financial sector, i.e. the rich and powerful, rather than the interests of the poor and marginalized. Community development, which leads to those with least power trying to assert some control over their lives, is unsurprisingly not favoured by those with a vested interest in the system as it is.

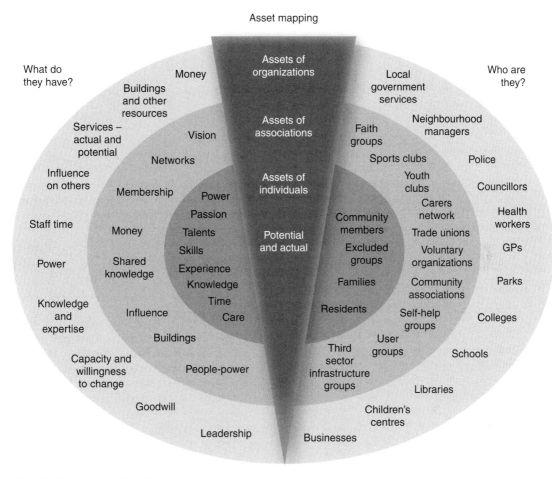

Asset mapping

What do
they have?

Who are
they?

Fig. 2.3. Partnership with individuals and communities – an asset-based approach.

Hence, community development has had a some-what chequered history across the world, with practice often falling out of favour with funders and those in power, when people become empowered and question the status quo. It does not fit comfortably as an approach with the current focus in many countries on achieving narrow targets around disease reduction and behaviour change, which originate with managers, funders and politicians, not with communities, and so has not been scaled up but remains a marginal activity in most countries.

The promulgation of the idea of the 'Big Society' by the Coalition Government in the UK is a good example of where the rhetoric (who could disagree with communities becoming more engaged with issues that affect them?) does not match the reality

of worsening living conditions, reduced services and widening inequalities. The challenge facing activists who believe in equity and social justice, is to reclaim ideas like 'community organizing', 'community engagement' and 'community empowerment', and use them to challenge hollow rhetoric and the imposition of 'top-down' approaches that have to grow 'bottom-up' if they are to be true to their real meaning and serve the interests of disadvantaged people.

Conclusions: Health Activism

Laverack (2004) sees social and political action as the end of the continuum of community empowerment, and much of this chapter has touched on ways in which community participation may involve such action; indeed Zoller (2005) coins the term *health activism* to imply 'at some level, a challenge to the existing order and power relationships that are perceived to influence some aspects of health negatively, or to impede health promotion' (Zoller, 2005, p. 344). Defined thus, health activism not only encompasses community development models of community participation, but it might also be seen as an example of a social movement, an attempt to build a new social order. More specifically, health social movements are defined as 'collective challenges to medical policy and politics, belief systems, research and practice that include an array of formal and informal organizations, supporters, networks of co-operation and media' (Brown *et al.*, 2004, p. 52), although we might wish to expand that definition to include health policy more broadly. Various typologies of health social movements (HSMs) have been offered, distinguishing them in terms of their focus; in health promotion, there has been interest in constituency-based HSMs such as the women's health movement, or grass roots-based organizations and community development projects addressing local health problems. However, formal alliances such as IBFAN (International Baby Food Action Network), which lobbies and advocates to promote breast-feeding, are examples of another type of HSM, as are groups demanding access to, for example, ART. Indeed, Zoller (2005) points out that, with a broader conceptualization of health, health activism may go beyond HSMs and incorporate action, for instance, on global poverty or the protests of 'los indignados' in Spain over the global financial crisis and political and economic responses. What is key here, however, is that all such movements,

and health activism, are evidence of the contribution that people make and their participation in forms of action that address health issues.

Summary

The central focus of this chapter has been the involvement of people and communities in promoting health, and we agree with Taylor (2007) who pointed out that health promotion that is imposed on people is rarely effective, and needs to be done not *to* people, but *with* and *by* them. However, such participatory approaches raise important issues for the practice of health promotion. Some of these issues relate to professional practice, models of working and the skills required, and these are explored further in Chapter 5. However, perhaps more importantly, we have seen that participatory approaches raise issues of power and control. Using the example of the poor health status of the Aboriginal peoples in Australia, Baum (2007) argues that efforts to improve health must recognize control as central, yet she points to other requirements too: our knowledge of the importance of control to health status (Marmot, 2004) suggests that policies should aim to encourage self-determination supported by resources that can make a difference. Linking social capital suggests a policy approach, which is trustful of communities, encourages them to do the right thing for their children and provides them with the infrastructure to create a health-promoting environment (Baum, 2007, p. 94).

Baum's reference to the resources, policies and infrastructure necessary for communities to promote health reminds us that action on the social determinants of health may well require communities to have a voice with people in positions of power, and support for their efforts in the wider policy arena. Indeed if the causes of health problems are to be found at the level of macro-social and economic policies (Pearce and Davey Smith, 2003), then we need to move beyond the community to look at such wider policies, the question of power, and their relevance for health (De Vos *et al.*, 2009). Therefore, the next chapter will explore healthy public policy and the policy process, with a focus on the importance of these for health promotion; however, in recognizing the role of people as health activists and stakeholders in relation to the policies that affect health, the question of participation and empowerment will remain a key issue.

Further Reading

Halpern, D. (2005) *Social Capital.* Polity Press, Cambridge, UK.

Ledwith, M. (2011) *Community Development: A Critical Approach*, 2nd edition. The Policy Press, Bristol, UK.

Ledwith, M. and Springett, J. (2009) *Participatory Practice: Community Based Action for Transformative.* The Policy Press, Bristol, UK.

Orme, J., Powell, J., Taylor, P., Harrison, T. and Grey, M. (2007) *Public Health for the 21st century. New Perspectives on Policy, Participation and Practice*, 2nd edition. Open University Press, Milton Keynes, UK.

South, J., White, J. and Gamsu, M. (2012) *People Centred Public Health.* The Policy Press, Bristol, UK.

3 Healthy Public Policy

Louise Warwick-Booth, Rachael Dixey and Jane South

This chapter aims to:

- demonstrate the importance of building healthy public policy;
- explain the differences between health policy, social policy and healthy public policy;
- explore the policy process;
- introduce key ideas from the policy analysis literature;
- show how ideology affects policy making; and
- discuss the role of advocacy within health promotion.

Introduction

This chapter will discuss the importance of 'healthy public policy' in relation to health promotion. The central role of healthy public policy within health promotion has been reaffirmed and redeveloped over the years since the Ottawa conference. Health promoters have consistently put health on the agenda of policy makers across all policy sectors and levels of government (Mohindra, 2007). The Jakarta Declaration (WHO, 1997b) listed a number of priorities for 21st-century health promotion, which were underpinned by multi-sectoral and partnership working, as well as a strong commitment to healthy public policy. The Mexico Conference (2000) described health promotion as a key part of public policy within all countries. The Bangkok Charter (WHO, 2005a) re-emphasized the importance of health promotion and called for global governance to address the harmful health effects of trade, marketing and specific products. The Health for All documents also clearly describe the importance of policy and healthy public policy remains central to health promotion both nationally and internationally (Green and Tones, 2010).

It is crucial that health promoters can make sense of policy processes if they are to be part of building healthy public policy. Therefore in this chapter, the policy-making process is discussed to illustrate its complexity, demonstrating how policy is made and shaped, debating what policy can achieve and discussing how policy can act as an instrument to effect change. The ideological basis of policy is also discussed, illustrating how different ideological positions are likely to result in a variety of outcomes for health-related policies. Policy sectors are identified and explained to show the ways in which many areas of policy relate to and influence health in both positive and negative ways. Agenda setting is touched upon, as part of the policy process, discussing stakeholders and how they influence policy. Advocacy as part of policy making is discussed, together with how health promoters can be advocates. The role of policy outside the health sector will be discussed, along with the importance of inter-sectoral collaboration. In short, the chapter attempts to offer a critical discussion throughout of the entire policy process, from how policy is made, who influences policy, the key players in world health policy and the implications of all of this for health promotion practice.

What is Healthy Public Policy?

'Healthy public policy' (Box 3.1) is policy that has a clear and explicit concern for health and so has arguably far broader scope than 'public health policy'. The World Health Organization (WHO) describes healthy public policy as being 'characterised by an explicit concern for health and equity in all areas of policy and an accountability for health impact' (WHO, 1988). Kemm (2001, p. 79) provides another definition; 'A healthy public policy is a policy that increases the health and well-being of those individuals and communities that it affects'. Within 'healthy public policy', the conceptualization of health is broad, along the lines of the social model of health discussed in Chapter 1, with a central feature of healthy public policy being to reduce health inequalities. Healthy public policy should improve societal conditions and create an environment that is more equitable and therefore results in more positive health outcomes.

The concern with healthy public policy partially emerged as a response to a perceived over-emphasis upon curative medicine and policy approaches adopting behavioural strategies (Kickbusch *et al.*, 1990). As we discussed above, the role of healthy public policy was stressed by the Ottawa Charter and elaborated on in Adelaide. It needs to be seen alongside the other four areas of action outlined by the Ottawa Charter. In tackling a major concern in westernized countries, obesity, for example, not only has it been recognized that an 'obesogenic environment' has emerged, but also the solutions lie beyond individuals and lifestyle changes. It is necessary in those countries with an 'obesity epidemic' to create supportive environments and therefore to develop transport policies which promote healthier ways of moving around, but also to use policy to control food advertising, to regulate the food industry, to develop school policies which promote healthier eating and exercise. It remains important too, to develop personal skills for healthier lifestyles and to develop a role for health services to help those who struggle with weight gain. 'Healthy public policy' thus could do a great deal to tackle what the WHO calls the obesity crisis.

There are many examples of already enacted healthy public policies. The Framework Convention on Tobacco Control (FCTC; Labonte and Laverack, 2010), which is the world's first global public health treaty, negotiated by the WHO in 2005, is a good example of a healthy public policy. This framework aims to support an internationally coordinated response to combating the use of tobacco. In the UK, the 2006 Health Act made it impossible to smoke in almost all enclosed spaces and workplaces across the country. This healthy public policy aimed to reduce exposure to second-hand smoke for workers and the general public, with the secondary objective of reducing overall smoking rates. Although the long-term impact has yet to be assessed, it has been argued that smoking-related diseases such as lung cancer and coronary heart disease will significantly reduce, and that smoking will gradually become less socially acceptable, further extending health benefits. A similar ban was introduced in Spain in 2010, with much the same goals, and a large number of African countries have followed suit (Tumwine, 2011). There are global examples that we would regard as healthy public policies, including the Kyoto Protocol on Greenhouse Gas emissions (Labonte and Laverack, 2010), which aims to reduce the levels of emissions at country level and so to reduce climate change and potentially mitigate against the many health effects that are likely to ensue with changing temperatures across the globe.

Whilst all of this sounds highly desirable, it remains incredibly difficult to predict the consequences of policies in relation to health, largely because their influence on health is indirect and often occurs through several complex and conflicting pathways (Kemm, 2001). Estimating the harm

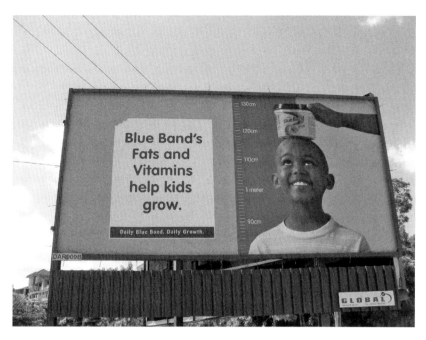

An example of food advertising.

and the benefits that arise from the implementation of policies is difficult and contested, with the harmful and beneficial impacts being likely to affect parts of populations and communities differently. Due to the inherent complexity of the policy process, health promoters need to remain concerned with the effects on health of policy perhaps designed for other purposes (Tones and Green, 2004). A new main road through a rural area of say, Nigeria, might enable people to access health care more promptly, but might also increase child pedestrian accidents or increase flooding of homes, where the highway is built higher than dwellings (as is often the case). Furthermore, governments may be reluctant to adopt healthy public policies on the grounds of costs and trade-offs; for example, there may be the loss of jobs if tobacco consumption decreases and this has to be compared with the gains of implementing healthy public policy. Moreover, many governments remain concerned with being perceived as a 'nanny state' that interferes in people's lives through the policy process (Joffe and Mindell, 2004). There are many areas of life that citizens regard as 'private' and not suitable for policy interventions. This might include the number of children a family decides to have – though in China the opposite was the case, where the government,

with its one-child policy, felt it could rightfully intervene!

Despite the complexity of using policy to promote health, there is evidence to show that healthy public policies *are* helping to reduce inequities, especially as we know that policies that increase wealth inequality are more likely to damage health (Wilkinson, 1996; Wilkinson and Pickett, 2009). In light of this evidence Labonte and Laverack (2010, p. 240) suggest a number of achievable healthy public policies for the future including:

- changes to global taxation to redistribute wealth because more equal societies have far better health outcomes across the globe (Wilkinson and Pickett, 2009);
- radical reform of current global policy-making organizations such as the World Bank and the World Trade Organization to increase world public spending on education, health care, water/sanitation and other interventions which promote equality;
- cancellation of poor countries' debts and fairer trade to allow the economies of poor countries to develop.

The key underpinning argument suggested by Labonte and Laverack (2010) is that a new global governance system is required, which is more ethical and rights-based, and this challenge remains for contemporary health promoters. Influencing policy and achieving the implementation of more equitable societies is a central tenet of health promotion practice, and this chapter suggests ways to do this by raising key questions about healthy public policy building.

What might be the pros and cons of using healthy public policy? Table 3.1 makes some suggestions.

The use of healthy public policy is also subject to critiques of 'health imperialism' because health is broadly defined and conceptualized as being affected by *everything* and therefore everything can be seen as 'healthy public policy'! Despite the issues with healthy public policy, health promoters remain committed to its greater use, as they remain engaged with putting health on the policy-making agenda and informing policy makers of the health consequences that result from the decisions they make. Consequently, 'more consistent attention to implementing healthy public policy, and amassing the evidence for it, are urgently required' (Joffe and Mindell, 2004, p. 968). Similarly, Sparks (2011) calls for the health promotion community not to be distracted by the critics of healthy public policy, pointing out the huge gains in lives saved due to policy measures: 'Those who make Nanny State claims may get attention but they are up against both the science and history of advancement in healthy public policy-making' (Sparks, 2011, p. 261).

Social inequalities and health inequalities are widely documented and very well evidenced. Furthermore, despite improvements in overall health in many high-income countries, inequalities persist. The 2008 Commission for the Social Determinants of Health emphasized the need to tackle the unequal distribution of power, money and resources. Previously Wilkinson and Marmot (2003) identified several key areas within countries that affect inequalities, all of which are amenable to change through the policy process:

- the social gradient;
- early life;
- stress;
- social exclusion;
- unemployment;
- work;
- social support;
- addiction;
- transport; and
- food.

The previous UK New Labour Government (1997–2010) introduced a range of policy approaches following the publication of a report by Sir Donald Acheson (1998), in which he argued that material disadvantage was the overall cause of health inequalities. Policy was developed to try to tackle inequalities, showing political willingness, but no additional funding was made available (Crinson, 2009). Despite the development of fiscal policies and more specific policies, evidence suggests that these interventions had little effect. Thomas *et al.* (2010) demonstrate that despite such policy, health inequalities have not reduced and in some cases have actually widened, showing that health inequalities are influenced by complex and long-term processes and therefore policy changes are unlikely to address such inequalities. Wilkinson and Pickett (2009) similarly argue that policy to address inequalities has previously failed, primarily because such policies do not tackle the root cause of the problem. Furthermore, Bambra *et al.* (2005) argue

Table 3.1. The advantages and disadvantages of using healthy public policy (adapted from Joffe and Mindell, 2004).

Advantages	Disadvantages
It is effective because it can encompass a whole population approach	Governments are often uneasy about its wider social and economic effects
The impact is felt across the whole population, and therefore it does not exacerbate inequalities	There are indirect costs and trade-offs especially for employment
The financial costs are usually very small and can on occasion be used to generate income through the taxation of unhealthy products	Libertarian reactions label the state as a 'nanny' and interfering with personal freedoms
It can also deal with hidden costs for example, road deaths can be reduced by decreasing car numbers as well as pollution	Implementation of policy to tackle health problems is still seen as a health service function despite a lack of evidence for this being the most effective approach

that, because of the neo-liberal basis of Western economies, inequality needs to exist as part of the social structure, and therefore any specific policies to tackle 'inequalities' are tokenistic because no government will support a policy process that permits the full implementation of radical redistribution and the creation of a more equitable society. (A socialist regime would take a different view.) Thus, policy purporting to tackle health inequalities is simply minor reform, and so does not deal with the macro-economic and structural causes of the problem. Bambra *et al.* (2005) argue that national-level policies to tackle inequalities also fail to consider the actions of global policy actors such as the WHO and the World Bank. The political content here clearly limits the formulation of effective health policy, ultimately 'the masking of the political nature of health, and the forms of the social structures and processes that create, maintain and undermine health, are determined by the individuals and groups that wield the greatest political power' (Bambra *et al.*, 2005, p. 192). Thus, the role of policy and its uses need to remain under critical scrutiny, as indeed do the strategies that are employed to build it.

Despite the criticisms of using the policy process to tackle inequalities, health promoters remain engaged with tackling inequalities in their daily work at the grassroots level. A European project (European Network for Health Promotion Agencies, 2001) called *The Role of Health Promotion in Tackling Inequalities in Health* produced a series of recommendations for policy approaches to tackling health inequalities at national and local level, as well as examples of good practice from across Europe. Experts recommended that health promotion strategies should be targeted at the socially disadvantaged as a mechanism to try to reduce health inequalities. The approaches suggested included:

- setting targets in relation to health inequalities;
- integrating health determinants in all policy areas that affect health;
- increasing people's participation, for example through community development approaches to health promotion;
- trying to improve access for everyone to health care;
- ensuring that all projects are both monitored and evaluated;
- carrying out health impact assessments of policy; and

- ensuring that good practice and research are disseminated.

Therefore, health promoters need to continue working on specific targeted initiatives to improve health, remain involved in research to build evidence around specific issues and ensure that they remain involved with strategies to build healthy public policy.

What is Social Policy?

Healthy public policy can be seen as a form of social policy and it is worth considering here what we mean by this. We are surrounded by social issues, some of which society feels there should be policies on – issues such as control of guns and knives, the age of consent for marriage, or human trafficking have all been subjected to *social* policy making. Other issues are more contentious as to whether they are suitable for policy making – whether women should be allowed to wear the hijab has been made into a policy issue in France, where women have been banned from wearing a full burka in public. In the UK, parents and other caregivers are barred from smacking their children. These two examples are more controversial, and some feel that they are 'private' matters and not conducive to 'social' policy making. So social policy topics are often mired in controversy and debate.

It may not always be clear what social policy is (Hudson *et al.*, 2008). Social policy can described as a field of activity decided upon and implemented by the government, a course of action and indeed a web of decisions rather than a single decision (Hill, 1997). The word 'policy' can be used very loosely in English, and Hogwood and Gunn (1984) characterize 'policy' in the following ways:

- as a label for a field of activity;
- as a statement of aspiration or purpose;
- as specific proposals;
- as (government) decisions;
- as formal authorization, as a programme;
- as an output(s);
- as an outcome(s);
- as a theory or model;
- and, finally, as a process.

Exworthy (2008) argues that the term policy is so widely used that is obscures meaning and that searching for definitional clarity can be confusing. 'Policy' can describe a set of written rules for dealing with bullying in schools – an 'anti-bullying policy' – or for sexual harassment at work; people might also use the term very casually, such as in 'it's our policy not to work on Saturdays', where this refers to custom and practice. Colebatch (2002) argues that *social* policy is concerned with order, authority and expertise. A simple understanding can be achieved by examining policy in terms of context, content, process and power (Walt, 1994). So 'social policy' is difficult to define and the scope of the field is extensive, typically covering social security, health, education, employment and housing. Furthermore, different nation-states adopt policies based upon various ideologies and principles so 'social' policies are by no means common to all nations (Esping-Anderson, 1990). Warwick-Booth *et al.* (2012) argue that policy can work in a variety of ways and hence affect health in both positive and negative ways. The policy-making process in which policy paths are determined is also complex and dynamic, itself subject to a range of influences from various groups and stakeholders who have an interest in directing policy.

What is Health Policy?

All countries would recognize the need for 'health policy', usually housed in a Ministry of Health and actually concerned with disease, illness and threats to health. Health policy is described by Nutbeam (1998b, p. 10) as 'a formal statement or procedure within institutions (notably government) which defines priorities and the parameters for action in response to health needs, available resources and other political pressures'. Health policy covers many diverse areas such as the provision of health care, policy to tackle specific diseases such as confinement for TB sufferers and policy to deal with specific issues and problems such as the right to die for the terminally ill and the reduction of incidences of teenage pregnancy. Many countries develop health policy to tackle particular areas of health, especially where those areas are neglected or given low priority. Mental health policy development for example, in Africa, is described by Gureje and Alem (2000), where policy development was used as a means to tackle the unsatisfactory mental health programmes in existence. Health policy is enacted through legislation but is distinguished from 'healthy public policy' because *health policy* more narrowly focuses upon health (care) services and the provision of programmes such as immunization, or screening (Nutbeam, 1998b).

'Health policy' can therefore be distinguished from 'social policies that affect health' – the situation is complex, as health is obviously affected by many policy areas, not just health policy per se. Thus, numerous areas of *social* policy determine health outcomes even if they are not intended to. Policy regarding crime, employment, regulation of industry and many other examples all impact on health even if that is not their primary intention. More centrally in the health area, many government activities such the taxation of products such as tobacco and alcohol, the regulation of air and water pollution, the safety of food and the working environment affect health and illness (Blakemore and Griggs, 2007). Joffe and Mindell (2004) argue that large health gains have emerged from a broad array of policies that often have not had health improvement as an objective at all. Thus, the provision of improved food supplies, sewerage and clean water resulted in the decline in infectious diseases (McKeown, 1979).

There are many more government actions that have played a part in improving health and not all of these are encompassed under the remit of *health* policy, but they could be called 'healthy public policy'. For example, transport policy can have massive health benefits. Within the UK, the introduction of compulsory seatbelt wearing for those travelling in cars was enshrined in law during 1983. This transport policy had clear health benefits by reducing the number of deaths in car accidents across the UK significantly. Moodie (2011) estimates that in Australia, 45,000 people have been

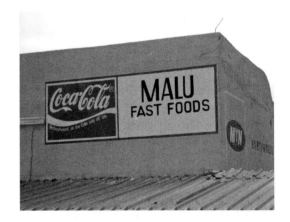

Changing food patterns have occurred across much of the globe, with the need to regulate the food industry.

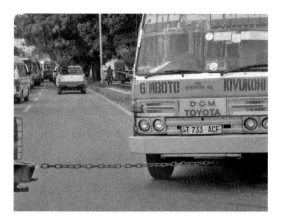

Transport policy has a major impact on health.

saved and 600,000 saved from serious trauma over the last 40 years due to seatbelt legislation. Conversely, the broader policy environment can be detrimental for health. For example, the use of pesticides for agricultural purposes affects health badly and has been well documented in South Africa (London and Bailie, 2001) and in The Gambia (Kuye *et al.*, 2007). Road building potentially leads to more pollution and higher levels of sedentariness. Roberts (with Edwards, 2010) argues that our increasing dependency upon the car for transport has been heavily influenced by social policy and has in turn shaped our bodies. We are now more inactive, obesity levels are rising and the environment is suffering. Thus, both our health and planetary sustainability are threatened as a result of social policy. Dixey (1998b) has argued that tackling child pedestrian accidents through new policy approaches to safety in the UK resulted in unwanted effects in terms of obesity and a curtailment of children's freedom to play. Furthermore, policies that enhance and increase inequality are likely to result in negative health impacts (Wilkinson and Pickett, 2009).

We can see that the field of social policy is a crucial determinant of health and this is now widely recognized in many conceptualizations. For example, Dahlgren and Whitehead's (1991) rainbow model frames policy as a determinant of health encompassed under general socio-economic, cultural and environmental conditions. In relation to terminology, 'healthy public policy' could be termed 'healthy social policy' and in this regard, we see 'public' and 'social' as interchangeable, and it

was an historical accident that the Ottawa Charter adopted the expression Healthy Public Policy. Whatever terminology is used, it is clear that the policy process is *political* and requires an understanding of who holds the ultimate power (Bambra *et al.*, 2005).

So far, we have discussed the necessity of healthy public policy as a tool to tackle health inequalities and the complex health problems facing all societies; we have also tried to disentangle health policy, social policy and healthy public policy. We now turn to the process of policy making.

How is Policy Formed and Shaped?

The policy process

Policy making is often conceived of in terms of a process or a cycle. This is a useful way of starting to look at policy as it breaks down the different stages of policy making. In addition, it signals that policy making is dynamic and about ongoing activity and change rather than focusing on set pieces such as legislation or formal documents. The policy process model can be used as both a descriptive (how policy *is* made) and a normative model (how policy *should* be made) of policy making. Sometimes the policy-making process is presented as a simple cycle very similar to programme planning stages, which includes goals, methods, implementation and outcomes (Spicker, 2006).

Rationalist models of policy making are predicated on the idea of policy makers having good knowledge of problems and being able to choose different options, enabling rational decisions to be made. Policies can be made, implemented and evaluated in a linear way as suggested in these eight policy steps (Box 3.2).

In the literature, there are a number of theories of policy making and thus different theoretical perspectives regard the nature of the processes at work in diverse ways and present the extent of conflict and consensus in policy development again in disparate ways. In 'real life', policies rarely proceed smoothly through the stages and some theorists point out the incremental, piecemeal and 'messy' way that policies are actually developed. Some of these alternative ways of seeing policy making are presented in Table 3.2.

The debate continues about how policy is actually made, hence the existence of these different viewpoints. Is policy making a rational linear process?

Box 3.2. The policy process.

1. Problem/state of society.
2. Agenda setting.
3. Issue processing/definition.
4. Selection of options.
5. Legitimation of options.
6. Allocation of resources.
7. Implementation.
8. Impact and evaluation.

(Adapted from Hogwood, 1987)

Table 3.2. Theories of policy making.

Theory about policy development	Explanation
Rationalist theories	• Policy making is a linear, sequence-based process in which a problem is identified and then solved, working through the stages of the process • This theory assumes that policy makers approach the problem rationally and go through the stages of the process logically
Incrementalist theories	• Policy makers never start with a blank sheet or perfect knowledge • Policy makers always react and respond to past policy change • Budget and resource decisions often result in incremental policy changes due to the constraints of shifting resources to and from different programmes and sectors • Policy change is always in small steps (incremental)
Marxist theories	• Policy is made by those in power to maintain the status quo • Power in policy making is held by those with money and business interests therefore policy is driven by them to meet their own goals
Network theories	• Policy is made by networks of actors who cluster together and focus upon specific interests • Networks can be formed when specific problems arise or they may already exist as part of dealing with ongoing policy problems
Pluralist theories	• Policy can be seen to emerge from the interaction of different parties at all stages of development and implementation • Colebatch (2002) refers to the horizontal and vertical dimensions of policy making to capture the pluralist aspects of policy making • Different groups hold brokerage positions and bargain for change according to their interests

Or is it much more complex and chaotic, dominated by certain groups and interests? Lindbolm described policy making in his seminal 1959 paper as the 'science of muddling through' and argued that there was a process of 'mutual partisan adjustment' (Parsons, 1995) in which policy making often occurs in a crowded arena where no single group is powerful enough to dominate the others. Consequently, policy emerges as a compromise between various interest groups who simply adjust their position to promote stability.

The role of evidence is described as increasingly important within policy-making circles and the emergence of evidence-based policy making has affected the policy process. It would seem self-evident that policy making should be informed by research and the 'best evidence', in the same way that 'evidence-based practice' has emerged to inform practice more generally (a theme which is taken up in Chapter 5). However, there can be so much disagreement about that 'evidence' that policy making is not possible or is fraught with disagreements. The state of evidence about climate change is an example where there is such a divergent range of views from 'experts' that any policy maker would not have clear direction but would instead have to proceed on the basis of selective interpretation of the evidence, on ideology and predilections. In UK policy-making circles, rejection of the 'evidence' about environmental causes of breast cancer has led to a lack of adoption of precautionary principles on this issue, in comparison to the USA, where policy has been used to address possible environmental causes of breast cancer (Potts *et al.*, 2007, 2008).

Solving social and health problems is thus very complicated. Policy analysts (Chapman *et al.*, 2009) have described 'wicked problems', which have the following characteristics:

1. Previously have remained unsolved, thus policy has repeatedly failed to tackle the issues.
2. There are disagreements about the causes of the problem and therefore debates about how best to address it.
3. The issue has a large scope and is connected with several other issues that are also 'wicked'.
4. The issue is difficult in the sense that it can never be claimed to be solved.
5. There is much complexity involved and so the issue or problem may be unpredictable.

All of these characteristics challenge traditional policy making which aims to resolve a (solvable) problem. The characteristics of a 'wicked problem' can be seen in health inequalities, poverty and social exclusion.

Identifying influencing factors

Debates remain about how best to analyse the policy-making process (Walt *et al.*, 2002), and there are many factors that serve to influence the process. Much policy analysis is concerned with developing an understanding of the relative influence of different actors in a process characterized by conflict, consensus and power imbalances. Most policies are shaped by a variety of factors although not all these influences will be visible or public.

Walt (1994) very usefully identifies a number of factors that influence policy:

- situational factors (such as politics and issues in the media);
- structural factors (relating to the organization of society and the political system of any given country);
- cultural factors (how society and individuals act and their value and belief systems); and
- environmental factors (events, structures and values that exist outside the boundaries of a political system but which can influence decisions within it).

Table 3.3 demonstrates these influencing factors in relation to the proposed changes to the provision of UK health care, specifically the re-organization of the UK National Health Service 2010. The UK Coalition Government published a White Paper called Equity and Excellence: Liberating the NHS on 12 July 2010. The paper detailed a major restructuring of the provision of health care within the United Kingdom, with the key changes being:

- general practitioners to take responsibility for spending and therefore hold their own budgets and drive demand for services;
- hospitals encouraged to become social enterprises rather than remaining within the NHS;

Table 3.3. Factors that influence policy change.

Factor	Example
Situational factor	• Increased costs and demands upon the NHS • Increasing management costs seen as a problem in removing funding from front line services, e.g. doctors, nurses and patients • NHS seen as bureaucratic and therefore inefficient • Media reports of various problems with the NHS
Structural factor	• Change in government – a Coalition Government with a different ideology came into power
Cultural factors	• NHS seen as an area in which political interference is unnecessary by many • Public satisfaction with the NHS remains high as reported in surveys, contradicting media reports
Environmental factors	• Global challenges to health care provision • Increasing costs of health care globally • Increased focus upon reducing costs, increasing efficiency and the importance of the market in providing public services (neo-liberal ideology)

- patients provided with more information, choice and the freedom to register with any GP that they want to;
- managers such as strategic health authorities and primary care trusts to be replaced by GP commissioners; and
- responsibility for public health to be passed to local authorities.

At the time of writing these changes have yet to be implemented after much opposition and criticism with many articulating fears that the NHS will be opened up to the private sector and become similar to the US health care system. However, despite opposition and demonstrations, the health bill detailing the changes already described was approved by MPs and will now go to the House of Lords (*BBC News*, 2011). Clearly there are many factors that influence policy change, and the above example is one in which many who oppose the proposed changes argue that ideology is the dominant driver of radical reform.

Values and Ideology

The role of ideology

Policy analysis needs to involve looking at the ideological perspectives, political ideas and values that inform policy development and shape policy structures. Ideologies are belief systems or sets of ideas that frame the way policy makers respond to problems.

> It is important to recognise here ... that ideological perspectives not only determine which policies we propose to develop or support but also influence how we view, and judge, policy developments that have already taken place.
>
> (Alcock, 2003, pp. 194–195)

Policy will always reflect societal, political and organizational values. These values may be expressed explicitly or conversely may be implicit in the policy. Political ideology includes assumptions for example, about where the responsibility lies for health – is health primarily the responsibility of the individual or of the government? Ideas about regulating behaviour and encouraging behaviour change are ideologically driven. Ideology is therefore an important aspect of policy-making because belief structures make certain policies possible. Consequently, political will has to be examined and viewed in terms of its ideological underpinnings. Table 3.4 gives a summary of key ideological positions and outlines how they influence policy. The table overleaf is a simplistic description to illustrate how ideology can inform and affect policy development, which then in turn impacts upon health outcomes. Policy is driven by a variety of actors and stakeholders holding different ideological viewpoints. Which ideology dominates is usually bound up with who holds the balance of power in the national or local government.

Who Makes Policy?

Policy actors and stakeholders

Policy actors are individuals, groups or organizations involved in policy making. The term 'stakeholders' is used to refer to any individual or indeed group with an interest in policy or those who are likely to be affected by policy. The study of policy actors is important in any policy area to gain an understanding of influences on policy formation and implementation.

Spicker (2006) gives three categories of stakeholders:

- organizations, agencies and individuals directly engaged in policy making;
- individuals on the receiving end of policy (service users and also staff); and
- citizens – in a democracy citizens have a stake in policy and are a source of political legitimacy; they might not be direct beneficiaries of a particular policy, but will be affected by it as a member of society.

Key actors vary depending upon the stage of the policy process – lobby groups may be successful at getting an issue on the agenda but will be less likely to be part of the implementation process. For example, Greenpeace have often gained media attention and headlines about specific issues by demonstrating, campaigning and taking direct action such as blocking the offices of oil companies and so may play a role in agenda-setting. However, this has not necessarily resulted in any policy change.

There are a number of policy actors with differential levels of power. There are global policy makers who are concerned with policies across the world, international policies made between nations and national-level policy from individual governments. Policy is also made locally for example at a regional level, within defined communities or

Table 3.4. Ideology and the direction of health policy.

Ideology	Key facets of the approach	Example policy
Conservatism	• Traditional order of society maintained • Recognizes inequalities but sees them as natural • Assumes that the role of the state should be minimal to avoid the creation of paternalism and welfare dependency • Values the private sector in service provision	• No policy focus upon dealing with health inequalities • Privatization of services including the provision of health care • Less public sector spending overall, with negative implications for such services • Increased inequalities
Liberalism	• Focuses upon freedom of choice and the importance of the individual • Individuals are seen as needing to behave responsibly • Neo-liberalism is a global economic approach scaling back the state and public spending and encouraging privatization	• Increased state intervention to control the market • Increased state intervention in relation to the provision of health care services • Individuals are responsible for their health • But neo-liberalism advocates reduced public spending, increased privatization and therefore increases inequalities
Socialism	• Broad ideology, with differing meanings • Originally associated with Marxism, and advocating revolution against the state • Contemporary socialism involves governments attempting to reform the state, and increasing state intervention in service provision	• Expansion of state involvement in public services including health care provision • Concerned with equality in both treatment and provision (the UK NHS was established upon the basis of socialist ideology)
Nationalism	• Rather than an ideology, this is a belief system • Nations should be self-governing, e.g. Scotland • Shared national identity is perceived as important in promoting social cohesion	• Difficult to say as the overall political context in which nationalism is employed will affect health • Scottish Health Policy has included more equalitarian policy within their NHS such as no prescription charge for everyone • Some nationalist approaches have been damaging for health due to cuts in public spending
Feminism	• There are a variety of different feminist approaches, e.g. liberals attempt to overcome discrimination via the legal system, whereas radicals focus upon the oppression within domestic relationships between men and women • Generally feminists are concerned with gender relationships	• Feminists draw attention to inequalities in health care provision in both diagnoses and treatment, arguing for changes in service provision
Environmentalism, 'Green ideology'	• Again this applies to a broad range of ideas • This school of thought focuses upon the global environmental crisis as well as the importance of the environment • Advocates sustainability and argues that policies should not damage the environment	• The environment and public health are seen as closely interconnected • The ecosystem should support public health rather than damage it • Policy should encourage sustainable development to reduce inequalities • Policy should encourage reduction in carbon usage and ecological footprints

organizations and enacted through local agencies. The following list shows the diverse range of actors who participate within the policy-making process:

- international agencies/policy-making bodies, e.g. the WHO, the United Nations (UN);
- government, local, federal or national;
- civil servants and local government officers, e.g. those who work in the department/ministry of health;
- professional bodies, e.g. doctors' organizations like the General Medical Council within the UK;
- trades unions, e.g. those who act on behalf of workers (in the UK, Unison is a trade union that acts for public sector workers);
- experts/advisory groups, e.g. the UK EAGA, the Expert Advisory Group on AIDS, which is a non-statutory public body that provides advice within policy circles about HIV/AIDS;
- interest or lobby groups, e.g. environmental groups such as Greenpeace, women's rights groups and anti-abortion campaigners;
- user groups, e.g. disability rights campaigners and mental health service users;
- non-governmental organizations (NGOs); and
- media.

Analysing the power that actors hold is necessary in relation to understanding both agenda setting and policy making. For example, Dean (2011) argues that the media in the UK has enjoyed an extent of power that has led to distortion of policy making and has actually undermined the democratic process. Professional lobbyists in many industrialized countries enjoy a level of access to policy makers and government officials that arguably has got out of hand.

It is useful to look at who is excluded as well as included in the policy process. Barrett *et al.* (2003) provide a fascinating case study of how the needs of people with disabilities were taken into account (or not!) in Leeds City Council's transport policy; the case study shows how disabled people are marginalized and excluded from policy making. The authors call for urgent changes given that policy making is dominated by large funded agencies and pays inadequate attention to the voices of those experiencing disability.

The role of the state/government

The state or government is an important player in the policy-making process; they deal with the provision of services, laws and regulations and distribution of resources.

> The modern state is a set of institutions comprising of the legislature, executive, central and local administration, judiciary, police and armed forces. Its crucial characteristic is that it acts as the institutional system of political domination and has a monopoly on the legitimate use of violence.
>
> (Abercrombie *et al.*, 2006)

Once elected, national governments can alter the direction of policy. The US and UK governments for example, have recently embraced the idea of 'nudging' as a policy directive. Nudging is discussed in more detail in Chapter 4, but briefly here, it can include a variety of approaches that aim to prod or gently move social and physical environments to make certain healthier behaviours more likely. Despite there being no precise definition of nudging and a lack of evidence to support it as a means to improve population health, it appeals to policy makers because it is low cost, it does not involve introducing legislation and it has been shown to work in some instances. However, 'nudging' as a policy measure remains contentious and it would have to take place across many policy sectors to achieve health improvements.

Policy sectors and inter-sectoral collaboration

We have seen that public health issues invariably come into a number of sectors outside of the health care policy sector. For example, the education, environment and employment sectors all affect health outcomes. Early policy analysis tended to focus on studies of public administration within specific ministries, but current policy analysis literature reflects interest in the horizontal dimension of policy making and the activities with and between different policy sectors because policy can support health in a number of ways, across a variety of policy sectors. In terms of analysis, the complex inter-relationship of numerous factors within different policy sectors (Tesh, 1988), and the development of inter-sectoral collaboration is what is of interest. Leeds Met played a leading role in early research on what makes inter-sectoral collaboration work well (Delaney, 1994). More recently, attempts have been made for example in Zambia, to show how inter-sectoral collaboration can help to develop alliances and advocacy to enhance maternal survival (Manandhar *et al.*, 2008).

Policy networks are another key part of the picture in terms of policy actors and stakeholders. They develop and exist due to interdependence between different organizations in order to meet goals and connections. A typology of networks is presented by Hudson and Lowe (2004, p. 131, adapting Marsh and Rhodes, 1992; Box 3.3).

Policy networks, organizations and communities vary in their ability to influence the policy process and this is context dependent, with more liberal democracies in theory facilitating more opportunities for participation within the policy process, compared with more authoritarian regimes (Walt, 1994).

What Makes Policy Happen?

Given the complexities of the policy process, an important question is what makes policy happen? Sutton (1999) draws together an extensive list of factors that facilitate the development of a policy innovation:

- new research, which clarifies the issues and the course of required action;
- the existence of good linkages between organizations and a history of lessons learned;
- a powerful person in authority becomes interested in a specific issue, influencing policy development in the area;
- the timing being right, for example with those in authority interested and new research being published at the same time;
- a crisis situation, which requires an immediate response;

- a dominant epistemic community that is an influential group, closely linked to policy makers able to get an issue onto the policy agenda;
- a general consensus within networks or organizations that change needs to be facilitated;
- a change in discourse resulting in different priorities and therefore a shift in policy direction; and
- change agents or networks of change drive forward new policy directions.

All of these demonstrate the complexity of the policy process at the development stage prior to the consideration of how any policy is to be implemented.

Implementation

Implementation is an essential stage of the policy process. Policies are not always implemented fully and there is often concern about the 'implementation gap'. Barriers to implementation include:

- practitioners – their levels of commitment, experience, attitudes to change, time available and perceived incentives act as barriers;
- resources – financial, staffing, facilities;
- policy overload and contradictions;
- policy not based on sound theory and understanding;
- organizational structures and reorganization;
- partners who aren't on board or who undermine implementation;
- lack of political will or leadership backing;
- poor project management;
- lack of community consultation and engagement;
- insufficient lead in time and unrealistic expectations; and
- poor communication and coordination.

Box 3.3. A typology of networks.

Type	Characteristics
Policy community	Stable, restricted membership, vertical interdependence, limited horizontal dimension
Professional network	As above but with shared goals of serving the profession
Intergovernmental network	Limited membership, limited vertical interdependence, extensive horizontal dimension
Producer network	Fluctuating membership, limited vertical interdependence, serves interest of the producer
Issue network	Unstable and large membership, limited vertical interdependence

---

More simply, Hogwood and Gunn (1984) group barriers to policy implementation:

- bad execution: non-cooperation or ineffectiveness of those implementing policy;
- bad luck: external factors intervene to prevent implementation, e.g. funding withdrawn; and
- bad policy: based on faulty information, poor reasoning and unrealistic assumptions.

Policy outcomes frequently differ from intentions and some policies result in unexpected spin-offs, both negative and positive. Policy analysts have attempted to understand implementation processes and offer solutions (see Parsons, 1995, for a good summary) and there are some interesting empirical studies in this area.

Theories of implementation can be broadly divided into three types:

1. Top-down models – for example, legislation such as taxation of unhealthy products in order to reduce consumption.
2. Bottom-up models – for example, community-led campaigns for speed restrictions in specific areas in order to reduce road deaths and injuries.
3. Models that seek to integrate both approaches – for example, community campaigns resulting in changes in legislation.

Top-down implementation

Analysts looking at implementation from a top-down approach focus on the policy inputs and the extent to which organizational or policy goals are achieved. Top-down implementation is strongly associated with rational models of policy making and the aspiration of better organizational structures and project management to improve implementation. However, there are many criticisms of rational approaches to policy making – in practice, it is rather messy and its outcomes are complicated social, institutional and political processes (Juma and Clarke, 1995). Clay and Schaffer (1986) suggest that policy is a chaos of purposes and accidents and their arguments certainly hold weight when the implementation of policy is examined. Gunn (1978) asks the question why is implementation so difficult? He argues that there are ten conditions required for 'perfect implementation' as follows:

- the circumstances external to the implementing agency to not impose crippling constraints;

- adequate time and sufficient resources are made available to the programme;
- the required combination of resources is actually available;
- the policy is based on a valid theory of cause and effect;
- the relationship between cause and effect is direct and there are few, if any, intervening links;
- dependency relationships are minimal;
- there is understanding of, and agreement on, the objectives;
- tasks are fully specified in correct sequence;
- there is perfect communication and coordination; and
- those in authority can demand and obtain perfect compliance.

These perfect conditions rarely exist within the real world and implementation does not simply occur from a top-down direction.

Bottom-up approaches to implementation

Bottom-up approaches are concerned with administrators and professionals who actually implement the policy and less with policy-making bodies. Emphasis is less on an implementation gap or failure to comply but the role of professionals and others in shaping policy. There is a focus on the study of professional power bases and the use of professional discretion. For example, Lipsky (1980) discusses 'street-level bureaucracy' and describes this as the decisions made by street-level (or 'ground-level') professionals. His analysis suggests that their routine and coping mechanisms to deal with both work pressures and uncertainties mean that policies may not be implemented as intended but according to the interpretation of those on the 'front line'. Hudson and Lowe (2004) suggest that policy outcomes are shaped at the point of final delivery, where individual workers have agency to drive and implement policy directives but also have the power to constrain that implementation. In our work on the implementation of policy regarding health-promoting prisons, prison staff are 'street-level bureaucrats' and, according to their inclinations, can block or enhance the implementation of a 'whole-prison approach' to health promotion (Dixey and Woodall, 2012). Studies have shown too, that prison staff disregard health promotion, frequently perceiving it as constituting additional work or something that is outside their professional remit (Bird *et al.*, 1999; Caraher *et al.*, 2002). This shows that public policy is not just about those in power administrating from the top down – implementation involves a range of players. Wells (2007) found that workers in a mental health team when implementing policy had to balance four tensions: they balanced political imperatives with local management agendas, professional and peer cultures in which they worked and finally their perceptions of perceived advantages that may result from implementing the policy. Wells' work (2007) provides a useful analysis in explaining why policy implementation is so complex and does not necessarily happen as policy makers envisage. Both managers and policy-makers may not scrutinize local-level implementation too deeply because of these complexities, as a way of deflecting any blame associated with negative outcomes (Wells, 2007).

Policy or Social Entrepreneurs

Catford (1998) has argued that health promotion needs social entrepreneurs to facilitate change. Social entrepreneurs share the same characteristics as commercial entrepreneurs but use their enterprise skills in the social arena. They have focus on vision and opportunity, the ability to convince and facilitate empowerment but this is coupled with a desire for social justice. The concept of social entrepreneurs has been linked to Kingdon's concept of a window of opportunity. Kingdon (1995) characterized the policy-making process as having three streams – policy streams, problem streams and political streams. Issues are placed on the policy agenda when all three streams come together. Then policy entrepreneurs are needed to utilize this opportunity. Policy entrepreneurs are involved in complex, interrelated social processes including the generation of ideas, problem framing, dissemination, strategic activities, lobbying and evaluation. Policy entrepreneurs when interviewed felt that whilst they were able to influence the flow of events, there were other factors and players who remained important (Roberts and King, 1991). Perkmann (2002) also analysed policy entrepreneurs in the context of the European Commission and argued that grassroots actors can engage in policy entrepreneurship and this is a necessary governance challenge. Craig et al. (2010) document how public health professionals can act as policy entrepreneurs to advance health-related goals when windows of opportunities open, with an analysis that focuses upon the development of a childhood obesity strategy in

Arkansas. Health promoters in practice then are able to use their knowledge within given windows of opportunities to facilitate policy change and the development of healthy public policy.

Strategies for Building Healthy Public Policy

Advocacy

A key strategy for building healthy public policy is that of advocacy, as recognized and discussed within the Ottawa Charter as one of three major strategies for achieving health promotion goals (WHO, 1986b). Advocacy can be defined in a number of ways and is used as a term in judicial systems, in individual casework, for example in mental health and in policy making. Smithies and Webster (1998, p. 105) define advocacy as:

> Advocacy is about people speaking up for or acting on behalf of themselves, possibly with the support of another person/group or 'advocate'. It is also about taking action to get something changed, in order to take more control over our lives.

Advocacy may be taken by or on behalf of both individuals and groups to create living conditions more conducive to health and healthier lifestyles (Nutbeam, 1993). Advocacy for health therefore is about protecting those who are considered vulnerable, empowering people and tackling inequalities. Health advocacy in the context of public health and health promotion is used to describe a process of support for health programmes and healthy public policy. Different types of advocacy can be seen in practice. For example, advocacy can be confrontational by challenging powerful commercial anti-health interests such as the tobacco lobby (Wallack and Dorfman, 1996), or it can be about mediating and negotiating between opposing groups and positions to try to achieve positive health (Nutbeam, 1993). Advocacy may also have a capacity building function, enabling individuals and groups to gain control over their lives and to improve their health by becoming effective policy advocates (Schwartz et al., 1995). Ultimately, advocacy in relation to policy is about trying to influence the policy-making process so that healthier legislation and healthy public policies are introduced and implemented. For example, the Bill & Melinda Gates Foundation advocates to raise awareness of less well-known and neglected diseases affecting lower-income countries because there is already much more political attention directed towards HIV/AIDS, TB and malaria. Smithies and Webster (1998) present a typology of advocacy to outline the different levels of advocacy that can occur. Table 3.5 outlines these types of advocacy levels and provides some health-related examples.

Carlisle (2000) also identifies four advocacy models: first, representational in which work is carried out on behalf of people; secondly, facilitational in which people are helped to represent their own needs; thirdly, confrontational in which powerful interests are challenged; and finally, advocacy can be in the form of acting as a conduit in order to mediate and negotiate between interests. She uses a conceptual framework to categorize advocacy based on two dimensions, whether the goals are empowerment oriented or protection/prevention oriented and whether the level is policy that addresses structural or individual-level issues. Advocacy is also associated with campaigning and includes a variety of methods such as individual casework, the use of the mass media/media advocacy, political lobbying, community mobilization and coalition building.

Advocacy in the policy process

Advocacy is often associated with agenda setting but can occur at different stages of the policy-making process, from international to micro-level policy making.

- Getting issues on the agenda. This can be through using the media or by directly lobbying politicians. The media is a useful tool in advocacy campaigns. For example, in Canada, the Manitoba Public Insurance campaigns demonstrate that media advocacy can be used to deal with alcohol and tobacco-related health issues (Asbridge, 2004).
- Changing public or policy makers' perceptions of issues. This is called issue framing; for example, is the real problem increasing rates of HIV or is it the poverty and powerlessness that leaves many individuals unable to negotiate safe sex?
- Presenting and lobbying for alternative options for policies (selection of options). This would involve presenting a number of solutions and options for how the problem could be tackled.
- Making sure policies are given a stamp of approval and are made official (legitimation)

Table 3.5. Types of advocacy (Smithies and Webster, 1998).

Type of advocacy	Explanation	Example
Citizen advocacy	People in the same community establish supportive relationships; this can be about addressing a specific problem or about protecting the vulnerable and giving them a voice	Local community volunteers ensuring that young people in the community are not ignored when large decisions are being made
Peer advocacy	This is support from individuals who have undergone similar experiences	Mental health service users working on behalf of other similar service users
Self-advocacy	This is about speaking up for yourself and making your views and wishes clear	Individual right-to-die campaigners try to challenge existing rules about assisted suicide within countries where this is illegal
Legal advocacy	People with specialist knowledge and training often represent others in a paid capacity within a formal setting such as a court or tribunal	The rights of patients to decide to refuse life-saving treatment can be legally agreed
Professional advocacy	People are paid, trained and employed to advocate on behalf of others	Paid organizations support people with learning disabilities in understanding the medical treatment that they are receiving
Staff advocacy	Workers in a specific organization advocate for each other as well as broader groups including service users	Accident and emergency staff may advocate for changes in traffic speeds to reduce accident admissions
Campaigning advocacy	This is often from issue-based groups who unite to raise awareness of specific problems	A community group forms to challenge the creation of a new waste disposal facility that is causing health concerns

because a policy has to be seen to be legitimate for it to move to the implementation stage.

- Mobilizing resources to implement policies (allocation of resources). Who will implement a policy and at what levels is implementation required? This is where gaps are often recognized as existing.
- Lobbying for improved implementation.

Involvement in advocacy – lobby groups

Many individuals and groups participate in the policy process by advocating for a specific policy outcome. Parsons (1995) contrasts policy communities with stable and restricted memberships and are highly integrated into the policy process and issue networks that have less stable, non-exclusive memberships and weaker points of entry to the policy process. There are many different lobby and interest groups, some known across the world such as Greenpeace and Oxfam. Others work on a more national level, for example the British Medical Association, which operates in the UK to lobby on behalf of doctors and medical students. There are also many lobby groups funded by commercial industry, and corporate campaigns are well funded, well coordinated and influential. This is cited as problematic by many because governmental regulations on lobbying are weak. For example, in the USA, the pharmaceutical industry has promoted profitable drugs deemed unsafe by their own research (Angell, 2004). The UK-based Portman Group is supported by drinks producers despite it being concerned with the social responsibility issues surrounding alcohol. The group is well placed to lobby, which it does effectively, leading many to suggest that it is not independent of industry and that UK policy is too heavily influenced by alcohol manufacturers (Harkins, 2010). In 2004, the alcohol strategy for England and Wales was produced, which ignored independent evidence calling for changes in alcohol pricing and availability. The Portman Group was cited in the final report as an 'alcohol misuse' group and thus has been cited as an example of successful pressure on the government from a powerful group that ultimately influenced how evidence was used to decide policy (Stevens, 2007). Similarly, in 2003 the sugar industry demanded that the WHO remove its planned healthy eating guidelines when they were about to be published. The guidelines were to recommend that sugar should not make up

more than 10% of a healthy diet. The industry had the power to demand that the US Congress would no longer fund the WHO if the guidelines were published (Boseley, 2003). The guidelines were not published.

There have also been successful health-benefitting changes made to the law despite heavy lobbying by industry, with health advocates and various other policy players mobilizing and campaigning for changes in corporate behaviour in order to improve population health (Freudenberg, 2005). Indeed, Wilson-Clay et al. (2005, p. 196) state that 'we have learned that a small group of committed individuals can gain access to lawmakers, participate successfully in the democratic process, and influence public health policy'.

Lobby and interest groups can differ on a number of dimensions. Their effectiveness can vary with issues and campaign tactics. Some key dimensions of interest groups are highlighted below.

- insider groups versus outsider groups;
- consensus building versus conflict generating;
- focus on a single issue versus involvement in a number of issues;
- covert lobbying versus open participation;
- formal mechanisms of involvement in decision making versus informal mechanisms of involvement; and
- use of legal methods versus the use of illegal methods.

Advocacy is also carried out through social movements, which have been a focus of much academic interest and are a prominent feature of 21st-century policy making. Some of the current social movements, such as anti-capitalist and environmental movements, have clear links to both health promotion and public health issues. For example, The Greenpeace Climate Change Campaign launched in 2010, encouraging the use of 'green' energy sources has the potential to mitigate against the many negative health effects associated with climate change. In the year 2000, climate change was estimated to have caused over 150,000 deaths worldwide (WHO, 2005b) and its health-related impact is likely to continue because the climate takes time to respond to change (Pope, 2008).

Barry and Doherty (2001) suggest that social movements have a collective identity but one that is fluid and provisional, are made up of groups and individuals linked in a loose network with a mix of formal and informal ties, protest and use (direct) action and pose a challenge to power bases.

Activism around health issues conducted through health-related social movements has been important in achieving social change. For example, in the USA, women's health activists have changed conceptualizations around women in gender, reproductive rights and treatments (Morgen, 2002). Similarly, AIDS activists have advocated for funding and research, as well as different treatment approaches (Epstein, 1996). Furthermore, self-care and disability activists have broadened health professionals' awareness of the capacity of lay people to be involved in their own health (Shapiro, 1993; Goldstein, 1999). However, within the literature, there are debates about how positive advocacy actually is, with several criticisms of the process. For example, Seedhouse (1997) argues that whilst health promotion and associated advocacy may be done on request, it is also carried out without intended recipients requesting it. Other critics of advocacy suggest that there is a contrast between the health promotion discourse of community participation and empowerment and the paternalism of the approach in constructing people as uneducated and requiring help from those who 'know better' (Wenzel, 1999, cited in Carlisle, 2000). Nevertheless, with health seen as an increasingly global issue and the influence of globalization described as important, advocacy at a global level by health promoters is important to influence the global policy-making environment.

Health promoters – a role in advocacy?

Advocacy has been identified as one of the key strategies and priorities of health promoters working in practice. A useful guide to how to do advocacy is provided by Sharma (no date). There are, however, different models of advocacy, as this chapter has already illustrated and it is not an unproblematic concept due to issues of representation, legitimacy, power and acceptable limits of state intervention. So as a practitioner, how do you decide to advocate? Using a rationalist approach, Maycock *et al.* (2001) propose an advocacy model to guide practitioners to make decisions about whether to advocate for a public health policy. The public health decision-making model has five questions:

1. What is the problem and is it significant?
2. Is it amenable for change?

3. Are the intervention benefits greater than costs?
4. Is there acceptance of the interventions?
5. What actions are recommended?

The reluctance of some professionals to become involved in advocacy is discussed within the literature. Galer-Unti *et al.* (2004) identify some common barriers and concerns about health education advocacy including, workers feeling that they were not 'activist', did not have time, did not know enough about advocacy, felt it would not make a difference or that the advocacy would not work.

In addition, values and ideological perspectives influence and underpin our professional practice. Fraser's (2005) four approaches to community participation summarize some of the positions held:

- anti-/reluctant communitarians and economic conservative approaches:
  - self-reliance and support for individual freedom;
- technical-functionalist communitarians and managerialist approaches:
  - pluralists – not challenging status quo;
- progressive communitarians and empowerment approaches:
  - focus on social justice and reform. Egalitarian, democratic and inclusive in orientation; and
- radical/activist communitarians and transformative approaches:
  - reject reform agenda; argue for redistribution of power/ resources.

Despite these complexities, Labonte and Laverack (2010) still argue for health promoters to become advocates for a new global governance system and says that although there are no blueprints for health promoters, there are steps that they can take and many strategies already exist within health promotion practice kits. Indeed, this is true of advocacy in general. Such steps include aligning with organizations and networks for the global movement for health and justice to develop a more powerful campaign for health promotion principles within the international arena; building partnerships that are empowering for health promotion, which use bottom-up approaches; entering current policy debates, either as individuals or via social movements; practising optimism as an act of political resistance.

Power, Policy and Partnerships

Given the range of actors involved in policy making and the number of sectors that influence health, inter-sectoral collaboration has been called for to achieve better health outcomes. Inter-sectoral collaboration refers to 'the collective actions involving more than one specialized agency, performing different roles for a common purpose' (Adeleye and Ofili, 2010, p. 1). Indeed, the Millennium Development Goals (MDGs) require inputs from a variety of sectors in order for targets to be achieved, showing the importance of such strategies for the delivery of improved health outcomes. However, there are numerous problems with such approaches: Adeleye and Ofili (2010) suggest a tripod of neglect when describing how inter-sectoral collaborations affect primary health care: often the non-health strategies are outside of the statutory control of the health sector, for example the provision of clean water; primary health care is not seen as significant in other sectors and health benefits tend to result by coincidence rather than as planned. For example, policy decisions are driven by politics rather than any perceived health benefits; collaboration projects between the health and non-health sectors are uncommon.

Despite this, partnership working and inter-sectoral collaboration do have the potential to bring about improvements in health and partnerships have been increasingly emphasized as a tool to deliver policy effectively within contemporary discourses.

Partnerships in policy

Partnerships can exist at any level of policy making from international alliances to groups working together at neighbourhood level. Partnerships can be inter-sectoral, inter-organizational and inter-professional (joint working). Some national governments have been keen to support partnership working, again demonstrating the importance of context for policy development. The previous UK New Labour government, 1997–2010, supported partnership working to develop policy in order to tackle cross-cutting issues, with the view that complex problems require multi-dimensional solutions. Indeed, there are many rationales for partnership working as it pools resources, attracts resources, can stop policy conflicts due to having common goals, can reduce competition, and break down barriers to implementation.

Despite these rationales, Dowling *et al.* (2004, p. 315) point to dearth of evidence on partnership approaches saying:

> Current policies advocate partnerships, rather than markets or bureaucratic hierarchies, as the preferred mode of coordinating organisations, services and teams. Although it might be assumed that this preference rests upon clear evidence of the superiority of partnerships in delivering welfare over other types of relationships, this does not appear to be the case.

They undertook a literature review on successful partnerships and identified that the dimensions of success vary according to the level of engagement and commitment of partners, whether partners hold shared vision and goals, whether environmental factors are conducive to partnership working, whether satisfactory accountability arrangements exist and whether there is clear leadership and management.

Yet many problems remain with a growing literature focusing upon processes within partnerships. Hudson (2002) identifies the 'Achilles heel' of partnership working, discussing barriers including professional identity, professional status and professional discretion and accountability. Despite the focus on sustainable 'partnerships' in the discourse of development, and its emphasis in funding calls suggesting that donor agencies value partnerships, there is little literature on the processes and operationalization of such types of collaboration (Jentsch, 2004). In terms of 'North/South' partnerships, Brehm (2001) suggests that whilst the financial power is held by the 'Northern' partner, there is little hope that a partnership can mean true equality and the sharing of responsibilities.

In relation to health promotion practice, partnerships are often termed 'healthy alliances' in which the notion of a coalition is often used, where policy actors come together to advance a shared goal. Douglas (1998) points out that healthy alliances are not 'natural alliances' but are driven by needs of health agenda. Indeed, there is no manual available to describe how to build healthy alliances and alliances need to be judged in context and on their own individual merits (Stern, 1990). Within the literature, questions remain about who holds the power within alliances and the processes of participation remain similarly debated. Despite this, participation within the policy process has been cited as increasingly important within recent discourses.

Participation and power

In recent years, citizen participation within the policy process has been labelled as positive and increasingly important. Participation was discussed in Chapter 2, and the role of active citizens will be taken up again in Chapter 5, but is discussed here in relation to participation in policy making. Bracht and Tsouros (1990, p. 201) provide a broad definition of citizen participation:

> The social process of taking part (voluntarily) in either formal or informal activities, programmes, and/or discussions to bring about a planned change or improvement in community life, services and/or resources.

Taylor (2003) defines four types of approaches to public involvement including consumerist approaches, representative approaches, interest group approaches and network approaches. Furthermore, involvement within both partnerships and the policy process is based upon a number of assumptions. First, participation is assumed to be a good thing. Some of the reasons advanced for public participation in policy making are that it:

- assists in targeting disadvantaged groups;
- widens inputs into policy and therefore results in more creative and innovative solutions;
- results in more responsive services targeted at needs;
- creates more ownership and involvement leading to more sustainable solutions;
- requires greater engagement for individuals to accept changes and support health improvement;
- brings benefits for individuals, communities and organizations; and
- is about democratic renewal in the sense that individuals have the right to be consulted.

The second assumption is that people want to be involved. However, involvement is complex and can be understood in different ways. Four categories of public involvement are identified by Taylor (2003): community leaders; initiators of activities and groups who are committed to and active in an issue or cause; participators in activities – individuals who join activities and support causes and events; and non-participators.

The third assumption is that community organizations and leaders represent the community. Some form of collective representation is necessary if participation is to be more than consultation. However,

the structures in communities may reflect and support established power relations, for example in relation to gender. Jewkes and Murcott (1998) carried out research on Health for All projects in England and found a mismatch between the ideology of participation and practical constraints. Barriers to participation meant that community representatives were often drawn from established voluntary sector organizations and there was a distinct risk of a voluntary sector elite participating, rather than the achievement of representation.

The fourth assumption is that power sharing can take place. Barnes and Walker (1996), in discussing the principles of empowerment, argue that power is not a zero sum and partnership models can exist where the empowerment of one group is not at the expense of another. However, there are more complex descriptions of how power operates within policy partnerships. Lukes (2005) describes three dimensions of power. First, the pluralist view of power where conflicts of (subjective) interest exist within policy making. This is associated with liberal ideology and moves to improve the quality of participatory processes with little critique of structural interests. Secondly, the inclusion of groups in policy making termed the 'mobilization of bias'. This is associated with reformist ideologies, with a focus on combating social exclusion and bringing disadvantaged groups into policy making. Thirdly, power is seen as an all-encompassing control that determines and shapes public wants and therefore demands in a political system. Powerful interests may not be visible in policy arenas as they remain hidden. This perspective is linked to radical ideologies and arguments to seize control and radically change the system.

These perspectives make for interesting debates given the centrality of advocacy and partnership working to health promotion practice, and they have ramifications for the skills of health promoters, which will be taken up in Chapter 5. One aspect of the policy process which health promoters have become involved in is health impact assessment, which is a process of assessing the impact of a policy on health. Lerer (1999), Lock (2000) and Kemm (2001) all provide useful discussion and practical guidance on how to carry out health impact assessments.

Global Healthy Public Policy

The final section of this chapter will consider the need for global healthy public policy making, given the processes of globalization. As health is increasingly conditioned and determined by both global processes and relationships (Yuill *et al.*, 2010) there are consequently global health problems and issues, which require tackling on a global scale. The need for global solutions has resulted in the development of global health policy organized through an increasing number of global actors shaping health policy, funding and provision (Davies, 2010). A number of large international organizations have made attempts to combat global health issues (Kaufmann, 2009), with many agencies working together in partnership and through alliances to deliver health-related programmes (Walt and Buse, 2006). Governmental and NGOs including the WHO, the World Bank, charities such as Oxfam, private foundations such as the Bill & Melinda Gates Foundation and large corporations such as pharmaceutical companies work globally to deal with numerous health problems. These actors drive the global health agenda and influence both priorities and resources (Davies, 2010). Thus global health priorities are defined through several policy actors (Table 3.6; Ollilia, 2005).

Table 3.6 provides a brief overview of the types of organizations that are working in the global policy arena and influencing policy. There have been a plethora of criticisms about the work that these organizations do and the overall impact that they have in relation to global health outcomes (Fidler, 2007). The ideological underpinnings of some of the organizations have been critically questioned (Macdonald, 2007) as have the lists of global health priorities determined by these actors (Ollilia, 2005). Global policy making is clearly aligned with industrial and trade policies arguably to the detriment of global health (Ollilia, 2005), and there are large, powerful transnational corporations working globally who have vested interests in specific policies, which are not always beneficial for health.

The huge growth of NGOs in the 1990s led to them being seen as a 'magic bullet' for resource-poor countries in terms of development, health and governance problems (Vivian, 1994). In Africa, they came to rival governments in terms of providing services, and indeed, when many economic sectors in Africa were in decline, they were seen as more capable of delivering development (Fowler, 1998). NGOs were also seen favourably as a corrective to the power of the major drivers of policy, the IMF and World Bank, which had forced structural

adjustment programmes which had fostered 'a congenial framework that legitimated an exclusionary approach to policy making' (Brautigam, 2000, p. 4). However, some argue that NGOs now have too much influence on policy making, especially where they are based in the global North and working in the global South (Manji, 2006). One category of organization missing from the table above is that which Chen *et al.* (2007) call Membership-based Organizations of the Poor, which attempt to promote the representation and inclusion, rather than exclusion, of informal workers (and most resource-poor countries are dominated by the informal sector), in policy-making structures. The People's Health Movement is an example of marginalized and indigenous people coming together to represent their own interests (Baum, 2001; People's Health Movement, 2012).

However, the role of global policy actors and associated governance has produced some health improvements and the establishment of the MDGs defined by the UN member states are an example of the positive role of global governance, as targets have been adopted in an attempt to deal with poverty, inequalities, health issues, environmental problems and global equity. The MDGs attempt to promote global collective responsibility for health threats and conceptualize health in the broadest possible sense by focusing upon poverty, preventable communicable disease and environmental degradation (Davies, 2010). Ultimately, all the targets are unlikely to be met and questions remain about who holds power within the global policy arena and how global partnerships and health alliances work in practice. Much more work is needed to assess how global policy makers are influencing health and whether this is positive or negative (Davies, 2010).

An example of how policy analysis can be used to understand how a particular policy came about is provided in Box 3.4.

In terms of moving on in the 21st century, health promoters have become more sophisticated in borrowing ideas from political science and using policy analysis in developing their policy work. De Leeuw (2010) and Hoeijmakers *et al.* (2007) have developed software and an 'expanded toolbox' for health promoters to enable analysis and mapping of policy networks and to understand the role of social and policy entrepreneurs, stakeholders and other participants. Guldbrandsson and Fossum (2009) have used Kingdon's multiple streams approach to understand

Table 3.6. Overview of global policy actors.

Organization	Remit
The UN	• A collective of several countries who formed an international organization to promote human rights and social progress; it has many specialist agencies including the WHO • Established 1948 • UN's specialist agency for health • Has the aim of attaining the highest possible level of health for all people • Has implemented many vertical programmes such as immunization • Implemented mass eradication programmes such as the successful smallpox campaign and the unsuccessful malaria eradication campaign • Has emphasized the importance of primary health care • Produces an annual report about global health
The World Bank	• Works like a bank in the traditional sense • Provides low-interest loans to low-income countries • Imposes policy conditions for repayment thus public sector reform is encouraged • 'Invests in people' • Has described health as an investment • Has encouraged the privatization of health care
The World Trade Organization	• Established in 1995, its role is to regulate trade • Promotes free trade • Has no specific health remit but trade of course affects health in many ways
International Monetary Fund	• Shaped the global economy since the 1940s • Encourages economic growth and stability • Stabilizes economies and reduces poverty • Responsible for much criticized structural adjustment programmes, which have resulted in less investment in health care in several lower income countries
Charities, NGOs and not-for-profit organizations	• Charities are funded via private donations • Each have their own remit and goals for example Oxfam helps people in crisis and aims to help reduce global poverty whereas Save the Children has a focus upon saving children, protecting them from harm and educating them
Aid agencies	• Aid Agencies are dedicated organizations aiming to distribute aid, which comes from a variety of sources • Many are governmental such as USAID, SIDA, EUROPEAID, and donate bilaterally from country to country • Aid is either humanitarian and used to respond to specific crises or developmental to help countries achieve economic improvements
Private foundations	• Legal organizations set up for philanthropic purposes • The Bill & Melinda Gates Foundation is the largest in the USA and is dedicated to finding innovative solutions to global health and development problems • Started the Global Alliance for Vaccines and Immunisation (GAVI) an independently governed initiative (Yamey, 2002)

policy windows and the operation of policy entrepreneurs in public health in Sweden. Meanwhile Rutten *et al.* (2011) have developed a model for health promotion policy called ADEPT in their attempt to move theory into practical steps. The model identifies the causal drivers that influence policy making and then explains the logic of events that can determine policy impacts. They claim that the model is of practical value to health promotion as 'it actually aids actors to influence the policy process' (Rutten *et al.*, 2011, p. 328), which of course is what it's all about!

Box 3.4. An example of policy making – smoke-free legislation in the UK.

The 2007 Health Act meant that all enclosed public places and all workplaces became smoke free. The Act became law on 1 July 2007, marking the end of a decade of politicking, which illustrates all the complexity of the policy-making process.

Walt and Gilson's (1994) policy triangle framework, where 'actors' are placed in the centre, can be used to analyse the way in which this policy came to fruition. The key actors in this case were the tobacco industry, which used its wealth to fund an organization called Forest, which campaigns for smokers' rights. It also mobilized the hospitality trade to make an economic argument that smoke-free legislation would cause huge losses for bars, restaurants and pubs. Other actors included the anti-smoking group ASH, which does not have large financial backing, the BMA (British Medical Association), Cancer Research UK, the British Lung Foundation, the Royal College of Physicians, the Trades Union Congress, the Charted Institute of Environmental Health, scientists and various government ministers and politicians. Arnott *et al.* (2007) show how this broad alliance, the Smokefree Action Coalition lobbied the Labour Government, illustrating how the various actors who are in agreement on an issue need to form strong alliances. Arguably, it was scientists who consolidated the argument by laying down strong evidence bases for legislation. Despite the Chief Medical Officer calling for such legislation in 2003, the Minister for Health, John Reid, an ex-smoker from a staunch working class background, stated strongly that he believed in a voluntary approach and would not support a ban.

The three corners of Walt and Gilson's model are made up of content, process and context. The content of the policy was to create smoke-free public spaces and workplaces, whilst the process in this case was to pursue legislation, and that process will be described here. The context of the smoke-free initiative takes into account the political landscape of the times; at that point, New Labour was espousing a 'third way' for politics, which meant an uneasy combination of neo-liberal economics with a social democratic, interventionist approach to public services (Leach, 2002). This meant, in the context of smoking legislation, a voluntary approach from industry but with a firm commitment from government to protect the public and workers from the dangers of second-hand smoke. In 1998, the Government itself had outlined the dangers of passive smoking in a White Paper (which is the precursor to an act of Parliament), with the uncompromising title 'Smoking Kills'.

By 2004, it was clear that a voluntary approach was not effective, with only 43% of pubs complying with smoke-free policies; that year, John Reid made a faux pas by claiming that working class people had few pleasures and that smoking was one of them. The media and public opinion were highly critical, and at the same time, a neighbouring country, Ireland, had introduced smoke-free legislation and it did not appear to be bringing about the economic problems forecast by the hospitality trade. The government responded by saying that it intended 'to shift the balance significantly in favour of smokefree environments' (DOH, 2004, p. 12). Reid, however, secured an opt-out for private members' clubs and pubs not serving food.

A turning point occurred with the appointment of a new Health Minister, Patricia Hewitt, who called for a complete ban. The way seemed to be set for the legislation to go ahead. However, John Reid still blocked this in the cabinet (the inner circle of ministers), and it was only when a House of Commons Health Select Committee (chaired by an MP who was a tobacco control advocate), reported on all the evidence, that further impetus was gained for the smoke-free cause. The health lobby swung into action to lobby MPs, though the tobacco and hospitality industries were also lobbying hard. Crucially, MPs were allowed a 'free vote', i.e. they did not have to abide by their party's line but could vote according to their individual inclinations.

This example illustrates the importance of individual actors with immense power to block or progress policy at the highest level and chimes with Parsons' (1995) point that the role of personalities and of actual people is a missing ingredient from policy analysis. The intense political debate became publicly prominent, though the Labour Government as a whole seemed ambivalent on the issue; this perhaps was one of the factors that led to a free vote being granted, which allowed those MPs who did feel strongly to assert themselves. The process (as in Walt and Gilson's model) was therefore an important factor.

Arnott *et al.* (2007) suggest that what really led to successful implementation of the legislation was the role of the health lobby, which managed to convince the public and media of the risks of second-hand smoke, and of the greater pleasure afforded by smoke-free leisure spaces. Cairney (2009) in addition, suggests that 'policy transfer' where policy makers are influenced by what is happening in other countries, was a key feature. This, together with the mounting 'hard' scientific evidence of the dangers to health, which began to outweigh the evidence on economic harm to industry, shifted the balance of power, enabling the window of opportunity (Kingdon, 1995) to be seized.

Summary

This chapter has established that policy is crucial to health and more particularly that healthy public policy is a central aspect of health promotion. Every sector of policy making, and all policies, therefore need to give consideration to health and how it might potentially impact upon health outcomes. Divergent views remain about how policy is, and should be, developed, enacted and implemented, and how the impacts of policy on health should be measured, as this chapter has illustrated. Debates about power and whose interests are served within the policy-making process remain ongoing. All of these debates have implications for health promotion practitioners and therefore health promotion practice involves advocating and becoming involved within the policy-making process.

The centrality of healthy public policy to health promotion thinking can result in those working on the ground feeling disempowered, as they are often not in positions where they *can* influence policy. They may be working in what is really a health education role. This does lead some to move jobs, and to seek a position where it is more possible to effect policy change. But what also could help is a shift in thinking, adoption of advocacy roles and developing a more holistic approach which *could* incorporate a contribution to healthy public policy making.

Further Reading

Baggott, R. (2010) *Public Health, Policy and Politics*, 2nd edition. Palgrave Macmillan, Basingstoke, UK.

Billis, D. (ed.) (2010) *Hybrid Organizations and the Third Sector: Challenges for Practice, Theory and Policy.* Palgrave Macmillan, Basingstoke, UK.

Davies, S.E. (2010) *Global Politics of Health.* Polity Press, Cambridge, UK.

Williams, P. (2012) *Collaboration in Public Policy and Practice. Perspectives on Boundary Spanners.* The Policy Press, London.

4 Communicating Health

RUTH CROSS, IVY O'NEIL AND RACHAEL DIXEY

This chapter aims to:

- consider models of communication and assess their relevance to health communication;
- suggest that health promotion must adopt participatory means of communication;
- critique top-down, 'banking' approaches to communication and education;
- assert the importance of health education and consider the idea of health literacy;
- explore and critique social marketing; and
- explore and critique psychological models of behaviour change.

Introduction

We asserted in the previous chapters that our view of health promotion is that of a social movement aimed at bringing social justice in health, and that it contains three broad areas of activity – working with communities, doing policy work and communicating about health. This chapter takes up the last of those three areas. The chapter first considers some of the models of communication that are now regarded as being too simplistic to understand the process of communication, but which were products of their time. Although they are now dated, they continue to influence the way that communication is perceived – as a one-way, top-down process of information transfer. Use of the latter has gained health education a bad name, as victim blaming and ineffective. Humanistic models of education are therefore explored, in an attempt to outline which ideas of education are truly helpful in bringing about empowered communities. Useful ideas from the counselling and psycho-analytic literature are also presented. This chapter thus explores the importance of health communication in promoting health and attempts to address some of the issues in communicating health messages. It will also critically look at theories about health behaviour, and how messages can be translated into behaviour changes. It covers social marketing and health literacy in relation to communicating health messages, as these have become part of the

modern public health discourse. Following the themes of the book, we assert that methods that involve communities and individuals, which are 'bottom-up', are essential in enabling people to take control of their own health.

Given the importance of health communication, the understanding of effective communication within health promotion has not really received the same attention as other health promotion theories and models. This is surprising, as communication is central to the success of any health promotion initiative. It is at the 'forefront of the achievement of health promotion objectives' (Corcoran, 2007, p. 1). Health communication is about communicating health messages that hopefully will help people to think about their health and the determinants of their health, and to change their behaviour if that is appropriate. It has been acknowledged that there is not a lack of health information; the problem is that health messages are inconsistent, uncoordinated and out of step with the way people live their lives (DOH, 2004). Health messages are often communicated in a top-down manner, which is not always appropriate, or the information is somehow 'lost in translation', is culturally insensitive or simply does not seem relevant to the people for whom the information is intended. It is clear through the philosophy of this book, that we adopt an assets-based view of people, not a deficits one – in other words we see people as resourceful and not as necessarily deficient. However, there are situations where people do need information from an expert, and there are examples where people do not have basic, correct information. How health promoters can provide such information in ways that are empowering is a conundrum that this chapter hopes to address. Moreover, there are obvious links between communication and some of the other key values outlined above, such as participation: 'before people of a community can participate, they must have appropriate information, and they must follow a communication process to reach a collective perception of the local situation and of the options for improvement' (Fraser and Restrepo-Estrada, 1998, p. 59). This chapter, more than others, crosses over into issues of health care, as well as of health promotion. Often one to one communication is with patients, and the need for patient education can be described as a neglected area within health promotion (Hubley, 2006).

Communication

Basic communication theories

Early health education assumed that a change in people's knowledge and beliefs would translate to a change in their behaviour. This perspective suggests that communication is unidirectional, uncomplicated, involving a linear flow of information from experts to individuals (Lee and Garvin, 2003).

Health practitioners often ask 'Why don't they listen?'. 'They' are the 'public' and health promotion has tended to have an obsessive emphasis on changing 'their' behaviour. The purpose of communication is therefore not only to deliver a message but to effect a change in the recipients' knowledge, attitudes, and eventually behaviour (Fletcher, 1973). The focus of effective intervention is often placed on the people who should be receiving health messages – did they get the message, and have they changed their behaviour? Evaluation tends to focus on the outcomes, on the impact of for example, a communication campaign, rather than on the process of intervention. The latter would involve asking searching questions: Am I an effective communicator? Have I chosen the right communication method? Was the design of the health messages appropriate? *Why* are our health messages not effective? Health messages are only considered effective when the audience has

acted or responded to a message in some way (Corcoran, 2007). Successful intervention is of course about the health promoters as much as the intervention itself. Having good communication skills as well as understanding the factors that influence the effectiveness of health messages is seen as essential to health educators and promoters. Later in this chapter, some of these skills at an interpersonal level are considered in more detail. First, we discuss theories of communication.

'In health education, communication is a planned process which is effective when the client attains certain goals' (Kiger, 2004, p. 84). This two-way communication concerns the exchange of meanings through a common set of symbols, a process that involves the transmission of a 'coded' message between a source and an audience, 'a process in which participants create and share information with one another to reach a mutual understanding' (Rogers, 1995, p. 17). Lee and Garvin (2003) argue that we should move beyond the traditional practices, the one-way information transfer toward a more useful and appropriate concept of information exchange – a two-way communication (Fig. 4.1). This is, of course, more consistent with participatory ways of working and with dialogue, rather than simply telling people what to do.

The development of communication theories

In its conventional wisdom about communication, health promotion has borrowed ideas from the longstanding study of communication as a discipline. At the beginning of the 'mass media' period, Lasswell (1948) developed the classic formula for communication (Box 4.1) – 'who says what to whom in which channel with what effect'. This formula is well known to those who subscribe to

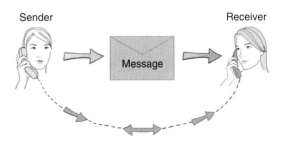

Fig. 4.1. Messages sent from the health promoter to the individual. It then goes forward and backward between the two.

Communicating Health

the transmission model of communication where communication is about the transfer of information from the source to the recipients.

This traditional linear model of communication is a one-way process where the main purpose is to transmit a message, and the purpose of effecting a change within the recipient is implicit. An historical perspective is essential here, as Lasswell was developing his ideas at a point when the power of fascist regimes was at its height, and the power of propaganda machines appeared terrifying. The persuasive power of the top-down communication message symbolized the power of mass communication.

The Shannon–Weaver model of communication (1949) (Box 4.2), another linear transmission model of the same period included a further element – 'noise', meaning anything which could interfere with the effective transmission of the message.

Traditional linear models of communication do not reflect the richness and dynamics of the process of human communication (Rogers, 1986). We now see communication more as a cyclical process (Corcoran, 2007), or at least a two-way process (Kiger, 2004), as theorized by Osgood and Schramm's model of communication (Steinberg, 2006) (Fig. 4.2). They saw communication as a circular process where messages are passed between coders and encoders (senders and receivers). The communication process is endless – the sender can become the receiver, and the receiver becomes the sender, both giving and receiving feedback and interpreting each other's messages. The interpretation of the message is the 'noise' in their model where messages can be misinterpreted by different coders and encoders. The meaning of the messages thus changes depending on who is decoding and encoding those messages.

Within health promotion, Green and Tones (2010) present a communication model (Fig. 4.3), which clearly showed the communication process and the reciprocal relationship between the sender and the receiver. The model shows how messages are encoded by the sender and decoded by the receiver. The message can be transmitted through a symbolic means such as a picture; iconic means such as a pink ribbon for breast cancer or red ribbon for HIV/AIDS or through an 'enactive code' such as an exercise involving participation. It also shows that memory and motivation have an influence on the interpretation of messages.

These models tend to view communication as a rational and technical process, and they are widely used in planning and developing health campaigns. McGuire's communication/persuasion model (1989) for example, talks of five 'input variables' – source, message, channel, receiver and destination – and there are many texts that elaborate on the most effective ways of manipulating these variables to maximize impact (e.g. Kreuter and McClure, 2004). Looking at this critically, two questions can be posed. First, is the process of communication a rational and technical process or an emotional, 'messy', complex set of processes? Secondly, is the idea of developing persuasive messages potentially dangerous and when does it become manipulation? The latter question is even more complex in a situation where knowledge needs are quite legitimate and where, in addition, health promoters *do* have an agenda – that is, we *would* prefer people to make healthy choices, not to smoke and so on. In other words, health promoters *are* interested in getting the message across, and in methods that result in people changing their health for the better. (Some of the

---

Box 4.1. The Lasswell Formula (1948).

Who (communicator) → Says what (message) → How (medium or channel) → To whom (receiver) → With what effect (impact).

Box 4.2. Shannon–Weaver model of communication (1949).

Transmitter (information source – giving a signal) → Noise (some kind of interference) → Receiver (message reaches destination).

---

ethical issues raised by communication methods are explored in more detail in Chapter 5.) So the whole area of what are appropriate and effective means of communicating about health is complex and difficult.

Educating 'the public' and communicating health messages

Many health care practitioners and indeed, members of the general public, view health promotion as providing information, or advice giving – a health education approach to health promotion (Naidoo and Wills, 2009). Gambling (2003, p. 68) writes, 'The aims of any health education programme are

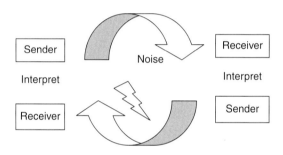

Fig. 4.2. Adapted from Osgood and Schramm's model of communication.

to improve knowledge about the [health] condition, increase health-promoting behaviours and enhance compliance with medication and treatment regimens'. The medical model thus sees the importance of information-giving, adherence to advice and in particular tends to assume that change in an individuals' knowledge, attitudes and beliefs results in the change of that person's behaviour. If the evidence is reliable enough, then the individual will act rationally and change should follow, as in the diagram in Fig. 4.4.

The assumption is that provision of information should be enough to 'empower' people, enabling them to make healthy choices and improve their health regardless of their social and environmental context. Thus telling someone to always sleep under an insecticide-treated bed net, or giving someone a diet sheet at a doctor's surgery, will inevitably produce changes. This is clearly fatuous. Evidence suggests that people do often know how to protect their health but cannot due to their material circumstances, or they have taken deliberate decisions not to act on the advice provided, or they do intend to act on the information but other factors intervene.

The one-way transfer of knowledge in health education, however, remains prevalent, and according to Lee and Garvin's view (2003) can be closely linked to the transmission of knowledge perspective in education (Pratt and Associates, 2005), where

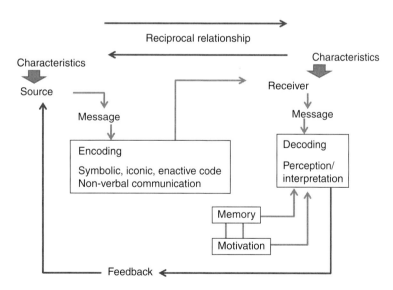

Fig. 4.3. Communication model (Green and Tones, 2010, p. 299).

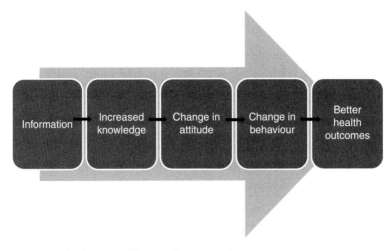

Fig. 4.4. Key assumptions underpinning health education approaches.

education is about imparting or acquiring knowledge from one person to another. Effective transmission of knowledge is content focused, based on the sender's expertise in the subject matter and their skills in delivering that content (Pratt and Associates, 2005). Using the acquisition metaphor as described by Sfard (1998), human learning is conceived of as an acquisition of something, gaining ownership over a body of knowledge. Knowledge is seen as a commodity, which can be applied, transferred and shared with others. The owner of that knowledge becomes privileged in some way, possessing something which others do not have (Sfard, 1998). This encompasses a 'deficit' model whereby the non-expert recipient of the knowledge is viewed as deficient in some way, which may, in turn, be described as a paternalistic perspective.

This one-way transfer of knowledge focuses on the individual message recipient and the scientific knowledge of the expert (Lee and Garvin, 2003); the health promoter is the expert who gives advice and information to the people. Many health practitioners do align themselves with this top-down approach to health promotion, but it is one of the reasons why health education began to be seen as victim blaming, resulting in the paradigm shift to 'health promotion'. If health promotion is about empowerment then we clearly have to reject this approach to education. And if 'knowledge is power' then we clearly have to think through what approaches to education, knowledge-transfer and health communication will truly empower individuals and communities. We also need to recapture the important place of education within health promotion. Health education is an integral part of health promotion and arguably there is an educative element in *all* efforts to promote health.

Moving to two-way, transformational education methods

Lee and Garvin (2003) argue that health practitioners must move from a monologue information *transfer* model of practice to a dialogue information *exchange* in order to reorient health communication practice. Likewise, Campbell and Cornish (2010, p. 1)

> ...distinguish between technical communication (the transfer of health-related knowledge and skills from experts to communities) and transformative communication (a more politicised process, where marginalised groups develop critical understandings of the social roots of their ill-health, and the confidence and capacity to tackle these).

The latter addresses the balance of power and control assumed by the 'expert'. This is particularly needed in public health where health communications tend to be firmly rooted in individual behaviour, ignoring the social context and the adaptive power of the people (Lee and Garvin, 2003). This way of 'doing' health promotion can be seen as similar to Freire's (2000) 'banking approach' to education, where the experts have a body of knowledge that they transmit to learners.

Freire believed that 'banking' approaches to education serve only to mould oppressed people to fit into the roles expected of them by society; the aim is to immobilize people. He believed education should be dialogical, similar to the social reform perspective we see in education (Pratt and Associates, 2005).

Earlier, Dewey (1916) argued that the purpose of education should not revolve around the acquisition of a pre-determined set of skills, but rather the realization of one's full potential and the ability to use those skills for the greater good. He believed that education provides a catalyst for personal and social change and development. Education is a problem-solving activity and it facilitates democracy. He considered education to be the key to empower people. Hence education would raise people's consciousness of health issues, so that they are able to make choices and eventually create pressure for healthy public policies (Naidoo and Wills, 2009), transforming society.

Dewey's humanistic and liberal approach shows that education can ultimately facilitate social change (Purdy, 1997). He challenged the authoritarian relationship between teachers and learners, arguing that schools should be run along democratic lines, which was a major challenge at the time to the hierarchical nature of schools, where children had little or no power. The teacher's role is not to transmit knowledge to passive students; rather, s/he should be a facilitator and guide, a partner in the learning process. Carl Rogers' humanistic view of education (Rogers, 1969; Kirschenbaum and Henderson, 1989) carries on this theme, asserting that we cannot teach another person directly, we can only facilitate his or her learning. Rogers is perhaps more well known for developing person-centred counselling, but his views on education have been equally influential, placing the learner in the centre of the learning process and promoting the dignity and self-efficacy of learners. These ideas have now been mainstreamed to a greater or larger extent in different parts of the world, but they were revolutionary when Rogers first introduced them.

Education and learning are social and interactive processes with the potential to bring about social reform, building a society of mutual respect (Freire, 2000). Freire was, of course, writing at a time when there was a dictatorship in his native Brazil and his 'pedagogy of the oppressed' aimed to give a voice to those who had no choice but to be silent.

He started by developing a system of teaching literacy, not merely teaching people to read and write, but at the same time developing their political consciousness, an awareness of their true position in the world. The main purpose of education is therefore to develop skills of enquiry in our social world, not merely to transmit what is known.

Dewey believed that education should strike a balance between delivering knowledge while also taking into account the interests and experiences of the student. This can be related to the participatory metaphor of Sfard (1998), which emphasizes togetherness, solidarity, collaboration and people in action in a constant flux. Thus in educational contexts, in order for education to be effective, content must be presented in a way that allows students to relate the information to prior experiences, thus deepening the connection with the new knowledge.

In health promotion, many of our learners are adults, implying that the principles of adult learning and of informal learning need to be understood. Adult learners are motivated to learn what they need to know, bringing with them their experience and knowledge; they tend to be problem-centred self-directed learners, driven internally to learn (Bach *et al.*, 2007). In adult education, according to Knowles (1980), the purpose is to enhance adult learners' ability to be self-directed in their learning. The educator's task is to facilitate learning, and prepare and share sufficient information and knowledge to help the learners participate in the learning process.

The humanistic view is that every human being is capable of looking at the world critically, in a 'dialogical encounter' with others. Education therefore needs to be based on dialogue, not curricula where people act *on* one another, but on people working *with* each other – a problem-posing education, a process of consciousness raising (Freire, 2000). Freire believed that through education, people can be liberated, see their oppression and act to change it. Through education, the learners' world is being 'decoded' so that they become aware of the oppressive forces that shape their lives; they would be able to gain power to transform these forces, to reflect on their situation, enabling them to take some control over their lives. Discussion and sharing experience help learners to explore diverse perspectives, recognize and investigate their assumptions, develop new appreciation for continuing differences, encourage attentive respectful listening, increase intellectual agility, help learners to learn the process and habits of democratic discourse, leading to transformation where we assimilate knowledge in a critical manner to become responsible decision makers (Mezirow, 1981). Unlike Dewey, Rogers and Knowles, Freire's view relates education even further to the social dimension of the education process and challenges the individualism of the humanistic perspective. Health promotion is therefore much more than educating the individual. It is about empowering, building skills, making conscious decisions and ultimately changing society.

The aim of education is thus to bring about social change in a collective manner, producing a better society. Health promotion teaching relates closely to the social reform perspective in education, learners are encouraged to look at the principles and values of promoting health. Probing questions are asked to provoke thinking. Learners are encouraged to question their practice. They are asked to critically discuss, analyse the literature and their practice, synthesize and apply their learning in practice.

Empowerment is central to health promotion, as is social change. If students are empowered to learn, to understand critically the beliefs and values of society, it is possible to bring about social change. Social reform is based on a constructivist approach to the understanding of the world (Pratt and Associates, 2005). Critical approaches in questioning the truth help to challenge the assumptions of knowledge and realities. Students learn through the reconstruction of knowledge and incorporating it into the social realities of their lives. The acquisition metaphor (Sfard, 1998), the one-way transfer of knowledge (Lee and Garvin, 2003) or the transmission perspective in education (Pratt and Associates, 2005) alone does not give power to the individual. As in health promotion, the top-down medical, educational or behavioural approach (Naidoo and Wills, 2009) to health promotion does not empower the people as we aspire to do in practice. Teaching based on the social change perspective enables learner engagement, encourages learners to critically look at their learning, relate their learning to their social context and thus helps learners to take action to change their lives.

Transformative or profound learning is where a 'shift' in the horizons of one's life world is experienced to the extent that it causes questioning of self-identity and has an impact on how the world is perceived, interpreted and acted on. Mezirow, a key thinker in understanding transformative educational experiences, asserts that in order for transformational learning to take place, learners have to intentionally want to learn from an experience; thus willingness to learn is a key aspect – transformational learning will not take place 'by accident' – the learner has to want learning to happen (Mezirow, 2003). This implies something about the 'attitude' that learners need to bring with them to the educational encounter. Earlier, Rogers pondered on the nature of 'significant' learning, whereby experiential learning can lead to self-actualization, where learners want to become more than they are. A related idea, of 'threshold concepts' (Meyer and Land, 2005) suggests that crossing a threshold can transform one's world view and/or cause a 'shift in perspective (that) may lead to a transformation of personal identity, a reconstruction of subjectivity' (Meyer and Land 2005, p. 376). Whereas most learning is not *that* transformational or profound, it can provide learning that is transferable, enabling the release of capacity for action in a range of spheres or new situations. This transferable learning may have transformative power. (Standing up and giving a talk in a village meeting *could* lead to having the confidence to stand up in the corridors of power such as a national assembly.)

In contrast to some of these ideas, Appiah (2006, p. 73) argues that the way that people 'move' is through 'just a gradually acquired new way of seeing things'. Whether people learn and develop through sudden leaps of transformation or more gradually over time, profound learning can take them to a crossroad, which Baxter Magolda (2001), as noted above in Chapter 1 on empowerment, says is essential in terms of 'becoming the author of one's own life'. This notion clearly links with empowerment, and has implications for the way that health promoters need to work to facilitate 'profound learning'. Health promoters can help people change their lives in less transformational ways, and a common phrase in health promotion is 'small steps', i.e. helping people to make small but significant changes, which are accumulative. We now turn attention to the characteristics of the messengers or educators.

The Communication Process as Conventionally Applied in Health Promotion

Hubley and Copeman (2008) present a model that clearly illustrates the characteristics of the four key components of the communication process – senders, messages, channels and receivers – with many factors within each component that could affect the effectiveness of health messages. They also include the feedback loop within their model to demonstrate the importance of feedback within the communication process. Conventionally, each of these components in the journey of messages from the senders through to the receivers need to be scrutinized in turn in order to improve the effectiveness of health communication. The discussion below (Table 4.1) uses the four components (senders, messages, channels and receivers) to frame an exploration and critique.

The senders

In any communication, the sender often assumes that they are a credible source and that they are doing everything correctly. However, humanistic education (which challenges the power dynamic between teachers and learners) and the newer models of communication (which stress the role of the relationship between senders and receivers of messages) have facilitated a move to understanding the role, credibility, motives and skills of the communicator or teacher. In simple terms, the focus has shifted from seeing the 'problem' as residing in the receiver (or learner), to seeing failures of communication as residing in the sender (or teacher). Fraser and Restrepo-Estrada (1998) cite experiences from Bolivia, Uganda and Algeria where a range of workers in health and agriculture had such poor

Table 4.1. The components within the communication process.

Senders	Who we are and how we communicate
	Our communication skills – verbal, non-verbal, written
	Interpersonal communication skills
	Do we listen to the message receivers?
Messages	Type of messages, simple or complicated, its appropriateness
Channels	Communication methods
	Mass communication
	The environment where the messages were transmitted
Receivers	Who are the audience – their literacy level, their state of mind, their views, their beliefs and their attitudes?

communication styles, were condescending, did not listen and were too theoretical, that their work could not be effective. Effective, reflective practitioners clearly will take time to reflect on their own communication styles, methods and effectiveness, though in practice, practitioners do not always take this time. This has led to health promoters finding useful a series of ideas, which help to illuminate the processes of human interaction.

Communication is a necessary process in any human relationship, and certainly is essential in the relationship between health promoters and the individuals and communities they work with. It is transactional, inevitable, purposeful, multidimensional and irreversible (Hargie et al., 1994). It takes place within (and is influenced by) the context, e.g. geographical location, time, relationships. Interpersonal communication is about face-to-face interaction that involves few people – a process by which information, meanings and feelings are shared by persons through the exchange of verbal and non-verbal messages (Brooks and Heath, 1985, cited in Hargie et al., 1994).

Credibility of the source of information is very important in health communication, with the perceived authority of the message source affecting the receivers' acceptance of the message. On a superficial level, gender, age and so forth may influence the acceptability of the message. The skills and style of communicating are obviously important, highlighting the need for communicators to be self-aware and to design and communicate messages in a way acceptable to the audience.

The Johari window (Luft and Ingham, 1955), is a useful tool in interpersonal communication, helpful for both community members beginning to question their status in the process of conscientization, and also for health professionals needing to consider how they come across to the community they are working with. Created by Joseph Luft and Harry Ingham in 1955, it consists of a four-paned 'window' (Box 4.3) representing open, hidden, blind and unknown areas. The lines dividing the four panes are like window shades, which can move as an interaction progresses. If you know yourself well and others know you, you are in a more open relationship with others. Through feedback from others and self-disclosure, you learn more about yourself. Being aware of your own strengths and weaknesses helps you to know more about yourself and your actions when you communicate.

The Johari window (Box 4.3) challenges the usual power relationship between health promoters and the groups or individuals they are working with. The top-down expert would not be expected necessarily to share their own thoughts, feelings and insecurities with their 'client' groups; a health promoter working in an open, dialogical way would need to do this if they were truly being transparent and honest in their dealing with the community.

Transactional analysis (Berne, 1964) is another approach to understand the psychological interpretation of how and why we act as we do when we interact with others (Box 4.4). It is useful to understand and be aware of the way we act when we are communicating with others. It draws on Freudian psychodynamic theory and was developed by Eric Berne. Berne identifies three observable changes in personalities – parent, adult, child – the three ego states within every individual's personality. At any given moment, each individual in a social situation will exhibit a parent, adult or child ego state. In each one of us, one state is more dominant than the others. We use these three states when interacting with others. Do we present ourselves as a parent when we deliver our health message, taking a paternalistic approach in imparting our knowledge, a top-down, medical or educational approach?

Or do we present our health messages in an emotional manner; behave like a child when we discuss important issues with clients? It is important that we know how we communicate with others, behave as an adult and treat others as adults when we communicate, taking a dialogical approach that empower the learner, an empowerment approach.

Within transactional analysis, it is suggested that we adopt four orientations towards other people and the world around us when we communicate (Harris, 2004). Health educators working from a top-down perspective can adopt the position of a controlling parent telling a child what to do, and implicitly from a 'deficit' position of 'I'm ok – you're not ok' (Box 4.5). Using these kinds of ideas to reflect critically on the communication process may help to increase understanding of why so many messages appear to 'fail'.

In terms of moving towards more empowering encounters between health workers and patients of people in the community, a number of attempts have been made to capture what creates that empowerment (Feste and Anderson, 1995; Kettunen *et al.*, 2001, 2003). Attention has also been given to the non-verbal communication of workers, which can communicate a clear and strong message – more than the message sender realizes (Kiger, 2004).

Box 4.3. Johari Window, adapted from Luft and Ingham (1955).

	Known to self	Unknown to self
Known to others	Free and open, known to others and self – the impression you know you are giving	Blind self – the impression you may be giving, unknown to yourself
Unknown to others	Hidden self – you know, but others don't, the part of you that you hide	Unknown self – both you and others don't know

---

Box 4.4. Transactional analysis, adapted from Berne (1964).

Parent	Nurturing, controlling	Feel and behave in ways learnt from mother, father, teacher, etc. It concerns taking responsibility or taking charge.
Adult	Rational	Observe, collect data, think, weigh probable outcomes of alternate course, make decisions.
Child	Feeling, intuiting, adapting	Feel and behave typically as a child; you experience strong feelings and emotions, create, have fun, adapt to or feel bad about the demands of more powerful people.

Non-verbal communication such as body language, facial expressions, eye contact, tone of voice and personal space can transmit messages that we did not intend to pass on – the blind self. Studies show that during interpersonal communication, 7% of the message is verbally communicated while 93% is transmitted non-verbally. Out of the 93% non-verbal communication, 38% is through vocal tones and 55% is through facial expressions (British Institute of Learning Disability, 2005). Often, we communicate our feelings about our views and attitudes via our body language, in conflict with our verbal message, a non-verbal leakage such as lack of genuineness or empathy (Green and Tones, 2010). Active listening is regarded as an essential skill of health promoters (Hubley and Copeman, 2008). Active listening demonstrates genuine understanding and empathy of the other's point of view, whilst the ability to show respect can help to build rapport and establish trust.

The channel and the message

Marshall McLuhan's famous dictum, 'The medium is the message', was coined as far back as 1967. He argued that, 'Societies have always been shaped more by the nature of the media by which men communicate than by the content of the communication' (McLuhan and Fiore, 1967, p. 1). The meaning for us is that the choice of medium used is more important than the message itself. He was writing at a time when mass media had arrived in the developed world. He wrote,

> The medium, or process, of our time – electric technology – is reshaping and restructuring patterns of social interdependence and every aspect of our personal life. It is forcing us to reconsider and re-evaluate practically every thought, every action, and every institution formerly taken for granted. Everything is changing – you, your family, your neighbourhood, your education, your job, your government, your relation to 'the others'. And they're changing dramatically.
>
> (McLuhan and Fiore, 1967, p. 1)

Clearly, these points are echoed in the 21st century by the arrival of electronic media, but whereas he wrote that the 'television generation is a grim bunch' (p. 126), the arrival of electronic technology is seen by many as allowing new forms of expression, a new pluralism and greater democracy. This will be returned to later in the chapter. These new media provide new means of communicating for those interested in health but rely on a degree of digital literacy.

A wide range of methods and channels are used to communicate health messages ranging from interpersonal, to groups and mass media, and at the individual, local, national and international levels. Examples are: face-to-face discussion or forms of counselling; written communication such as leaflets and posters; participatory arts such as drama, role play, storytelling, games and songs; and mass communication through television, film, radio, newspaper, mail shots, billboards and digital communication such as the Internet, podcast, YouTube and mobile phone. This list is by no means exhaustive. Studies of successful health communication suggest that a combination of channels contributes to success (Laverack and Dap, 2003).

Health communication is a goal orientated activity – the designer's goal is to prompt active thought in what they presume is a passive audience. Well designed messages *can* motivate people, who then will actively seek, attend and process messages. For example, unexpected or discrepant content can trigger active thought in a passive audience, e.g. outlining fat content on the menu in a restaurant (Maibach and Parrott, 1995). For education to be effective, participatory learning is needed to promote learner engagement and enhance the understanding and acceptance of health messages, enabling people to internalize and act on the message to suit their needs and make changes according to their situation. Thus although a great deal of energy and resources have gone into mass audience campaigns, their effectiveness can be questioned. Recently, the use of celebrities by the mass media

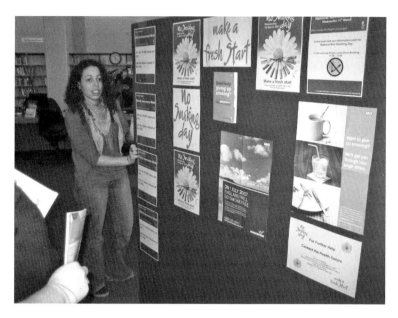

Do these kinds of messages work?

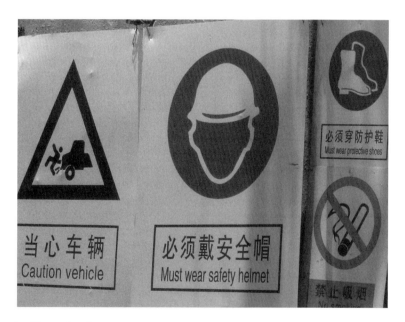

How effective are health warnings?

has become a popular and useful way of attracting attention, encouraging people to be actively involved in health activities, doing what their admired personalities want them to do. Many examples have shown how celebrities raise the profile of health issues. For example, Bob Geldof seriously shamed world leaders over their neglect of world hunger through his 'Feed the World' campaigns in 1984 and 1991 and, more recently in the UK, the celebrity chef Jamie Oliver has led a crucial campaign not only highlighting the need for healthier food in schools but also showing how it could be achieved. Whether these campaigns do effect sustainable change is a moot point.

The receivers

As health communicators, it is often said that it is essential to understand the 'audience' – the individuals and communities worked with – to understand their knowledge levels, their beliefs and, more importantly, their constraints – the barriers they are facing when making health choices. The design of the messages, the methods in communicating the messages need to be acceptable, bearing in mind the characteristics of the audience, the situation they are in, their demographics as well as psychographics. For example, people often want information when they have become ill but how can health messages be designed to suit patients' needs in hospital, and is it a good time to promote health when they are ill? Is it unrealistic to expect people in poverty to be able to act on healthy eating advice and to choose 'healthy' food? Their age, gender, cultural background, their ability and disability, their mental health state, literacy levels, their living and work environment, all need to be taken into consideration.

It is generally agreed that health care provision should be culturally appropriate, and so should health communication. It is worth unpicking the wide-ranging label of 'culture'. Culture can be defined as: 'the learned, shared, and transmitted knowledge of values, beliefs, norms and life ways of a particular group that guides their thinking, decisions, and actions in a patterned way' (Leininger, 1991, p. 47). However, 'culture' is a complex concept, more often assumed than assessed (Kreuter et al., 2003). Health promotion materials that are designed for a population-based health education programme may not always be culturally appropriate for the numerous possible cultural groups and sub-groups in any given society. Often health promotion materials are translated and adapted to different cultural groups from the mainstream health promotion materials rather than specifically developed for a particular group or population (Larkey and Hecht, 2010). Further, individuals within 'cultures' are not all alike.

Messages cannot be 'free' of cultural perspectives but it is obviously important to understand what cultural perspectives are shown. Reflecting the values and norms of a particular audience, specifically designed narrative-based health promotion programmes such as storytelling, drama, soap operas and radio broadcasts can be used to produce culturally grounded health messages (Larkey and Hecht, 2010). Kreuter et al. (2003) discuss the five strategies often used to ensure culturally appropriate health education material. These are: (i) peripheral strategies where materials are packaged to appeal to a given group; (ii) evidential strategies where the relevance of the health issues is directed to a particular group; (iii) linguistic strategies where materials are translated to the group's language; (iv) constituent-involving strategies where experiences are drawn directly from members of the group; and (v) socio-cultural strategies where health issues are discussed in the context of the broader social and cultural values and characteristics of the intended audience. Targeting the needs of the audience can also be seen in 'audience segmentation' as in social marketing strategies as discussed later in this chapter.

The theme of lay knowledge, which runs through this book, is also pertinent here. Popay et al. (1998, p. 619) suggest the need to explore lay knowledge about everyday life, and the nature and causes of health and illness in particular, as 'narratives which have embedded within them explanations for what people do and why – and which, in turn, shape social action'. These studies all have implications for those engaged in promoting health, and suggest the need, at the very least, for what has been called 'cultural sensitivity' in messages about health (e.g. Krumeich et al., 2001). But they also suggest something more. In the case of many of the studies, the respondents live in a context where they are surrounded by the messages of the last few decades about personal responsibility for health, and the role of individual behaviours in maintaining health and preventing disease. If they do not respond to these, it is surely not a question of a 'knowledge deficit'. As we have seen, many lay accounts of health and illness often recognize those factors that are stressed in medical accounts, but these ideas coexist with other accounts of health and illness, and lay epidemiology offers an example of this, with Bury (1994, p. 28) pointing out that 'people rationally assess official information and apply it to their lived experiences on an on going basis'. Bury argues that such rationality applies in the face of what are often simplified messages; for example, even to say 'smoking kills' is a message that may

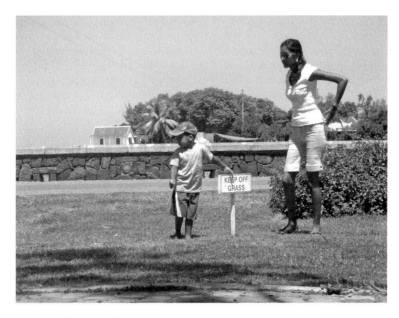

People don't always do what they are told!

well be treated with some scepticism when we see smoking centenarians around us. His suggestion is to introduce a more negotiated element into health promotion, which recognizes the over simplification of much advice, and the complexity of people's lives. For instance, it is important to realize that health is not the only consideration in people's lives.

Mass Media Communication

The growth in the use of mass media to influence people rose to prominence in the propaganda campaigns of the Second World War (Grant, 1994). It has since been widely used as a method in transmitting health messages to the public particularly to promote behaviour change. Seventy-five per cent of the population cite the media as their most important source of health information when making health care decisions (Barker *et al.*, 2006), demonstrating that we are living in a media-driven society and fuelling the idea that mass media is a powerful agent of communication. It can be argued that the media has a medical approach to health issues, with their interests mainly on newsworthy topics to attract public interest. Coverage is about the prevention of ill health rather than the promotion of good health. It relates health promotion to lifestyle problems and the unhealthy influence on health,

e.g. tobacco, alcohol, fast food, selling health rather than giving choices to the people.

In general, mass communication media for health promotion can be categorized into four different types (Corcoran, 2007). They are:

- audio-visual broadcast media such as television, radio;
- audio-visual non-broadcast media such as video, CD, DVD, self-help packages;
- print media such as newspaper, magazine, leaflets, mail shots, billboards; and
- digital media such as Internet, YouTube, mobile phones.

Mass media is one-way communication where messages are transferred from the source to a presumed receptive audience. The message is impersonal and direct feedback from the audience can be difficult to obtain. Mass media can have a strong influence on the public's perception of health issues (e.g. the perception in 1998 in the UK that the MMR injection can cause autism and irritable bowel syndrome). Once the message is broadcast, the interpretation is left to the receivers, with no control over this by the communicators. Conventionally, health promoters see many advantages in the use of mass media, and are influenced by the putative success of commercial advertisers. Mass media can reach a large number of audiences in a very short space of time. However, there is no guarantee that the message will reach the target audience or that it will be understood, despite careful planning of the timing, location and type of media. Although it is expensive to produce a short media message, considering the size of audience it can reach, it could be argued that it is relatively cheap.

Mass media in itself cannot change the structural, political and economical factors that influence health. However, it can be an effective strategy if it is supported by appropriate policies (Wakefield *et al.*, 2010). It is a useful method in raising awareness of health issues. It cannot provide face-to-face support or teach psychomotor skills, e.g. cooking skills, and cannot be regarded as an effective education tool. Short repeated health messages, which are reinforced regularly, can be useful as a constant reminder and have more impact, but can only convey simple information rather than complex information. It does help to place health on the public agenda, stimulate public debate and create pressure for policy changes, particularly where grassroots community organizations are involved. It is debatable that mass media is an effective method in changing people's behaviour without other enabling factors. Evidence suggests that mass media can only be effective if used as an integral part of a campaign where multiple interventions are used (Wakefield *et al.*, 2010). The provision of supporting services to the public is an important element to support mass media health promotion. For example, when encouraging the public to stop smoking it can limit the impact if smoking cessation services are not available.

It is commonly asserted that 'mass' media is now becoming a misnomer, as the possibility of capturing mass audiences is reduced by the proliferation of channels and outlets (Abroms and Maibach, 2008). Broadcasting can be reconceived as narrowcasting, although globalization has also produced a contraflow to this trend, with events being shown in many countries simultaneously, and the same products (TV shows for example), being shown around the world. The longest running radio series in history, *The Archers*, started in 1951 and is still broadcast today; it aimed to educate farmers in the post-war period in the UK, and in the 1950s, two out of three adults listened to its 15-minute broadcasts (Fraser and Restrepo-Estrada, 1998). More recently, *Shuga* was shown all over Africa in 2010; a television drama with an overt didactic element, about the lives and loves of a group of young students in Nairobi, it was seen by 60% of Kenyan youth, and 90% of these said the show had an impact on their thinking (Singh, 2011).

Communication Theories relating to Mass Communication

One of the earliest models relating to mass media is the 'direct effect' model or the 'hypodermic needle' model, where media has a direct influence on the public, like a needle injecting a message into the people. The propaganda campaigns in the Second World War were based on this model. However, Mendelsohn (1968) saw mass media messages as an 'aerosol spray' model, where some of the spray hits the target and most of it drifts away. One of the limitations of this was demonstrated by the 'uses and gratification' theory in which it believed individuals interact and select messages that suit their own needs (Blumler and Katz, 1974).

Lazarsfeld and Merton (1955) identified three conditions for the effectiveness of mass media:

1. Monopolization – limited opposition of the messages in the media.
2. Canalization – messages are consistent with audience's existing motivation, it tells people what they want to hear.
3. Supplementation – it is supported by interpersonal influences, emphasizing the role of the change agent.

This links to Katz and Lazarsfeld's work on the two-step model of communication. Katz and Lazarsfeld (1955) incorporated the interpersonal aspect of communication into their work and developed the two-step flow model where mass media information is channelled to the 'masses' through opinion leaders to a wider population. The opinion leader acts as an enforcer to clarify, strengthen and enforce the importance of the message. It is suggested that individuals are more influential than the media: as Rogers (1983) points out, the first step is a transfer of information only, and it is the second step that provides the transfer of influences. It is this influence that encourages the reception of messages showing that interpersonal communication has a superior effect on influencing changes as compared with mass media. It is also worth noting that opinion leaders are not the only people who receive information from the mass media and that they also receive information through other channels (Windahl *et al.*, 2009). This also demonstrates the lack of control in the communication process from the health communicators' point of view.

The two-step flow model laid the foundation for the study of the Diffusion of Innovations (Rogers, 2003). The principle is that an innovation (the message) can be communicated through certain channels (e.g. opinion leaders) over time among the members of a social system. The model was originated from Rogers and Shoemaker's (1971) communication of innovations theory, which emphasizes the important role of the change agent and interpersonal communication. The process demonstrates a slow initial uptake of the innovation, how it then gathers momentum and slows down again when saturation is reached, creating an S-shaped curve (Tones and Green, 2004).

The process of the adoption of any message goes through five stages (Rogers, 2003):

- knowledge – exposure to the message and developing understanding of it;
- persuasion – the forming of a favourable attitude to the message;
- decision – commitment to the adoption of the initiative;
- implementation – applying it to practice; and
- confirmation – reinforcement of the message based on positive outcomes.

The success of adoption depends on the encounter of the adopters through each stage of the process, e.g. the quality and comprehensiveness of knowledge obtained; the credibility of the information source; the acceptability of the innovation in the social system; the persuasiveness of the message; the factors influencing decision making in taking up the innovation; how easily can it be implemented and the support provided after the implementation of the innovation. The communicator as the change agent plays an important role in the adoption process. It is acknowledged that the message becomes stronger when the adopters become the change agents themselves (Rogers, 2003). The principle of homophily also suggests that people can easily be influenced by others who are similar to themselves (Windahl *et al.*, 2009). This can be linked to peer education, where people accept health information readily from their own peers. It also reinforces the strength of interpersonal communication over the mass media channels.

Peer education

Peer education is a health promotion method used widely, particularly in programmes relating to young people's health. However, it can equally be useful elsewhere. Peer education has been defined as the sharing of information, attitudes or behaviours by people who are not professionally trained educators but whose goal is to educate (Finn, 1981) and where peers from the same societal group educate each other (Svenson, 1998). It has proved useful in promoting behaviour change (UNAIDS, 1999). Behaviour change theory such as social learning theory (Bandura, 1986) underpins the idea, as the peers learn through observation and modelling. It also links to the use of behaviour models as discussed later in this chapter as well as Diffusion of Innovation (Rogers, 2003), where health messages are passed to the target group via their peers. Many believe that peer education is key to behavioural change (UNAIDS, 1999).

Through the use of peers, the process helps to reach so-called 'hard to reach' groups in the community. Messages from peers are more acceptable and credible. However, a review from the EPPI centre (Harden *et al.*, 1999) suggested that evidence for the effectiveness of peer-delivered health education is limited. Monitoring and evaluation is needed to provide evidence for effectiveness. Complementary activities such as improved service provision, policy and structural changes are also important to provide a supportive environment for its success. Recent work has begun to identify the factors needed for successful peer-led interventions (Cornish and Campbell, 2009).

There is some caution in the use of peer education particularly relating to sustainability. Young people will grow up and move on, or prisoners who operate as peers might move back to the community. In health promotion work with young people, they grow up and move on after a period of time. Therefore, recruitment and selection is continuous. Ongoing training as well as supervision and support are essential for effectiveness and sustainability. If peers are not well supported through the process, it would be unacceptable from an ethical point of view (Milburn, 1995). Some evidence exists to show that peers gain a lot from being engaged in this way (Tones and Green, 2004).

People's media – traditional and popular media

Consistent with our view in this book, those methods that mean most to people themselves and that they feel most comfortable with will probably have a greater success in enabling people to think about their health, to understand the determinants of health, to move away from a purely medical model of health and so have the greatest chance of bringing about desired changes to people's lives. These methods are likely to be 'bottom-up', participatory, and ultimately, empowering. There is a range of methods that are close to the people who produce them – songs, stories, dramas, proverbs and oral histories – but they could also include people's attempts to produce written materials, magazines and radio broadcasts, i.e. methods that are mediated by technology. Examples abound of initiatives that have attempted to work alongside people, with groups or whole communities, to communicate about health. 'Community Arts for Health' projects have gained increased attention in the last 20 years or so and have been shown to increase social cohesion and community networks, thereby increasing social capital; they can attract and engage young people and other marginalized groups, and they can produce personal change (South, 2005). These methods not only enable two-way communication, but the process of producing the communication materials can also be participatory.

Mda (1993) provides a thorough analysis of the role of popular theatre in achieving development goals in a book that, though written nearly 20 years ago, has stood the test of time in terms of principles. The work of the Marotholi Travelling Theatre Company in Lesotho, he argues, facilitated six processes: it (i) revitalized people's own forms of cultural expression; (ii) led to intra-village and inter-village solidarity; (iii) enabled community discussion and community decision making; (iv) provided a two-way communication process with inbuilt feedback; (v) led to conscientization; and (vi) mobilized people in support of national development. Likewise, Linney's (1995) practical manual shows how people can be involved in developing materials for health communication, particularly pictorial materials, using an empowerment paradigm.

Under this heading, we could include popularly watched television programmes, or soaps, which often have a health story as a deliberate instructional means. The South African *Soul City* falls into this category, and this has proved to be an effective multimedia initiative tackling a range of health issues. *Tribes*, a show made in Trinidad and Tobago, used social networking and word of mouth to arrange showings in homes without televisions. Although it was only seen by 8% of young people, it did raise important issues about HIV testing. It is part of the Staying Alive initiative launched in 1998. To quote its publicity material,

> The Emmy Award-winning campaign consists of documentaries, public service announcements, youth forums and web content. Staying Alive provides all its television programming rights-free and at no cost to third party broadcasters globally to get crucial prevention messages out to the widest possible audience. The Staying Alive campaign has a long term partnership between MTVNI, UNICEF, UN agencies, governments and foundations. MTVNI is also an active member of the United Nations-supported Global Media AIDS Initiative (GMAI) and the Global Business Coalition on HIV/AIDS, TB and malaria (GBC).

It thus illustrates the use of multimedia and the partnership between major players in the global health arena.

At a much more local level, in The Gambia two terms that make sense to local people and have entered the health communication discourse are *Fankanta* and *Bantaba*. Both concepts are based on traditional values and practices and have been harnessed in new ways.

The 'Fankanta' initiative originated to highlight reproductive health in a country with high rates of fertility and maternal mortality, especially where over the last decade attention on family planning programmes has decreased worldwide. Although family planning is a big issue in The Gambia, it cannot be discussed openly or in public, on the radio or television. Needing to clear misconceptions surrounding family planning, a nationwide survey in 1996 assessed people's perceptions and suggestions for improvement. The results led to the Fankanta initiative. *Fankanta* is a Mandinka word meaning 'planning for the future', and is an acceptable euphemism for family planning. Since 1997, Fankanta has two components – 'Support for family planning' and 'HIV/AIDS and STI control'. Traditional leaders, community health workers, women's support groups and youth associations are strongly involved with its participatory approach involving negotiating intervention principles with partners to obtain consensus. Fankanta includes culturally sensitive strategies and gains the active participation of religious leaders. As an expression that stresses the importance of thinking about the future, it has resonance with the idea of sustainability, deferred gratification and thinking about the implications of actions on others.

The 'Bantaba' approach, derived from the Mandinka word meaning a meeting ground or a 'conversation' at community level, where community members meet to discuss community issues and concerns, was initiated by a new model of health communication otherwise called 'Operation 2010' undertaken in communities by multidisciplinary health field workers. Bantaba creates a forum for community members to discuss pertinent health issues, share positive experiences and lessons, and encourage positive changes. This community forum helps to mobilize influential community leaders to take charge of promotion of health in their localities. Thus the Bantaba approach is a community-driven behaviour change strategy based on the principles of participatory appraisal and finding solutions to health problems important to communities, with health workers facilitating. It is a tool for empowerment by enhancing communication, analytical, problem-solving and health skills.

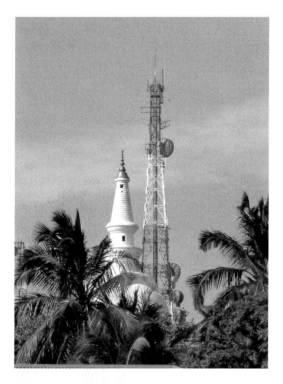

New technologies: a radio mast sits alongside a temple in Sri Lanka.

Electronic/digital communication

The past decade has seen the growth of World Wide Web, providing unprecedented access to information (Bach *et al.*, 2007), enabling services such as online shopping and banking, and allowing new ways of social networking and virtual communities. The new media have also been used as means of mobilizing dissent, coordinating protests and generally bringing more power to the people. In this year of the 'Arab spring', mobile phones, social networking and other digital means have been key instruments in bringing down repressive governments. The radical Chinese artist, Ai Wei Wei writes:

> China is at a very interesting moment. Power and the centre have suddenly disappeared in the universal sense because of the Internet, global politics, and the economy. The techniques of the Internet have become a major way of liberating humans from old values and systems, something that has never been possible until today.
>
> (Obrist, 2011, p. 6)

The accessibility of the new media is bringing about new ways of sculpting the social world, challenging the status quo, and thus it is not surprising that repressive regimes close down networks when feeling threatened. The social media enable people to network in ways that were impossible only a few years ago, and to have control over their messages. These methods have been harnessed such as by the website *Pesky People*, which demands better access to facilities for people with disabilities, and by coalitions to stop the cuts to welfare services in the UK (van der Zee, 2011). These new media provide a voice and visibility, allowing the non-powerful and marginalized a space in which to counter the dominant media culture (Lievrouw, 2009). In an era where involvement in conventional politics has waned, the new media have led to a different kind of political activism, rousing in some, the optimism for a different kind of democracy (Papacharissi, 2010). The huge amount of blogging and Internet-based activism demonstrates that people and communities are not disinterested in current issues, politics and social affairs. Electronic communication has engaged some groups that hitherto have been perceived as 'hard to reach' in terms of health communication. These include men in developed countries who conventionally have been reluctant to seek health information. Conrad and White (2007) provide a useful guide on how health promoters can work effectively with men. There are many websites dedicated to particular illnesses and conditions, where people can share their own experiences, their struggles and successes in getting treatment, and thus to provide social support.

Whilst there remains a major 'digital divide' between those with electronic and mobile technology, these technologies are moving fast. The ability to access information becomes an important source of social capital and aids social cohesion and communication (Bach *et al.*, 2007). A survey on Internet use found that 93% of health seekers went on the Internet to look for information about a particular illness or condition, more than any other route in accessing health information (PEW, 2000). Modernizing the NHS in the UK was one of the objectives of the previous Labour Government. Their document – Information for Health – An Information Strategy for the Modern NHS 1998–2005, aimed to give 'the people of this country the best system of health care in the world, providing information which is accessible when and where it is needed' (NHS Executive, 1998, p. 3). The Information Strategy would enable NHS professionals to provide seamless care to improve the public's health. Since the Information Strategy document in 1998, information for both the public and health care professionals has much improved, e.g. The NHS Information Centre, NHS Direct.

The use of mobile phones in health promotion has been increasing in the last few years, for example in Chlamydia screening in the UK. Hazelwood (2008) found that using text messaging on mobile phones helped her in the management of eating disorders. Lester *et al.* (2010) also found that patients who received SMS mobile phone text support had significantly improved treatment adherence compared with the individuals in their control. Mobile phones might be effective tools to improve patient outcome in resource-limited settings. However, further comprehensive study is needed to maximize health gains. There are also other points to consider, e.g. network coverage in rural areas. In addition, not everybody can afford or have the access to a mobile phone.

The rapid growth of electronic communication is undoubtedly to be welcomed and exploited. However, consideration must be given to sections of society who are being left behind in the information technology revolution – the 'digital divide' – including older people, those with little formal education, people who do not understand the dominant languages used on the Internet, the socially disadvantaged, those with visual, hearing or physical impairments, and the 'technophobes'. The accessibility, affordability and availability of broadband can also pose problems in

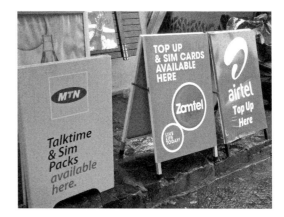

Mobile phones have spread dramatically throughout the world.

ensuring equity of access. Last but not least, health literacy and information security is another issue in the use of these new technologies.

Summary

So far, we have looked at the process of communication and woven in aspects of educational theory. We have attempted to challenge the conventional wisdom of the communication theories so readily adopted in health promotion, and to show how they can very often be top-down. We have also attempted to show that far from merely being 'victim blaming', health education is an essential part of health promotion. People have needs for information and for knowledge and learning. However, given the failure perceived by some, of health education to achieve health gains, recent years have seen the introduction of other means of communicating about health. Thus social marketing has come to prominence as an alternative to health education, and more recently the concept of 'nudge' has gained attention. We would argue that it is not health education per se that is failing. Rather, it is unrealistic to expect educational methods to achieve health gain in the absence of supporting measures such as healthy public policy and the other 'planks' of the Ottawa Charter. 'Health literacy' has also risen as a 'new' concept whereas some would argue that this is one aspect of health education. Health literacy, and motivational interviewing will be discussed as two current terms within health promotion, and we also include a consideration of the more dominant theories of individual behaviour change. Conventionally, it is held that 'successful' communication strategies need to be underpinned by theory, and so these theories are explored and their utility assessed.

Social Marketing and Health Promotion

The rise of 'social marketing' – the use of marketing principles to sell social goods – within health promotion has received mixed reviews. Its chief proponent, Richard Manoff, applied marketing techniques to family planning, nutrition and other health practices back in 1965 (Manoff, 1985), and Fraser and Restropo-Estrada (1998, p. 54) suggests that the health sector 'has used social marketing more than others'. French (2007, p. 24) argues that social marketing is increasingly emerging as a dominant approach to promoting health and that it provides an alternative to what he refers to as the 'paternalistic professional-dominated approaches to population health improvement', which have characterized health promotion (specifically in the UK context). Alternatively, Werner and Sanders (1997, p. 29) assert that social marketing 'often comes closer to brainwashing than awareness-raising' and 'does not give people the opportunity to make their own decisions and take autonomous action'. It is diametrically opposed to Freire's

open-ended, problem-solving approach and thus resembles his 'banking' approach to education; social marketing does not enable people to make the first, crucial decisions about what types of communication activities could be useful for them (Linney, 1995). Green and Tones (2010), like Griffiths *et al.* (2008), take a more pragmatic approach and conclude that health promotion and social marketing remain distinct, with social marketing having an important place within health promotion and that the two working together increases the potential for effectiveness. Reynolds and Thorpe (2009) see it simply as a set of project management tools rather than being embedded in a particular ideology, and as a useful means to change travel behaviour for example, as exemplified by Worcestershire's 'Choose How you Move' initiative, which aimed to change how people use cars in an attempt to combat global warming.

Arguably, a key aim of both health promotion and social marketing is behaviour change and the encouragement of healthier choices. Each also takes into account people's circumstances and attempts to gain insights into what people need and want. Green and Tones (2010) argue that social marketing, like health promotion, is also concerned with tackling the wider determinants of health. A key question for Green and Tones (2010), then, is

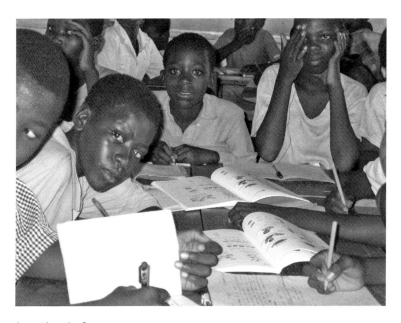

A banking approach to education?

Chapter 4

Box 4.6. Case study: Using social marketing to increase the use of insecticide-treated bed nets in rural Tanzania.

Armstrong *et al.* (2001) carried out a study looking at the effects of a large-scale social marketing programme to promote the use of insecticide-treated nets (ITNs) in rural Tanzania in order to improve child survival. ITNs were introduced over a period of 2 years to a population of nearly half a million people. The effectiveness of this intervention was determined by examining child survival rates using a case control approach. Questionnaires were also used about ITN use and factors mitigating against this.

The social marketing strategy used included the following elements:

● involvement of private and public sectors;
● community sensitization meetings;

● baseline research; and
● locally branded ITNs, locally available (subsidized).

Alongside these, a 'comprehensive information, education and communication campaign was developed and implemented' (p. 1242).

Child survival rates improved by 27% compared with baseline figures. Uptake of ITNs increased from 10% to 50%. The authors estimated that the use of ITNs 'prevented 1 in 10 child deaths at that time' (p. 1241). They therefore concluded that social marketing is effective in promoting ITN use with subsequent implications for malaria control.

'is social marketing an alternative to health promotion?' (p. 387). This raises a further question about what, if anything, are the differences between the two? For this, we return to the underpinning values of health promotion. Here we see a clear contrast between the emphasis on empowerment in health promotion and on the achievement of behavioural goals in social marketing. There is also arguably a difference in approaches – health promotion being committed to bottom-up ways of working and social marketing arguably working in more prescriptive, top-down directive ways – although Lefebvre (1997) argues that if people are kept at the centre then the result is bottom-up ways of working. In addition, Naidoo and Wills (2005) argue that health promotion faces a dilemma when employing social marketing techniques because using advertising strategies necessarily means using images that are most likely to be effective and these tend to be those associated with consumer culture. They propose that the difficulty is that consumer culture promotes stereotypical ideas, many of which are inherently 'unhealthy'.

The cost–benefit analysis that takes place in social marketing is the same as that described within certain behaviour change models (for example the Health Belief Model), which refer to a value-expectancy mechanism. These models (described later in this chapter), are often used to plan, implement and evaluate health promotion programmes (Wills and Earle, 2007). Box 4.6 provides a case study of the use of social marketing in Tanzania.

The advocacy mechanism within social marketing is employed differently to that in health promotion. Green and Tones (2010) argue that in social marketing advocacy is more likely to be done on behalf of people rather than involving them in the process. Further challenges to health promotion values are the strong persuasive element in social marketing and the ultimate emphasis on the individual, which emphasizes personal responsibility for health (Naidoo and Wills, 2005). However, supporters of social marketing would counter this and highlight the 'voluntary' nature of our consumer behaviour (Hastings and Stead, 2006), the implication being that power and control about decision making ultimately lie with the individual. This claim becomes tenuous if we consider the powerful influences of marketing and advertising processes on our subconscious decision making, after all for example, how often do we end up buying things that we don't really need?

For a comprehensive overview of social marketing and public health read French *et al.* (2010).

The notion of 'nudge'

Nudging people is an idea that also has parallels in marketing approaches, and has individualistic, Western origins. The notion of 'nudge' is becoming more and more influential in the UK and, specifically, its influence on public health policy is increasingly evident. In 2008, a book was published about the concept of 'nudge', written by two professors from Chicago (Thaler and Sunstein, 2008).

Underpinning the concept of 'nudge' is a set of assumptions essentially to do with making whole populations change or modify their behaviour (Marteau *et al.*, 2011). These include the idea that small changes in our immediate environment or context can 'nudge' (or encourage) us to behave in different ways and/or make different choices. Thaler and Sunstein (2008) argue that relatively small changes can have a large impact on the way in which people behave and the choices that they make.

'Choice architecture' is a related term and is about designing environments and contexts (even situations) in order to alter people's decision making and behaviours. Choice architects are therefore people who have 'responsibility for organizing the context in which people make decisions' (Thaler and Sunstein, 2008, p. 3). This is a strategy that we can appreciate works well in marketing and advertising. The label 'choice architect' can be applied to many different people in different types of roles. This idea can also be applied to public health and health promotion. The premise is that we can design environments with the aim being to 'nudge' people to make the healthier choice by default. Choice architecture may also be about the removal of choice (through for example, legislative or penal measures).

Nudge and choice architecture are about unconscious processes for the most part. Marteau *et al.* (2011, p. 263) state that this is to do with an 'automatic, affective system that requires little or no cognitive engagement and is driven by immediate feelings and triggered by our environments'. As Marteau *et al.* (2011) argue, this strategy is one that is widely used by the advertising industry.

There are several difficulties with nudge as a concept, however. First, it lacks a clear definition (Marteau *et al.*, 2011). Secondly, it is difficult to find evidence in health to support 'nudge', although intuitively it appears to make a lot of sense and we do know, from marketing for example, that it does work. It is also difficult to isolate 'nudge' as a single causative agent in behaviour change. Thirdly, there are conceptual and philosophical challenges. Thaler and Sunstein (2008) argue that the concept of nudge (nudging people towards making decisions that are better for them) is 'libertarian paternalism' – 'libertarian' to do with the position that people should be free to do what they like. The meaning of the word 'paternalism', they argue, becomes different when it is preceded by the word 'libertarian'. This, they argue, modifies it to mean

'liberty-preserving' (p. 5). A paternalistic position is justified from the point of view that it is 'legitimate … to try to influence people's behaviour in order to … make their lives healthier' (p. 5). The question here then is does the means justify the end? The notion of 'liberty' (freedom of choice) is undermined by the inherent contradiction in the manipulation of the unconscious mind. If we are being nudged to behave in certain ways and make decisions that we otherwise would not have made then we aren't really free to do as we 'want'. This whole idea brings us back to a fundamental foundational principle in health promotion – that health is something to be highly valued and something to attain or strive towards. The direct implication of this is that there is a set of behaviours and choices that are deemed to be either 'good for us' or 'bad for us' (right or wrong) (Crossley, 2002) and that there are people that know better about what we should be doing. 'Nudging' people towards changing behaviour is based on the premise that we know what people want and that this is 'better health and longer life' (Hastings and Stead, 2006, p. 141). This is paternalism in action. It is also evidence of 'healthism', which is another general critique of health promotion. Fourthly, as well as being an infringement on individual liberty, some may even go as far as to argue that 'nudge' is an infringement on human rights. By definition, it takes away rights to behave in certain ways assuming inherent flaws in human judgement. Fifthly, in terms of health promotion, nudge also raises questions to do with empowerment. Arguably, rather than enabling people to take control of their health and their lives, choice architecture takes control away and puts control in the hands of the architects. And finally, the ethics of nudging may also be questioned. 'Nudge' appears to align itself with manipulative, coercive and persuasive ways of working, which are contrary to some of the underlying principles of health promotion that would suggest that using such approaches is unethical.

Health Literacy

'Health literacy' has become an increasingly important concept in health promotion. There appears to be general agreement in the literature that health literacy concerns the level of understanding required to make sense of health information, as well as an ability to subsequently act 'correctly' on that information (i.e. make the right decision as a result of understanding it).

In the *Health Promotion Glossary*, Nutbeam (1998b) links health literacy to participation and argues that access to education and information is key to empowering individuals and communities. Nutbeam (1998b, 2000) clearly links health literacy to health education highlighting the importance of it for promoting health and argues that it is a key outcome of health education. Nutbeam defines health literacy as representing 'the cognitive and social skills which determine the motivation and ability of individuals to gain access to, understanding and use information in ways which promote and maintain good health' (p. 10). So, for Nutbeam, health literacy isn't merely about being knowledgeable about health but it is also about being able to put that knowledge into positive effect for health gain. However, a person may be fully cognisant about an aspect of their health yet still choose to make unhealthy choices – does this then render them 'health illiterate'?

Nutbeam (2000, p. 263) also proposes three levels of health literacy:

- **Functional (or basic) Literacy**: sufficient basic skills in reading and writing to be able to function effectively in everyday situations.
- **Interactive (or communicative) Literacy**: more advanced cognitive and literacy skills, which together with social skills, can be actively used to participate in everyday activities, extract information and derive meaning from different forms of communication as well as to apply new information to changing circumstances.
- **Critical Literacy**: more advanced cognitive skills, which, together with social skills, can be applied to critically analyse information and to use this information to exert greater control over life events and situations.

These different levels highlight the empowering nature of health literacy as they give a clear indication of what someone who is health literate has the capacity to *do* as a result. This typology also emphasizes the need for basic levels of literacy as a basis for developing *health* literacy, which is an extremely important factor given that low levels of literacy remain a global issue (especially for women; Berry, 2007) and a key factor in inequalities in health. In his paper Nutbeam (2000) makes reference to the fact that health literacy has been around for some time (albeit under the umbrella of 'health education') and he uses the phrase 'new oil into old lanterns' in recognition of the 'repackaging' within health literacy of familiar terms such as health

education and empowerment. However, Tones (2002) argues that additional theorizing around the term 'health literacy' is unnecessary and that the various ways in which it is used within the health promotion literature increases the confusion surrounding it. Nevertheless, it seems that the term health literacy is here to stay and it could be argued that it provides a practical shorthand way in which to refer to the more complex ideas that are being discussed here. Certainly, health literacy has received increasing attention globally and in health policy and practice (Nutbeam and Kickbusch, 2000).

In a relatively recent paper revisiting the concept of health literacy, Peerson and Saunders (2009) argue that health literacy remains a confusing concept, not least because it is hard to define and therefore to measure. Yet there still appears to be a number of studies that have tried to do both. Various different scales have been produced in order to try to measure health literacy but it is argued that these need further testing and refinement (see Peerson and Saunders, 2009, for a summary). In addition, Peerson and Saunders (2009) argue that we need to better understand the role of motivation and activation in health literacy and use this to inform health promotion.

Corcoran (2011, p. 160) defines health literacy as 'the ability to locate and understand and act upon basic health information'. By definition then health literacy is linked to general levels of literacy (the ability to read and write), which can help or hinder people's health (Nutbeam, 1998b). This is very important for the way in which messages about health are communicated. Corcoran (2011) argues that there are several ways in which written health information might be designed to make it more readable, understandable and more likely to be acted upon.

In addition, Hubley and Copeman (2008) highlight the importance of the concept of 'risk', arguing that people need to have an understanding of the risk associated with different behaviours, which requires being cognizant of facts and figures including percentages. Perhaps then, we should also be thinking about a notion of 'risk literacy'? However, research on lay ideas about perceptions of risk show that developing literacy around risk might be a complex affair. For example, Davison *et al.*'s (1991) study of lay ideas about 'candidacy' and coronary heart disease risk shows that lay people are often well aware of risk communication, and risk factors such as lifestyles are often cited as important in causing disease. However, such awareness does not extend to a wholehearted acceptance of official medical thinking and advice. Rather, what Davison *et al.* (1991) suggest is that such thinking has to be married with people's own ideas and experiences and that what needs to be developed is a 'lay epidemiology' that acknowledges that not all those who behave 'unhealthily' get ill, and not all who get ill have demonstrable 'risk' factors. In addition, ideas about risk and disease have been explored in terms of, for example gender and heart disease (Emslie *et al.*, 2001), social class, smoking and ill health (Lawlor *et al.*, 2003), and ethnicity and heart disease (Grunau *et al.*, 2008).

Visual literacy has been highlighted by Linney (1995), who argues that, whereas in rich countries children and adults are exposed to many pictures, enabling them to develop visual literacy, this may not be the case in poorer countries or in rural areas. Bradley's research (1994) shows how pictures can be misinterpreted, but they are commonly used in health communication with the presumption that they *will* be understood.

In addition to 'risk literacy' and visual literacy, Berry (2007) argues that computer literacy is now viewed as included in general health literacy. Rapid increases in technology and the ever-expanding Internet mean that the way in which information is presented and accessed is undergoing huge changes, resulting in a move away from a reliance on paper-based sources of health information. Arguably, this means that 'health literacy' is necessarily becoming an expanded concept. Skills in finding accurate, reliable and up-to-date information using information technology are just as important as knowing what to do with it once it has been accessed. Ishikawa *et al.* (2008) highlight the importance of this in their research on health literacy in Japanese office workers. They found that workers with higher levels of health literacy were more likely to report better health-related and coping behaviours than those with lower levels. Robinson and Robertson (2010) also demonstrate that this is an issue that will need to be further considered as technology advances and impacts on the way in which information is communicated. This requires the 'user' to possess and hone certain IT skills, which are becoming increasingly important to health literacy.

There are many studies, which demonstrate the disadvantages and potential negative effects of a lack of health literacy, however it is defined and measured. This is a key argument for its significance in promoting health. However, there appears to be some further distinction in the literature about the nature of health literacy. Pleasant and Kuruvilla (2008) argue that it is possible to differentiate between two different approaches to health literacy – the 'clinical' approach and the 'public health' approach. The 'clinical' approach has historically focused on promoting better communication between patients and health care professionals in order to promote compliancy, imposing a deficit model on the patient (lack of knowledge or understanding as being primarily problematic). The 'public health' approach, in contrast, connects health literacy to health promotion, education and empowerment. Pleasant and Kuruvilla (2008) conclude that a combination of both approaches is needed to be fully effective in promoting public health. However, both approaches have implications for research and practice. For example, a more clinical approach will lead to more diagnostic ways of trying to measure health literacy.

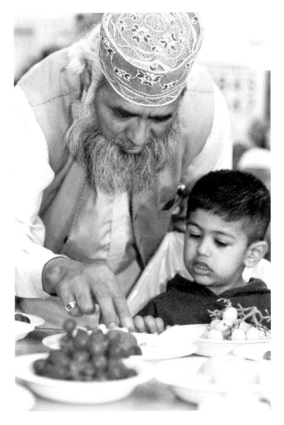

Learning from others.

Zarcadoolas *et al.* (2005) define health literacy as 'the wide range of skills and competencies that people develop to seek out, comprehend, evaluate and use health information and concepts to make informed choices, reduce health risks and increase quality of life' (pp. 196–197). This covers many different things, from being able to listen effectively to being able to access information through mobile technology. One of the key features would appear to be the ability to adapt to changes over time – changes in the ways in which information is communicated and reproduced as well as the ability to discern what is most important at any given time.

Motivational Interviewing

Motivational interviewing is one approach trying to effect behavioural change at an individual level using a face-to-face mechanism (Hillsden, 2006). Its central purpose is to encourage exploration of reasons to change behaviour, which may not have been dwelt on before (Bennett and Murphy, 1997). Motivational interviewing, initially developed as a strategy for working with people with addictions, was first described by William Miller, and has been further developed by Miller and Rollnick (Hillsden, 2006). It is increasingly used within health promotion, as a strategy designed to influence behaviour at the individual level in relation to 'problematic' health behaviours. Miller defined motivational interviewing as follows: 'a client-centred, directive method for enhancing intrinsic motivation to change by exploring and resolving ambivalence' (Miller and Rollnick, 2002, cited in Hillsden, 2006, p. 75).

It is apparent from this definition that the concept of ambivalence is central to motivational interviewing. Ambivalence has only relatively recently come into play in contemporary health promotion. Hillsden (2006) argues that it is this

that distinguishes motivational interviewing from other types of approaches to behaviour change, based on more traditionally medically or disease-focused approaches. Maio *et al.* (2007) highlight the importance of ambivalence as an obstacle to healthier behaviour. Different factors such as freedom of choice, stress and habit formation influence feelings of ambivalence towards health behaviour change. The challenge therefore, is in designing health promotion activities, which tackle ambivalence and encourage change.

What is significant about motivational interviewing (and consistent with the underpinning principles of health promotion) is that the 'client' is seen as an autonomous person with the right to choose to change or not. The concept of motivation is central to motivational interviewing. Motivation is to do with what makes us take certain actions or behave in a certain way (or not). Different types of motivation have been identified in the literature. The importance of the concept of motivation is highlighted by Green and Tones (2010, p. 117) in the Health Action Model where the 'motivation system' is depicted as one of four interacting systems determining health behaviour. The motivation system consists of four kinds of motivation – values, attitudes, drives and emotional states (affect) (Green and Tones, 2010). Motivation may also be defined as being 'intrinsic' – 'based on feeling of pleasure, pride or enjoyment brought about by participating in an activity' – or 'extrinsic' – 'based on external factors such as appearance, conformity or norms' (Marks *et al.*, 2005, pp. 418–420). Hillsden (2006) identifies three essential components of motivation as conceived within motivational interviewing – readiness to change, the importance or value placed in change and confidence in the ability to change. Hillsden also outlines a set of principles for motivational interviewing (as detailed in Box 4.7) and states that a key

---

Box 4.7. Principles of motivational interviewing.

1. Expressing empathy – this refers to showing acceptance of where a person is.
2. Developing a discrepancy – this is about establishing the difference between where a person is and where they would like to be (or get to).
3. Rolling with resistance – this refers to accepting (on the facilitator's part) the fact that resistance is

likely to occur (on the client's part) and having strategies to deal with it when it does.
4. Supporting self-efficacy – this refers to supporting the client in the belief that they have the capacity to effect change.

(Adapted from Hillsden, 2006)

---

strategy in motivational interviewing is 'change talk'. 'Change talk involves the client expressing personal advantage of changing behaviour, optimism for change, intention to change and the disadvantages of change' (Hillsden, 2006, p. 78).

Motivational interviewing has similarities with 'brief behavioural counselling' (which might also be referred to as 'brief behavioural intervention'; Steptoe *et al.*, 2003) and 'health coaching' (Palmer *et al.*, 2003). Although some may argue that motivational interviewing and health coaching differ, there are many similarities and it is gaining in popularity (Palmer *et al.*, 2003). Palmer *et al.* (2003, p. 93) offer a 'tentative definition' – 'health coaching is the practice of health education and health promotion within a coaching context, to enhance the well being of individuals and to facilitate the achievement of their health-related goals'. The similarities with motivational interviewing are evident here. Palmer *et al.* (2003) also emphasize the links between health coaching and more 'traditional' health education approaches. Certainly, both motivational interviewing and health coaching will involve a level of health education to some degree.

Motivational interviewing draws on a range of psychosocial theory relating to behaviour change including step change theories and Bandura's ideas about self-efficacy. It has distinct parallels with the Transtheoretical Model (Prochaska and DiClemente, 1983) and, as the Model does, motivational interviewing highlights the importance of the person's 'readiness to change' and may provide an incentive for moving through the key stages of change identified within the Transtheoretical Model (Miller and Rollnick, 2002). In terms of the underpinning principles of health promotion as outlined by the Ottawa Charter (WHO, 1986b) we can see that motivational interviewing can help to build on and develop personal skills as well as enabling practitioners to work in more empowering ways with the client at the centre of the interaction (in the 'driving seat'). The focus then is away from 'telling' people what to do and much more towards facilitating the process of change if and when appropriate.

Motivational interviewing appears to have been effective in enabling behaviour change at an individual level in relation to a range of health-related issues including smoking cessation (Colby *et al.*, 1999) and physical activity (Brodie and Inoue, 2005). However, there are a number of critiques about motivational interviewing, which are worth attention. A key challenge is that motivational

interviewing starts from the position that health itself provides a key motivation for change (Hillsden, 2006), but this is not always the case for everyone. The focus at the individual level fails to take into account the wider social determinants of health and the macro-factors, which impact on, and influence, behaviour at an individual level.

We already know that brief interventions can be effective in increasing consumption of fruit and vegetables (Steptoe *et al.*, 2003). Steptoe *et al.* (2003) set out to measure the effect of using brief behavioural counselling in general practice on consumption of fruit and vegetables in adults from a low-income population. The intervention was based on the Stages of Change model and comprised two one-to-one individually tailored consultation sessions. The intervention was shown to be effective as determined by subjective and objective measures.

One of the difficulties in establishing an evidence base for motivational interviewing in health promotion is that, as Hillsden (2006, p. 81) argues, it is 'quite common for people to refer to an intervention as MI because it is loosely based on MI principles'. Rubak *et al.* (2005) carried out a systematic review and meta-analysis to establish the effectiveness of motivational interviewing. They concluded that it was more effective in scientific settings than traditional advice giving in the treatment of a range of behavioural problems but that future research was needed, which clearly identifies exactly *how* motivational interviewing is carried out and includes direct/objective measures, as well as qualitative perspectives. Motivational interviewing may be carried out on its own, or in conjunction with for example, a subsequent course of treatment. This also has implications for how we measure effectiveness. In addition, it may be carried out at the individual level or within groups. There are a number of studies reporting the effect of motivational interviewing in different contexts and with reference to a range of different 'health issues'. For example, Burke *et al.* (2003) carried out a meta-analysis examining the efficacy of motivational interviewing in relation to reducing drinking levels and reported a positive outcome; however, this effect was specific to a clinical setting. A literature review conducted by Branscum and Sharma (2010) concluded that motivational interviewing was effective in reducing alcohol use in heavy drinkers but this is not supported by findings from a meta-analysis by Lundahl *et al.* (2010), which failed to find significant findings specific to motivational interviewing when used on a range of addictive behaviours including alcohol use. So the evidence for effectiveness is not conclusive.

For more in-depth information about motivational interviewing, see Chapter 5 'Motivational interviewing in health promotion' in MacDowall *et al.* (2006).

Central Components in Behaviour Change

A number of models of behaviour change have been developed over the years, which can aid our understanding of health behaviour and behavioural choices at an individual level. The purpose of this section of the chapter is not to go into great depth about these types of models but instead to provide an overview of them within the context of health communication. (Individual models of behaviour change have been explored in detail in the wider literature, so the reader is encouraged to look elsewhere for this.) One of the most important roles that behaviour change theory plays in health communication is to provide a theoretical foundation for the design, implementation and evaluation of public health and health promotion activities. In addition, theory can be useful in determining what works, or is effective, in health communication and behaviour change (as well as what does not work).

A number of different factors influence health behaviour and behavioural choices. Some of these exist at the individual level. The philosophical underpinnings and value base of health promotion exhort us to examine wider social determinants and factors in order to account for health-related behaviour. Nonetheless, behaviour change models can be useful and they may enable us to take account of individual factors when planning health promotion interventions and communicating for health. The roots of behaviour change theory are within a number of different fields, most notably psychology but also ecology and philosophy. Behaviour change is complex. One of the difficulties of trying to provide a representation of it via theoretical means is that 'one size does not fit all'; however, there have been several useful attempts to capture the different variables involved in the process at an individual level. The most 'influential' models will be briefly described here in relation to the different variables identified as important in health behaviour. These have been selected on the basis that they are most frequently applied and researched within the wider literature. This discussion will therefore include reference to

some of the central constructs and processes presented within key theories including the Health Belief Model (Rosenstock *et al.*, 1988), the Theory of Planned Behaviour (Ajzen, 1988, 1991), Protection Motivation Theory (Rogers, 1975, 1983), the Transtheoretical Model (Prochaska and DiClemente, 1983) and the Health Action Model (Tones and Green, 2004). The variables selected for discussion (as deemed particularly salient to the area of 'health communication') include beliefs, motivation, stages of change and behavioural intention.

Beliefs

The concept of beliefs (or 'perceptions') is very important to behaviour change and is a central construct in several behaviour change models, most notably the Health Belief Model, which is built primarily around a set of beliefs deemed important in influencing behavioural outcomes. Beliefs can exist about a range of different things and have a direct influence on health-related behaviour as well as whether or not someone is likely to change. Beliefs are discussed here specifically in relation to perceptions of 'threat', perceptions of 'benefits and barriers' and perceptions of 'control'.

Beliefs about the *threat* of an illness as a mechanism for providing an incentive to act to avoid it are reflected in the Health Belief Model (labelled 'perceived susceptibility' and 'perceived severity') and Protection Motivation Theory (labelled 'severity' and 'vulnerability'). 'Threat perception' is important in communication for behaviour change. The assumption is that if a person believes themselves to be at risk of becoming unwell as a result of their current behaviour, they are more likely to want to change it. A great deal of health promotion messages have previously been predicated on this assumption, although this approach has had mixed results.

The Health Belief Model developed initially to explain and predict screening behaviours (Abraham and Sheeran, 2005), also focuses on beliefs about the advantages and disadvantages of taking action (changing behaviour). These are labelled 'perceived benefits' and 'perceived barriers', respectively. This 'cost/benefit' analysis process is also reflected in the Protection Motivation Theory. The assumption here is that an individual engages in a rational and thoughtful decision-making process whereby they 'weigh-up' the pros and cons of taking action and make a decision accordingly (normally in the direction of the action that yields the greatest benefits and least costs). The Transtheoretical Model refers to this as 'decisional balance'. Health promotion and public health communication, which highlight benefits over cost, may therefore be more effective in promoting behaviour change. Many of the models presented assume that people carry out a cost/benefit analysis when they are deciding whether to change their behaviour. The adoption of an economic framework here implies that someone will take action when the advantages (or benefits) outweigh the disadvantages (or costs). This degree of rationality has been contested in the literature. Experience tells us that behaviour may result from unconscious processes, emotion and impulsivity, none of which resonates with a rational cognitive process.

Beliefs about personal capacity to take action are also important and feature (albeit in different guises) in several of the models of behaviour change under consideration. In the Theory of Planned Behaviour, beliefs about control are represented in the variable 'Perceived Behavioural Control'. 'Self-efficacy' was also later added as a variable to the Health Belief Model and, some argue, is not dissimilar from perceived behavioural control. In essence, both concepts refer to the extent to which someone believes they are capable of taking action (changing their behaviour). Self-efficacy has its roots in Social Learning Theory (Bandura, 1986) and is closely related to constructs such as self-esteem. The 'coping appraisal' variable within Protection Motivation Theory also shares some similarities with self-efficacy, and perceptions about control and self-efficacy also feature as a construct within the Transtheoretical Model (Sutton, 2005). Beliefs about control are important in health behaviour and the research shows that people with higher levels of self-esteem generally fare better health-wise, particularly when it comes to mental health (Marks *et al.*, 2005; Straub, 2007). Again, however, research on lay beliefs about control indicates that they are complex, with many aspects seen as beyond the control of individuals (as we saw in Chapter 1).

Motivation

Motivation is an important construct in behaviour change (hence the stress on motivational interviewing as a technique). Many different factors can impact on motivation to change behaviour. These may be crudely separated into two main areas – 'internal' motivation (from *within* the individual) and external (from *outside* of the individual, or existing within the wider socio-politico-economic environment) motivation. Motivation is a central construct in Protection Motivation Theory, implied within the Health Belief Model through the variable 'cues for action' and is taken into account in the Health Action Model in relation to the construct of 'self' (personality). Regarding health communication, how messages are designed might have an impact on internal motivation in terms of changing the way in which someone thinks about something. Equally, a message about health may be viewed as 'external' motivation. Either way we do know that, in order for change to occur, there needs to be some motivation for action at the individual level.

Stages of change

The Transtheoretical Model is probably the most well known model, which incorporates the concept of 'stages' or phases of behaviour change. Central to this idea is that people move through different stages towards changing behaviour. In the case of the Transtheoretical Model, there are five key stages: pre-contemplation, contemplation, preparation, action and maintenance. This is a more descriptive way of looking at behaviour change. In terms of communicating for health it is clear that, as Sutton (2005, p. 224) argues, 'different factors are important at different stages'. This means that the design of interventions intended to move an individual from one stage to the next may vary considerably depending on which stage they are at. The assumption is of linear progression through the stages. However, there is 'room' for relapse within this framework whereby someone may 'go back' a stage or more. The acknowledgement of relapse, a very important factor in health-related behaviour change links to a key feature in motivational interviewing.

Behavioural Intention

Intention is another variable that features strongly in some of the behaviour change models. The focus on behavioural *intention* is often at the expense of providing an explanation for, or account of, behavioural *outcomes*. The assumption tends to be that an intention to change behaviour leads to the behavioural change, or at least that this is more likely if intention is present. A great deal of research has been done, which examines the factors influencing behavioural intention. Of course, intending to behave in a certain way does not necessarily mean that the actual behaviour will occur – we are not talking about a linear and non-complex process. Many different factors will impact on the point between behavioural intention and actual behaviour. The Theory of Planned Behaviour and Protection Motivation Theory are both examples of models that include 'intention' as a key component and that assume a direct link between the two. Behavioural intention also features centrally within the Health Action Model. However, this model goes further to consider what will influence the move from intention to actual behaviour change. It therefore takes into account the wider environment, existing skills/knowledge and constructs of the 'self' (Green and Tones, 2010) as influencing forces, which the other two models fail to do.

Critiques of behaviour change models

A number of critiques of the key behaviour change models have been offered within the literature.

These are nicely summarized in Box 4.8, adapted from Warwick-Booth *et al.* (2012).

There are a number of things that impact in health behaviour at the individual level that are not taken into account within mainstream behaviour change theory. These include factors such as resilience, resistance and voluntary risk-taking. In addition, this whole field has come under some criticism from some at the more critical ends of health psychology and public health, where the very idea of 'health behaviour' is challenged framing it instead as 'social practice' (Mielewcyzk and Willig, 2007) and advocating that the focus should be on the wider social, political and economic context rather than at the individual level (Marks, 2002a). These wider factors are often seen by psychology as benign 'background factors'. However,

> Put simply, roads, railways, freezers, heating systems, etc. are not innocent features of the background. Rather, they have an active part to play in defining, reproducing and transforming what people take to be

---

Box 4.8. General critiques of models of behaviour change.

The models tend to…

- focus at the individual level and not on the wider determinants of health (social, political, environmental, etc.) and so they tend not to account for factors outside of the individual, which influence behaviour;
- put the emphasis on the individual (a 'reductionist' approach) (Bunton *et al.*, 2000) and 'objectify' human experience in contrast to a holistic approach (Tones and Green, 2004);
- promote individualism and individual responsibility for health (Airhihenbuwa and Obregon, 2000); and
- view individual actions or behaviour in isolation from the actions or behaviour of others (Hubley and Copeman, 2008), neglecting to consider social influences.

They tend to neglect the role of…

- past behaviour and habit (Sarafino, 2002; Albery and Munafò, 2008; Thirlaway and Upton, 2009);
- affect ('emotion') (Roberts *et al.*, 2001; Lawton *et al.*, 2009); and
- culture and cultural context (Lin *et al.*, 2005).

They tend to neglect the fact that…

- processes of behaviour change take time and significant change cannot take place over a short

period (Ramos and Perkins, 2006) and they also over-simplify processes of behaviour change (Abraham and Sheenan, 2005; Berry, 2007).

In terms of research, a number of difficulties have been highlighted including…

- problems defining individual constructs (Bunton, 2002);
- limited predictive utility (Abraham and Sheenan, 2005);
- a weak relationship between intention and behaviour – Stevens (2008) argues that other factors should be explored, i.e. environmental factors;
- a lack of standardization across constructs in experimental design (Conner and Norman, 2005) – it is difficult to compare the results of studies that 'test' out the theories because they often use different methods and inconsistent ways of measuring the different components of the models;
- they tend to have been developed in specific contexts which can lead to a 'Western', patriarchal bias;
- much of the research using the models relies on self-report measures, which have limitations; and
- whilst many of the models draw upon aspects of sociological, psychological and anthropological theory they tend to neglect political and economic theory (Hubley and Copeman, 2008).

---

normal ways of life. The key insight here is that the material world and related systems of production and provision are important in organising, structuring and sometimes preventing certain practices.

(Shove, 2010, p. 2)

Newer paradigms of conceptualizing health behaviours will be alluded to in Chapter 6; Shove (2010, p. 3) suggests

Much of the conventional literature supposes that behaviours are subject to external drivers like price and persuasion, or that they are obstructed by 'barriers'. This implies a linear relation between factors and effects and supposes that 'outside' forces bear down on behaviour. Although very familiar, interpretations of this kind are incapable of capturing or describing the forms of mutual adjustment, adaptation and accumulation involved in shaping and changing the repertoires of 'doings' that, in combination, constitute contemporary ways of life.

She suggests that, in terms of understanding everyday life, we need to develop radically different theories.

Whilst there are limitations to existing behaviour change theory, it is important to try to understand and explain behaviour change through, among other things, the development and testing of theoretical models. This is because we can then influence how we plan, implement and evaluate health promotion activities or 'communicate' with people to improve and promote health.

For further, in-depth information about the models that have been referred to here, please see the following:

- for the Health Action Model, see Green and Tones (2010); and
- for the Health Belief Model, Protection Motivation Theory, Transtheoretical Model and Theory of Planned Behaviour, please see Conner and Norman (2005).

Summary

This chapter has attempted to take a critical look at some of the assumptions about health communication, such as that mass media is a useful means of getting health messages across, or that theories of behaviour change drawn from psychology necessarily help us to understand people's behaviour. Much of the theory about communication in health promotion relies on the 'classic' theories of one-way communication and, as such, these are out of step with the 21st century, where networking as a means of communication has

taken over from hierarchical, 'expert'-led means. These one-way methods are authoritarian in that they vest the authority in the communicator, and we have suggested that methods need to be found that are interactive, empowering and helpful, rather than top-down, failing to build in feedback and serving to further the agendas of the health promoters without fully understanding the health-worlds of the individuals and communities involved. These means will be dialogical and people-centred, and thus people need to be involved in each stage of developing health messages. Furthermore, health education need not be victim blaming, and some of the attempts to rehabilitate 'health education' have only served to confuse the arena, such as by introducing 'new' concepts that are essentially the same as the old. Differing ideological perspectives inevitably lead to different views on the adoption of practices from commerce, such as social marketing, but, taking a pragmatic approach, we have shown that there are places where some of this may be appropriate. The dominance of behaviour change approaches within health promotion and the adoption of theories from psychology has been critiqued, and the fact that these are Eurocentric and provide only partial understanding is taken up again in Chapter 6.

These views present challenges for health promoters and health educators and may cause pause for thought in terms of established ways of working. Most health education materials for example, are produced with no involvement of the individuals and communities for which they are intended, on the assumption that the expert, whether a dietician, nurse, rehabilitation worker or any other, will 'know' what people want, and ought to know. Given the importance of knowledge, and the need for effective, evidence-based approaches, these established ways of working need to be scrutinized.

Further Reading

Barlow, D. and Mills, B. (2009) *Reading Media Theory: Thinkers, Approaches, Contexts*. Longman, London.

Berry, D. (2007) *Health Communication: Theory and Practice*. Open University Press, Maidenhead, UK.

Freire, P. (2005) *Pedagogy of Indignation*. Paradigm Publishers, Boulder, Colorado.

Kamalipour, Y.R. (2007). *Global Communication*, 2nd edition. Cengage Learning (formerly Wadsworth), Belmont, California.

Thirlaway, K. and Upton, D. (2009) *The Psychology of Lifestyle: Promoting Healthy Behaviour*. Routledge, Oxford, UK.

5 Practising Health Promotion

RACHAEL DIXEY, JAMES WOODALL AND DIANE LOWCOCK

This chapter aims to:

- explore the role of the settings approach to health promotion and the need for organizational change;
- discuss the importance of evidence-based practice and evaluation;
- describe some of the ethical issues in practising health promotion;
- suggest a means of overcoming the top-down/bottom-up tensions in practice;
- explore the need for developing partnerships between civil society, NGOs, private and public sectors; and
- outline the skills and competencies of health promoters practising in the 21st century.

Introduction

It is clear from the preceding chapters that health promotion is not short on vision or strategy, and health promoters have developed practical ways of implementing those visions and ideas. This chapter does not have the 'answers', but does aim to make some suggestions about how steps can be taken to implement the vision.

It should be clear that we believe that top-down, programmatic approaches to change are not likely to be effective in tackling the complex, real-life problems that health promoters want to address. Such approaches also do not bring about sustainable development or sustainable, long-lasting solutions. There are no universal prescriptions or 'quick fixes' to the health problems facing the global community. What we do want is transformational change, in individuals, communities, organizations and governments – nothing short of transformational change will produce the desired redistribution of power required to bring about equity in health.

Later in this chapter, we suggest that the evolving, new, relationships between the private sector, governments, the non-governmental or 'third sector', and civil society might be one way to move towards creating the kind of societies that people prefer to live in. There needs to be a move away from 'interventions' and a move towards working *with* people to implement change. If people are put at the centre of the change process, and if the way to transform communities and organizations is to develop networks based on cooperation, then there are clear implications for the professional-community relationship and for the skills required of health promoters. The skills and competencies of health promoters are discussed below, together with some ideas about what needs to happen in terms of taking on leadership roles for the health promotion agenda. The roles of professionals – 'experts' – is challenged by moving away from top-down approaches and raises questions about the relationships between professionals and communities.

There needs to be practical ways of overcoming the top-down/bottom-up dichotomy, with new ways of working that properly reflect the 'messy' real life problems and the equally messy types of solutions required, which can be contextualized to the needs of specific situations and cultures. It cannot be the case that 'one size will fit all', and therefore ways of working need to be flexible, adaptable and adopt an action learning or action research approach.

To achieve a healthier society, we suggest that there must be: involvement of communities and citizens; healthy public policy building; and the development of organizations and organizational cultures towards health (Fig. 5.1).

The ways in which citizens and communities can be involved are described below in the examples of

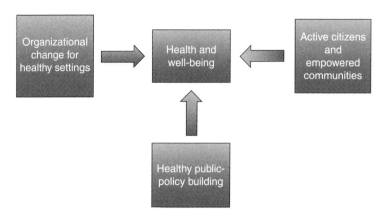

Fig. 5.1. Building blocks to create a healthier society.

the People in Public Health Project, community health champions and the roles of community-based organizations in solid waste management. Some suggestions for ways in which organizations can contribute to producing healthier societies is also discussed.

Health promotion in its brief history has also not been short on rhetoric and idealism, and disagreements about the 'best' ways of working. We would assert that a hefty dose of pragmatism will help the implementation process; given that there are many routes to the same goal, what is important is that the journey begins. In this regard, we suggest that settings approaches offer one practical way to 'do' health promotion, and one section of this chapter therefore discusses in detail the strengths and weaknesses of this approach.

Evidence-based practice and the importance of evaluating health promotion work are also explored in this chapter as essential aspects of health promotion practice. Evidence-based practice and evaluation are linked in as much as the latter feeds into an understanding of what works and what does not, which then forms an evidence base. 'Research into practice' is another important activity, given that much health promotion research aims to 'make a difference'. Another section of this chapter considers ethics in health promotion work, although there is also a thread of ethics and exploration of the value base of health promotion work throughout the book. This chapter includes some examples of health promotion, which we consider showing aspects of good practice and which might be of interest to illustrate 'good' health promotion on the ground.

This chapter therefore focuses on ways of working, and includes sections on: working in settings;

working to change organizations; developing evidence-based practice and skills in evaluation; working ethically; working with active citizens and the third sector (or NGOs); working in ways that resolve the top-down/bottom-up conundrum; and the skills and competencies of health promoters. These sections are not in any particular order, except working in settings is logically followed by a section on organizational change, evidence-based practice and evaluation are linked, and the final section is in that position because it considers all of the rest in terms of what it means for the skills of health promoters. More simply, the chapter considers where health promotion can take place (in settings), and how we should work as effective promoters of health.

The Settings Approach to Health Promotion

General support for the settings approach is such that it is now firmly considered a crucial element of public health strategy at local, national and international levels (Dooris, 2004; Dooris and Hunter, 2007). The idea of promoting health through 'settings' has become a popular approach within health promotion practice, reflected through the diversity of global interventions now being implemented in schools, workplaces, universities, hospitals, etc. As an approach to 'doing' health promotion, the settings approach has provided practitioners with a tangible way to promote health, primarily because social systems have a huge bearing on people's lives and because they provide a distinct location for intervention.

However, despite the considerable strides made in practice, the theoretical framework underpinning the settings approach has not always been made explicit and a variety of words have been used, as shown in Box 5.1. Similarly there have been difficulties in evidencing the outcomes of settings intervention and some have therefore suggested that the approach has been legitimized more through 'an act of faith' than through robust research and evaluation (St Leger, 1997, p. 100). There are certain exceptions to this, e.g. the establishment of an evidence base for health-promoting schools (South and Woodall, 2011).

The underlying premise of the settings approach is that investments in health are made in social systems where health is not their primary remit. Fundamental to this is the belief that health is produced outside of illness (health) services and that effective health improvements require investment in social systems (Dooris, 2004). This was espoused in the Ottawa Charter, which argued that health was not primarily the outcome of medical intervention, but an ecological concept that embraced the interplay between social, political, economic and behavioural factors (Dooris *et al.*, 1998): 'Health is created and lived by people within the settings of their everyday life; where they learn, work, play and love' (WHO, 1986b, p. v).

Consistent backing by the WHO through the late 1980s and 1990s (WHO, 1986c, 1991, 1997b, 1998a, b) saw ecological views of health promotion, delivered through the settings approach, gain increasing momentum.

Proponents of the settings approach, like L.W. Green *et al.* (2000, p. 23), have suggested that settings can be conceptualized as both:

1. Physically bounded space-times in which people come together to perform specific tasks (usually oriented to goals other than health).

2. Arenas of sustained interaction, with pre-existing structures, policies, characteristics, institutional values and formal and informal social sanctions on behaviour.

This provides added scope to the WHO's (1998b, p. 19) definition of a setting for health:

> The place or social context in which people engage in daily activities in which environmental, organisational and personal factors interact to affect health and well-being…where people actively use and shape the environment and thus create or solve problems relating to health. Settings can normally be identified as having physical boundaries, a range of people with defined roles, and an organisational structure.

Despite useful definitions and guidance being put forward within health promotion discourse, there remains some ambiguity as to what actually constitutes a 'setting'. Institutions such as hospitals, prisons, schools and workplaces, where a hierarchical system exists, are clearly distinct from settings that have informal, flexible and open structures, such as homes, communities, cities and islands (Poland *et al.*, 2000; Whitelaw *et al.*, 2001; Dooris, 2004). Galea *et al.* (2000), in their paper on healthy islands in the Western Pacific, attempt to provide some clarity by proposing a hierarchy of settings. They distinguish between contextual and elemental settings, explaining that:

> Elemental settings are contained within a broader contextual setting. Thus, a city may contain important elements, e.g. schools, hospitals and markets. Elemental settings directly affect the life of the people who live within them; they only affect others indirectly. (p. 170)

Similarly, Barić (1998) sees health-promoting settings made up of health-promoting units – operating somewhat like 'Russian dolls' (Dooris, 2006, p. 5).

Box 5.1. The settings approach: etymology.

A range of terminology has been used to denote settings-based approaches to health promotion. 'Health setting', 'health-promoting settings', 'settings for health', 'settings for health promotion', 'the settings approach' and 'the settings-based approach' are all terms commonly in use (Richmond, 2009). Whilst the semantic differences may seem trivial, the terms do carry different nuances (Richmond, 2009). Denman *et al.*

(2002), for example, have drawn attention to the subtle semantic variations between organizations labelled as 'health-promoting settings' and those categorized as 'healthy settings'. Dooris (2006) notes the difference between a 'health-promoting setting' and a 'healthy setting', proposing that the former has a greater focus on people and a commitment to ensuring that the setting takes account of its external impacts.

Commentators, like Hancock (1999), have argued that the settings approach has been one of the most successful strategies to emerge from the Ottawa Charter. However, others have been less supportive of the approach and have claimed that the settings approach is simply a re-labelling of traditional health education (Wenzel, 1997). In moving away from this conceptualization, Barić (1992, 1993, 1994, 1995) has consistently advocated the necessity to distinguish between 'health promotion in a setting' and a 'health-promoting setting'. Barić notes that 'health promotion in a setting' refers to any institution that has some kind of health promotion or education as part of its activities (Barić, 1992, 1993, 1994). In contrast, a 'health-promoting setting' reframes health promotion as an integral part of the organizational infrastructure (Barić, 1994; Corcoran and Bone, 2007) and includes:

- the creation of a healthy working and living environment;
- integration of health promotion into the daily activities of the setting; and
- creating conditions for the setting to reach out into the community (Barić, 1993, p. 19).

This thinking represents a shift in merely aiming various forms of health education at those who conveniently interact in a particular location (King, 1998; Paton *et al.*, 2005). Instead, a 'health-promoting setting' adopts an ecological approach in which the whole environment and culture is committed to promoting health in a coherent and integrated manner (Tones, 2001).

The Settings Approach and the Current Variability of Practice

In practice, variability of activity under the rubric of settings-based health promotion exists. Johnson and Baum (2001, p. 286), for example, highlighted a variety of interpretations in the meaning of a health-promoting hospital. They suggest that:

> Some hospitals do little more than move beyond providing health information and education to patients, while other initiatives achieve a significant re-orientation of their activities and institute significant organizational reform supported by strong policy and leadership.

This issue is not limited to hospitals, as variation of practice seems to exist across settings. However, variations in activities may arise from the extent to which organizations aspire to, or are able to achieve the 'ideal' (Tones and Green, 2004). Often, practical limitations hinder the development of a settings approach including:

- translating the philosophy of the approach into tangible activities;
- competing forces acting against the health agenda;

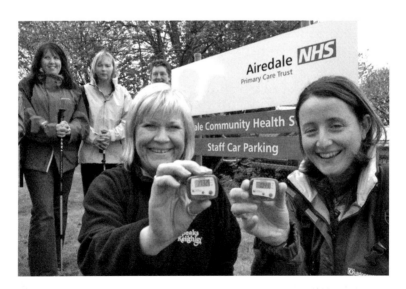

Workplace health promotion.

- problems associated with health promoters being perceived as credible agents of change; and
- limitations in support structures, e.g. finance, time, training, expertise (Whitelaw *et al.*, 2001).

Whitelaw *et al.* (2001) have created a typology of settings activity. This consists of five types of settings-based activities and is presented in Table 5.1. The typology rests on the way health problems are framed and solutions are identified. For example, at one end, the solution and problem lie with the individual (passive model); whilst in contrast, the comprehensive/structural model views the solution and problem within the setting. In the passive model, for instance, the setting assumes a subordinate role within which traditional forms of education are employed.

Joined-up Settings

Clearly, people connect with a range of settings throughout their lives and this can occur either in a concurrent or consecutive nature. Children, for example, may spend their time in the school, family and community settings (concurrently), whereas offenders may spend time within a prison setting and then resettle back into the community (consecutively) (Dooris, 2006; Dooris and Hunter, 2007; Dooris *et al.*, 2007).

A criticism of the settings approach is that it can only address individuals in certain organizations and not the whole person whose life may 'straddle' different settings and organizations (Naidoo and Wills, 1994, p. 165). It is important to understand lay people's meanings of places and spaces (Gustafson, 2001) and to incorporate them into settings approaches. Similarly, people's lives are not as compartmentalized as the settings approach would suggest and often many problems experienced in one setting are often deep rooted in another (Poland *et al.*, 2000; Dooris, 2005). Clearly, health does not acknowledge boundaries – it crosses a range of settings and situations (Dooris, 2001; Dooris *et al.*, 2007). By focusing on settings in isolation from the wider perspective, there is a danger that the approach fosters 'insularity and fragmentation' (Dooris, 2006, p. 5). Addressing alcohol issues in only one setting, for example, may be relatively futile. Eakin (2000) notes that alcohol dependency can stem from workplace settings (e.g. drinking 'cultures' in certain industries), but also from other settings, such as marital strain and stress in the home and family setting. However, in promoting the Wellness@Work scheme, Bull *et al.* (2008) state that 60% of the UK population spend an estimated 60% of their waking hours at work, making the workplace a good place to develop collective action for health.

Writers in the area have recognized that the focus needs to not only be on the setting itself, but on the spaces in between them (Barić and Barić, 1995; Dooris, 2004, 2005). Mullen *et al.* (1995)

Table 5.1. Overview of the 'types' of settings-based health promotion according to Whitelaw *et al.* (2001, p. 346).

Setting type	Description
'Passive' model	Both the problem and the solution lie with the behaviour and actions of the individual. Setting plays a passive role only providing access to population group. Traditional health education activities are at the heart of the work.
'Active' model	The problem lies within the behaviour of the individual; however, the solution is broadened to encompass features of the system in which the individual exists.
'Vehicle' model	The problem lies within the setting, the solution in learning from individually based projects. This is still focused on topic-based activities but does so with an expectation of moving beyond individual behaviour change to impacting on broader settings features.
'Organic' model	The problem lies within the setting, the solution in the action of the individuals. This approach focuses on strengthening collective participation, the focus is not on tangible health gains but reflects a desire for improved ethos or culture within the setting.
'Comprehensive/ structural' model	Both the problem and the solution lie within the setting. This approach sees that individuals are powerless to make any changes therefore enduring change can only come from within the system. The emphasis therefore targets broad settings policies and bringing structural change.

similarly point out the limitations in our understanding concerning the relationships 'between settings'. Resources and investment must be developed between work in different settings and the gaps between them bridged (Dooris, 2004). Dooris and Hunter (2007), for instance, note that settings initiatives should move away from operating on 'parallel tramlines' (p. 118) and should instead link with other settings, thereby moving beyond the physical boundaries towards a more 'orchestrated approach' (King, 1998, p. 129).

Challenges

The settings approach has offered health promotion a conceptual base that has allowed practice to be pursued across a far wider scope (Whitelaw *et al.*, 2001). Whilst the settings approach is now recognized as an important means to tackle health inequalities, there remain some concerns about the effectiveness of settings initiatives.

Workplaces as Settings

Whilst some cynicism is allowed concerning whether businesses and workplaces really are embracing a health agenda for altruistic reasons or because it will simply lead to greater productivity and better public relations, it can be seen that workplaces do have an interest in maintaining the health of their workforce, and many *have* made changes to the way their organizations operate. Initiatives in England, such as the Health@Work awards, developed by the NHS Plymouth Public Health Development Unit (PHDU), through its Business Health Network, has helped workplaces to implement healthy living policies (Griffiths and Reynolds, 2009). As people do spend so much of their time working, the way that workplaces are run provides huge possibilities for people to make changes to their lives. A number of countries in South-east Asia such as Singapore, Thailand and Korea have stressed workplace health promotion, and 'workplaces' are relatively easy to identify in countries at a certain level of 'development'. However, much of the available work in countries of the Global South lies in the informal sector, or informal economy, where normal legal protection in terms of health and safety, pay and conditions is lacking (ILO, 2006). The importance of this sector to a country like Tanzania, for example, was estimated by Mukangara and Koda (1997), to contribute

30% of Tanzania's GDP in 1997, and offered employment to 56% of the urban population. Chen (2007, p. 7) estimated that 'informal employment broadly defined comprises one-half to three quarters of non-agricultural employment in developing countries' and in sub-Saharan Africa as a whole the figure was 72%. Not only is this informal economy very significant, it is also gendered, with women making up 60–80% of the informal workforce in developing countries (UN, 2006). To make changes in this informal sector would require colossal efforts and may compromise the advantages in terms of employment opportunities. Ways to overcome some of these issues are to develop settings that do make sense in these contexts, such as 'healthy markets' and also to adopt other approaches, such as working with particular groups of people, such as street food sellers – in other words, to accept that a settings approach cannot address all issues.

The Potential Exclusion of Marginalized Sections of Society

Whilst the original policy references to settings typically concerned environments such as cities, schools, workplaces and hospitals (Barić, 1992; DOH, 1992), this was a narrow view of a setting. Consequently, early settings-based approaches only managed to focus on 'legitimate sites of practice' (L.W. Green *et al.*, 2000, p. 25) by focusing on large-scale, identifiable and easily accessible organizations. The danger was that, if this had continued, it may have potentially exacerbated health inequalities (Speller, 2006; Dooris and Hunter, 2007) by failing to consider groups who are found outside of these formal organizations (for example, the unemployed, illegal immigrants, children who truant from school and the homeless).

As the settings approach has developed, it has stimulated practice in 'non-traditional' arenas (Poland *et al.*, 2000; Tones and Tilford, 2001). For example, there has been a surge of activity under banners such as: health-promoting universities and further education colleges (Dooris, 2001; Dooris and Thompson, 2001; Whitehead, 2004; Doherty and Dooris, 2006), healthy marketplaces (WHO, 2004), healthy nightclubs (Bellis *et al.*, 2002), healthy stadia (Crabb and Ratinckx, 2005), health-promoting sports clubs (Kokko *et al.*, 2006), healthy farms (Thurston and Blundell-Gosselin, 2005), health-promoting emergency departments (Bensberg

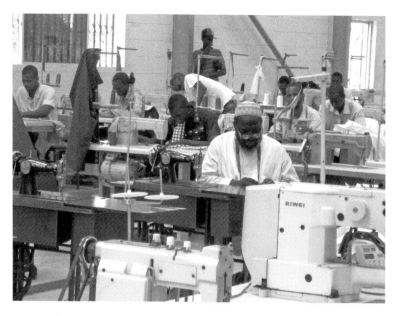

Formal workplaces are not that common in Africa – a factory making garments in The Gambia.

and Kennedy, 2002), health-promoting general practices (Watson, 2008) and, in predominantly African-American communities, healthy beauty salons and hairdressers (Lewis *et al.*, 2002; Corcoran and Bone, 2007; Linnan and Ferguson, 2007). Furthermore, the concept of health-promoting prisons (DOH, 2002; Whitehead, 2006; Woodall and South, 2011) has emerged despite the possible tensions between the core values of health promotion and imprisonment. Box 5.2 outlines the emergence of the health-promoting prison.

This continued shift towards focusing attention on 'non-traditional' settings will undoubtedly offer those once marginalized by a settings approach to have some contact with professionals to address key determinants of their health (Poland *et al.*, 2000). The challenge ahead seems to be that those working within health promotion must continue to consider emerging settings to tackle health issues.

Evaluation

One major drawback to settings-based health promotion has been the paucity of high-quality evaluation leading to 'an uneven and under-developed evidence base' (Dooris *et al.*, 2007, p. 335). The healthy cities project is a notable example. Regardless of the commitment and support from

the academic community, very little research evidence has been generated of its success, with outcome evaluations proving particularly difficult (Baum, 2002; de Leeuw and Skovgaard, 2005). School settings are an exception, as the evidence base tends to be stronger and more robust in comparison with other organizations (Corcoran and Bone, 2007; Richmond, 2009). This has been facilitated, to some extent, by the standards and criteria developed for the 'health-promoting school' and other key texts (e.g. Barnekow *et al.*, 2006), which have arguably made it easier to conduct evaluative studies.

Clearly, a settings approach provides researchers and academics with a number of unique challenges in regards to evaluation. The distinctiveness of many settings means that conducting randomized controlled trials and other experimental methods are very difficult (L.W. Green *et al.*, 2000). These methods on their own would also tell us very little about the processes of the intervention (Poland *et al.*, 2000). This has also been noted by Downie *et al.* (1996, p. 90):

> The tendency to strait-jacket health promotion into models of biomedical evaluation focussing on outcomes ignores the creative, developmental components of health promotion and leads to a loss of opportunities to learn about approaches.

Box 5.2. The emergence of health-promoting prisons.

Prisons are not necessarily in the primary business of promoting health (Smith, 2000), but do provide an opportunity to access marginalized groups. Those entering the criminal justice system have been often been subjected to a lifetime of social exclusion, including poor educational backgrounds, low incomes, meagre employment opportunities, lack of engagement with normal societal structures, low self-esteem and impermanence in terms of accommodation (including bouts of homelessness) and relationships with family members (Social Exclusion Unit, 2002). Research has also consistently demonstrated that the prevalence of ill health in the prison population is higher than what is reported in the wider community.

The notion of a health-promoting prison emerged in the mid-1990s under the guidance of the WHO. Commentators argue that the health-promoting prison should include all facets of prison life, from addressing individual health needs through to organizational factors and the physical environment (de Viggiani, 2009). The Ottawa Charter is a useful framework to envisage these facets of prison life and has been used by others to map health promotion work in prisons (Ramaswamy and Freudenberg, 2007; Woodall and South, 2011). Its application is demonstrated below.

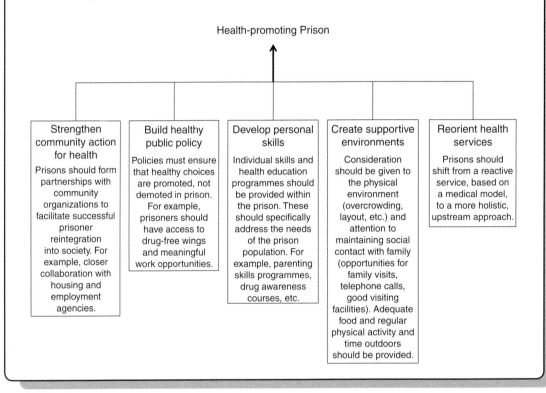

Reductivist methodologies may simply be inappropriate for measuring the success of settings initiatives, especially if researchers are asked to demonstrate positive health gains, which may be subjective and culturally contingent. Webb and Wright (2000) challenge researchers to view health promotion research with a postmodern lens, encouraging a re-consideration about the role of a single truth and embracing multiple narratives that reflect a range of perspectives. Furthermore, the problem of evaluation is not only a methodological and epistemological challenge but also a practical one. As an example, a prison setting can be a difficult environment to conduct research and may require intensive human resources especially when following-up prisoners to gain post-release data (Crundall and Deacon, 1997; Grinstead et al., 2001). This is partly due to offenders leaving prison lacking residential stability and not wanting any further contact with activities associated with the criminal justice system

(Freudenberg, 2007). Time is also an important factor when evaluating settings-based projects, as sufficient time is needed to consider systems change and organizational development. Yet, time is often a 'rare commodity' in health promotion programme evaluation (Kickbusch, 1995), where rapid, measurable success is frequently prioritized over determining longer-term achievements.

Dooris (2005, 2006) has outlined the main challenges that have inhibited the generation of a convincing evidence base. First, the funding structures for evaluative work are often focused on specific diseases and risk factor interventions. This would run counter to a comprehensive settings-based evaluation. Secondly, the heterogeneity between and across settings, coupled with the diversity and understanding of the approach, creates issues in transferability of research evidence. The 'conceptual variances', 'pragmatic influences' and differences in the 'size and type of setting' (Dooris, 2005) make building a substantive view of 'what works' challenging. Finally, there are problems with evaluating ecological and whole system approaches. Dooris, for instance, makes the valid point that if the settings approach is about integration within organizations, it can be argued that the greater the success, the more difficult the evaluation becomes. Therefore:

> Integrative approaches allow the language of 'health' to recede – and as the work becomes mainstreamed and the effectiveness of organization development becomes more apparent, 'health promotion' as an entity becomes more remote.

> (Dooris, 2005, p. 59)

Baríc and Blinkhorn (2007) concur, as they see embedded health promotion and health education within organizations as a logical outcome of the settings approach. This leads to health promotion losing its professional identity as it develops into the core work of organizations. This makes health promotion difficult to assess or evaluate since it becomes integral to the function of a setting. Perhaps the ultimate evaluative indicator will be when health is so firmly embedded into the structure of organizations and settings, the qualifying term 'healthy' or 'health promoting' is no longer required (Tones and Green, 2004).

Organizational Change

The settings approach throws into sharp relief the need for organizational change. The Bangkok Charter stated that *all* sectors and settings should advocate for health, invest in sustainable policies, actions and infrastructure to address the determinants of health, build capacity for policy development, develop leadership in health promotion and build strong partnerships with public, private, NGOs and international organizations and with civil society to create sustainable actions. If all sectors of government and all possible settings (schools, workplaces, sports stadia, clinics, cities, islands and so on) are to embrace the health promotion agenda, then radical change is. required. There is a lot of literature on organizational change, but John Kotter's work is often the first cited (Kotter, 1996). His steps to organizational change are in Table 5.2.

It would also be possible to adapt some of the individual behaviour change models to organizations – for example the stages of change model outlined in Chapter 4. Griffiths and Reynolds (2009) provide practical steps for organizational change in terms of embracing environmental issues, which include those that would help employees to be healthier, such as healthier transport plans. In terms of being change agents, Arneson and Ekberg (2005), in their study of empowerment in the workplace, found that when employees engaged in problem-based learning, with a non-directive facilitator, they developed an ability to reflect and be more self-aware, gained more self-direction and felt more empowered such that they experienced greater psychological control over decision making.

If organizations are to change, we would argue that they need to become 'learning organizations'. Learning organizations are defined as those that facilitate the learning of all their members, continually transforming themselves (Pedler *et al.*, 1991; Burgoyne, 1992). In short, a learning organization is one where 'people continually expand to create the results they truly desire, where new and expansive patterns of thinking are nurtured, where collective aspiration is set free, and where people are continuously learning how to learn together' (Senge, 1990, p. 3). This is in contrast to many organizations that rely on historical ways of doing things, are resistant to change, rely on hierarchies where most do not have to think about strategic direction and where people are not seen as intellectual capital to be harnessed for the development of the company or organizations. Pedler *et al.* (1991) outlined 11 dimensions of a learning organization, and this has been adopted in a number of different spheres with attempts to measure the

Table 5.2. Kotter's steps to organizational change.

Establish a sense of urgency	For leaders to commit to lead organization change, there must be some recognition that change is needed and important
Create a guiding coalition	A group of organizational leaders must buy in and commit to the change process, and represent the key stakeholders in terms of position, power, credibility, expertise and leadership
Develop a vision and strategy for the specific change	A shared vision for exactly what the change will look like and a strategy for how to get there must be developed that can inspire organizational members
Communicate the change vision and strategic plan	In order to utilize the vision and strategy, they must be communicated effectively throughout the organization
Empower individuals for action	Leaders must facilitate organizational members' abilities and engagement in the change initiative. This may require specific training and requires management styles, which clear the path for individuals and support their taking action
Generate short-term wins	Building in visible, unambiguous, related successes to support and reinforce the attainability and momentum for change
Consolidate gains and produce more changes	Leaders need to continue to monitor and support the change effort with further wins to help continue to drive change and prevent relapse back into old patterns
Anchor the new change in the culture	As positive change happens, leaders must explicitly tie the changes to 'who we are'

extent to which an organization is a learning organization (de Villiers, 2008). A useful guide to learning organizations is provided by Serrat (2009), from which Fig. 5.2 is taken.

In addition, as single organizations are not especially conducive to learning, they need to develop networks. In today's complex world, most organizations already have partners, or work with others in a supply chain analogy. The WHO (1998b) in its health promotion glossary, defines a network as 'A grouping of individuals, organizations and agencies organized on a non-hierarchical basis around common issues or concerns, which are pursued proactively and systematically, based on commitment and trust'. Networks function to exchange knowledge, to learn and to move agendas forward synergistically and in ways that would not be possible working alone. Increasingly, networks operate across the boundaries of private, public, voluntary or third sector, and with community involvement. The role of health promoters in facilitating organizational change and leading networks is discussed later in this chapter.

Changing does not necessarily need an infusion of cash, but thinking of new ways of working. Becoming a health-promoting school, a health-promoting workplace or a healthy market could have resource implications but could also achieve much simply by organizing and thinking in different ways. Organizing

schoolchildren or workers to pick up litter for example, does not need cash, but would considerably enhance the environment, reduce litter-based health problems and also provide exercise! The director of a major NGO in Tanzania realized that, on field trips, her driver did not have anything to do whilst she was in a community meeting; much of his time was effectively spent waiting around. He was encouraged to train as a peer educator, so that whilst she was engaged, he was too – talking to men in the community about health issues. He was keen on this development and is also learning IT skills (personal communication). This organization is therefore creating an environment where employees are stimulated and supported to learn (personal communication). Senge (1994) suggests that if organizations are to do things differently, and move from traditional, authoritarian organizations that control their workers, and are resistant to different ways of doing things, they need to develop in five areas:

1. Motivating individuals to learn, and to make the connections between their personal aspirations and the needs of the whole organization.
2. Challenging deeply rooted 'mental models' ('drivers are meant to drive, not talk to people').
3. Building long-term commitment in people by sharing the vision.

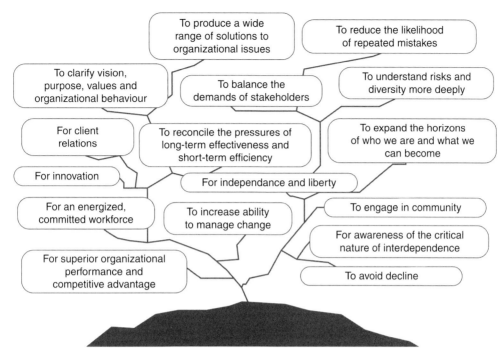

Fig. 5.2. Why develop a learning organization? (From Serrat, 2009.)

4. Developing dialogue so that people create genuine teams where they can think together.
5. Developing whole systems thinking – which essentially integrates the previous four points.

Although Senge could be criticized as being optimistic about such sharing in a capitalist global economy and the fact that he ignores the power relations (and salary differentials!) between staff, there are important points that health promoters can take into their practice.

The role of health promoters in leading change is discussed below, but we now turn to a key dimension of working in health promotion, that of evidence-based practice.

Evidence-based Practice and Evaluation

Evidence and evaluation are of significant importance in underpinning the practice of health promotion. Increasing reference is made to the concept of evidence in the WHO health promotion declarations (Groot, 2011). Some commentators would argue that health promotion will be judged entirely on 'its ability to demonstrate in a scientific way that it is an effective field' (McQueen, 2001, p. 261). Evidence-based health promotion can be defined as the 'explicit application of research evidence when making decisions' (Wiggers and Sanson-Fisher, 1998, p. 126). If practitioners are *successfully* to effect change, then they should draw on existing evidence to enhance logical decision-making processes. Practitioners can use evidence in order to make decisions about a variety of key questions including: What are the *nature* and *determinants* of a health issue? What is the most appropriate approach that should be undertaken to address these determinants? What are the processes of *how* programmes should be implemented? Are programmes considered successful (Raphael, 2000)? In some contexts, the word 'evidence' conjures up notions of law courts and scientific forensic forms of evidence in order to support judgments about innocence or guilt. But the nature of what actually constitutes 'evidence' within health promotion is hotly contested and so raises questions about epistemological foundations underpinning different research methodologies (MacIntyre and Petticrew, 2000; Kelly *et al.*, 2002). Simplistically, the nature of evidence takes the form of qualitative and quantitative forms of data (Brownson *et al.*,

2009). The epistemological debates about the nature of evidence are outlined in the sections below. The same epistemological discourse underlies *how* to evaluate health promotion activity (Rootman *et al.*, 2001). Evaluation can be defined as 'the systematic examination and assessment of the features of an initiative and its effects, in order to produce information that can be used by those who have an interest in its improvement and effectiveness' (WHO, 1998b, p. 3).

Evaluating empowerment approaches to promoting health exemplifies the difficulties of effective evaluation. Although the term 'empowerment' is frequently used, the availability of high-quality research that demonstrates its success for improving individual health and well-being is fairly minimal (Woodall *et al.*, 2010). Hubley (2002), amongst others, comments on the disappointing number of evaluations demonstrating that empowerment has occurred. This is perhaps not surprising given that empowerment is a 'fuzzy' concept and problematic to measure (Green and South, 2006). Measuring the impact of empowerment on a community level is very difficult, not least because of methodological difficulties and the fact that the experience of being empowered may occur sometime after the 'intervention' (Baistow, 1994). A review by Woodall *et al.* (2010) found few published instances where empowerment approaches had made a difference to the actual health and well-being of communities. This is arguably because long-term health effects at a community-level are difficult to measure and because there is limited research on the benefits of community participation (South and Woodall, 2010). Despite the difficulties, it is essential that the pursuit of effective evaluation is prioritized.

Evidence-based practice and evaluation are explicitly linked through the health promotion planning cycle (Green and South, 2006, p. 5), in which evaluation of health promotion programmes feeds into the evidence base about *what types* of approaches are successful (or not) and *under what conditions* these effects happen. Knowing the answers to these types of evaluation questions ultimately strengthens the practical decision-making processes about what types of strategies should be implemented and whether successful projects can be translated into different settings and contexts.

In the following sections, the epistemological debates about the nature of evidence and the approaches used to evaluate health promotion practice are developed. Given that health promotion activities should address the wider social, environmental and economic determinants of health and be focused on 'upstream' rather than 'downstream' approaches, it then follows that of particular importance are programmes that feature action at community and policy level (Warwick-Booth *et al.*, 2012). Programmes at these levels of action are discussed to illustrate principles of both evidence-based practice and evaluation. Information about how practitioners can implement change by: (i) evaluating health promotion initiatives; (ii) using existing evidence base within their own practice; and (iii) developing and enhancing the evidence base to support health promotion is discussed.

Epistemological and Methodological Issues Surrounding the Nature of Evidence and Evaluation

Epistemology is concerned with how knowledge is derived and what type of approaches we use to uncover knowledge. Evidence-based practice in health promotion originally borrowed epistemologies and frameworks developed for evidence-based *medicine* in the 1990s (Sackett *et al.*, 1996). Positivism, which underlies principles of evidence-based medicine, privileges objective factual knowledge by drawing on quantitative methodologies and design. Simply put, positivism defines reality only in terms of what is observed objectively and can be measured through our physical senses. Quantitative design such as experiments, cohort studies and case–control studies are used to answer questions about cause and effect. This question of cause and effect is central to both evidence base of effectiveness of interventions and evaluation of health promotion initiatives. For example, we may wish to know if a health promotion intervention (cause) is effective in producing positive health outcomes (effects). One particular experimental design, the randomized control trial (RCT), has been heralded as the 'gold standard' and forms the basis of the type of evidence considered the most prized sitting at the top of a hierarchy (Box 5.3). The RCT forms the foundation of evidence-based medicine and clinical decision making and has been adopted by many western countries. More latterly, hierarchical approaches to grading of evidence have been adopted by agencies such as US Preventive Services Task Force and National Institute for Clinical and Health Excellence in the UK.

The RCT is considered methodologically strong to assess cause and effect relationships and evidence of the effectiveness of interventions because of several features embedded in its design. The basic principles of an RCT design are that a sample is randomly allocated into either a comparison (control) group or an intervention group, but only the intervention group receives the intervention that is being assessed. This randomization attempts to ensure that both groups are similar in their characteristics, for example age and gender structures. This is important because if the characteristics of these two groups are different at the outset then any difference in effects (outcomes) between the groups at the end of the trial could be a result of the inherent differences between the groups at the outset of the trial. Any potential confounding factors that lead to changes in outcome will affect both the intervention and comparison groups equally and therefore any differences in outcomes can be attributed more confidently to the intervention.

The over-reliance and prioritization of RCTs as the strongest form of evidence has been heavily criticized especially within the context of health promotion as it applies principles, developed within the natural sciences and clinical settings, to social settings that cannot be easily controlled in an experimental fashion (Green and Tones, 1999; MacDonald and Davies, 1998). It is important to note that despite these criticisms some commentators contend that experimental design and principles allied to positivism are useful frameworks within social sciences and naturalistic settings (MacIntyre and Petticrew, 2000). Epistemologically, social constructionism underpins criticism of positivist approaches to evidence. Social constructionism 'is the view that whatever any individual believes, is true is true for him or her' (Marks, 2002b, p. 14). Within this school of thought, knowledge is subjective and constructed by the social world in which we live. Knowledge is derived from interpretation and meaning about events that exist in the social, cultural and political world. There is no single 'truth' as stated within positivist traditions, but different perspectives about truth are accepted and valued. Qualitative research methodologies and methods are strongly associated with evidence generated within social constructionist paradigms. Unlike positivists the questions posed by social constructionists tend not be ones of cause and effect, such as 'is an intervention effective?', but are concerned with how members of society (social actors) experience and give meaning to their world. Questions about *how* interventions lead to effects can be addressed by utilizing qualitative methodologies and methods. Pawson and Tilley (1997) refer to the black box of evaluation in which is contained the *processes* that lead to change. Health promotion places emphasis on valuing the perspectives of lay people who are the most important recipients of health promotion activity and therefore central to its practice. In addition, methods allied to action are empowerment and community development, which at the very least aim to place power and control of their health within the reach of lay people. Constructionist epistemologies, by acknowledging the valid multiple narratives of different perspectives, have the capacity to respect the accounts of lay people. Indeed some would go as far as to say that lay people have expertise and only they can give valid data on their experiences and lives (Popay *et al.*, 1998; Prior, 2003). By drawing on qualitative forms of evidence, 'black boxes' can be illuminated bringing a richer picture of events and processes to practitioners and policy makers in their evidence-based decision making.

Using different forms of evidence to address different evidence-based questions is well received within health promotion circles. This *pragmatic* approach (Marks, 2002b; Petticrew and Roberts,

2003) to utilization of differing forms of data in evidence-based practice and evaluation has led to the development of typologies of evidence (Table 5.3) rather than the hierarchical approach previously presented (Muir Gray, 1997; Petticrew and Roberts, 2003). There is a growing movement to synthesize different forms of evidence (Dixon-Woods *et al.*, 2004) and indeed several systematic reviews have been published that do not frame a review question of effectiveness but do frame questions about what is already known about an issue. For example, what is known about the facilitators and barriers to healthy eating? Shepherd *et al.* (2001) systematically reviewed and synthesized quantitative surveys, qualitative narratives and intervention studies in order to answer their initial review question rather than simply appraising RCTs.

Using pluralistic pragmatic approaches where 'the relative contributions that different kinds of [design] and methods can make to different kinds of research questions' (Petticrew and Roberts, 2003, p. 529) should be recognized and accepted in order to develop evaluation frameworks and research evidence to underpin decision making. It is clear from the typology in Table 5.3 that the nature of evidence is contingent on what research questions are posed. Many sources of evidence are often required to address complex initiatives. Rigorous evidence of outcomes may be evidenced using RCTs but evidence of how those outcomes were achieved and under what conditions and contexts they can be replicated is likely to come from qualitative data. Practitioners need to consider what they wish to find out and then draw on appropriate methodologies, designs and methods to address the issues.

Marks (2002b) provides an excellent and much fuller discussion of the epistemological and methodological considerations of evidence used within public health.

Being an Evidence-based Practitioner

Two strategies exist for health promotion practitioners wishing to draw on research evidence to support their decision making. First, in some countries, national agencies have been commissioned to find, appraise, synthesize and produce evidence 'briefings' aiming to update practitioners in easy to digest bite-sized chunks largely focusing on what the most effective strategies to produce improved health outcomes are (Speller *et al.*, 2005). However, while this is a solid development to tackle the translation of evidence into practice, it is unlikely to address all the concerns of practitioners. In addition, within a developing countries context, culturally relevant evidence may not be published or widely disseminated. Systematic reviews tend to be undertaken on issues specific to western health priorities and where relevant systematic reviews do exist; it may not be possible to implement interventions because of limited resources and infrastructures available to practitioners (McMichael *et al.*, 2005). The second strategy necessitates building capacity for practitioners to find and appraise evidence themselves and apply it to their own practice. Muir Gray (1997) and Brownson *et al.* (2003) outline the steps and skills in the process of evidence-based decision making (Box 5.4).

Table 5.3. Example of typologies of evidence.

Research question	Type of research design					
	Qualitative	Survey	Case–control	Cohort study	RCTs	Systematic reviews
Effectiveness – does it work?				+	++	+++
Processes of delivery and implementation – how and why?	++	+				+++
Safety – good versus harm	++	++				+++
Cost effectiveness – it is worth buying for health gain produced?					++	+++
Appropriate – is it the right service?	++	++				++
Satisfaction with service or policy	++	++	+	+		+

Box 5.4. Steps and skills in the process of evidence-based decision making.

1. Ability to *frame* evidence-based questions.
2. Ability to *find* evidence that addresses the stated questions.
3. Ability to *assess the quality* of the evidence.

4. Ability to *determine* whether the results of the research can be *transferred* to the practitioners' local context and client group.
5. Ability to communicate and disseminate evidence to other practitioners.

Framing Evidence-based Questions

The overwhelming majority of existing evidence pertains to questions of effectiveness of interventions but as we have suggested in the typology of evidence, not all questions of interest to practitioners relate to whether an intervention works. Practitioners implementing initiatives are concerned with what are the best ways of working with different partners, sectors and clients. Commissioners of health promotion interventions may be interested in framing questions about which interventions are most equitable, acceptable and accessible to clients and therefore more likely to be effective (Rada *et al.*, 1999).

Searching for Evidence

Evidence can be in the form of practical experience and may not be published. However, these forms of evidence are not thought to be reliable or robust enough to be used for rational decision making (Box 5.3). Typically, a body of evidence is needed to make sound judgements. If half the existing evidence is not found, then it is not possible to make balanced decisions about evidence. Evidence that underpins decision making is likely to be obtained via academic databases such as Social Science Citation Indices and the Science Citation indices or PubMed. Specialist evidence databases such as the Campbell Library of Systematic Reviews give full details of completed and ongoing systematic reviews in education, crime and justice, and social welfare; Evidence for Policy and Practice Information (EPPI) Centre and Cochrane Database Systematic Reviews contains the full text of regularly updated systematic reviews of the effects of health interventions carried out by the Cochrane Collaboration. Grey literature such as paper-based reports that are not available electronically are also potentially useful sources of evidence. An excellent guide about how to search for evidence can be found in Craig and Smyth (2002).

Appraising Evidence

This step in the process is important as practitioners should be able go beyond what the descriptive findings of the research state to a more critical understanding of the *methodological* rigour about how the research was designed and conducted. If research is poorly designed and implemented the findings themselves are untrustworthy, whatever findings are presented. Criteria and checklists to assess different types of evidence have been developed in order to provide systematic and consistent judgements to be made about the methodological quality of the research undergoing assessment (Rychetnik *et al.*, 2002; Critical Appraisal Skills Programme, no date).

Transferability of Evidence into Local Context

To assess whether existing evidence can be transferred to other settings and situations, detailed descriptions of the design, development, delivery and context of an initiative should be available. It may be that interventions that are effective and acceptable in one setting or context, may fail in another. Context refers to the social and cultural environment and the particular political and organizational system in which the research takes place. Wang *et al.* (2005) have developed a useful set of questions (e.g. are the characteristics of the target population comparable between the study setting and the local setting?) to aid judgements to be made about transferability of initiatives.

Dissemination of Evidence into Practice

Crucial to the processes of evidence-based decision making is communication of existing evidence to practitioners who can rationally make judgements about what strategies should be used to undertake health improvement and how they should be implemented. Research indicates that resources designed to disseminate evidence-based information are unlikely to facilitate change in decision making unless they are linked to a knowledge management process that includes practitioner engagement (Armstrong *et al.*, 2007). Innovative work has involved practitioners and service users being actively involved in the development of evidence-based guidelines to promote and support breast feeding. This approach 'allowed a transparent, accountable process for formulating recommendations based on scientific, theoretical, practical and expert evidence, with the added potential to enhance implementation' because of the strong engagement with practitioners and service users (Renfrew *et al.*, 2008, p. 3). This type of approach involving relevant stakeholders is considered a principle of good practice.

On a positive note, whilst many challenges face implementation of evidence-based decision making, research has shown that capacity building projects can be successful and lead to improvements in decision making processes. In an innovative, ambitious programme, the US Centers for Disease Control and Prevention (CDC) developed a Data for Decision-Making (DDM) Project implemented in four countries. The CDC facilitated identification of important health problems, development of implementation plans, in-service training programmes for mid-level policy makers and other relevant practitioners (Pappaioanou *et al.*, 2003).

Evidence-based Policy Making

As suggested in the introduction, existing evidence clearly informs us that in order to address health inequities and increase life expectancy for those countries that have poorer health outcomes, we need to tackle the social, environmental, economic and political determinants of health. This necessitates acting at policy and community level. Unpicking processes about *how* a policy is implemented and whether it can give rise to evidence of effectiveness is complex. It has been suggested that policy and community action cannot be evaluated to produce an evidence base because the causal chain leading from the policy (cause) to health outcomes (effects) is not straightforward and many other policy interventions are also

acting on populations. Teasing out single attributable effects is problematic. Asthana and Halliday (2006) analysed 125 systematic reviews and concluded that the current evidence base favours those interventions based on individual lifestyle factors and educational approaches. However, the evidence base for interventions addressing the wider determinants of health via policy making is much weaker. Nevertheless, systematic reviews do exist about policy and community action. For example, the health effects of volunteering (Casiday *et al.*, 2008), interventions that aim to increase employee participation or control (Egan *et al.*, 2007) and the effects on health and health inequalities of partnership working (Smith *et al.*, 2009) have all been assessed using systematic review approaches. Bambra *et al.* (2010) also provide a systematic review of evidence where social determinants have been the focus of action. Within the context of developing countries, some optimistic commentators contend that the evidence-based global health policy movement has taken many important strides with the development of organizations such as the Evidence to Policy initiative (E2Pi), which aims to help narrow the gap between evidence synthesis and practical policy making in global health (Yamey and Feachem, 2011). An interesting study highlighted that policy makers were persuaded by surprising forms of evidence such as *timely stories* especially if they were combined with scientific evidence. Where academics and researchers were able to produce stronger evidence for health improvement and financial reductions in governmental departmental budgets, the evidence was more likely to be persuasive and actioned (Petticrew *et al.*, 2004). It is this type of research that will enable a stronger interplay between academics, policy makers and practitioners.

Evaluative Culture in Health Promotion Practice

Wimbush and Watson (2000) reiterate that differing stakeholders will have different evaluation questions and that these will be addressed by drawing on appropriate epistemologies, methodologies and methods.

Given the previously stated link between evaluation and evidence, it is important that health promotion develops a stronger evaluative culture in which practitioners embed process, impact and outcome evaluation at the outset of their programmes. The epistemological and methodological debates about how to evaluate have already been discussed earlier.

Nutbeam (1998a, p. 30) provides one framework for defining the outcomes associated with health promotion activity such as education, social mobilization and advocacy. These activities are linked to: the immediate health promotion outcomes (programme impact measures); the intermediate health outcomes (modifiable determinants of health); and the desired long-term health and social outcomes (reductions in morbidity, avoidable mortality and disability, improved quality of life, functional independence and equity). Green and South (2006) also provide practical frameworks for the practitioner wishing to embark on rigorous evaluations of initiatives including more complex community-based programmes. Dissemination of evaluation evidence is crucial: (i) if good practice is to be translated across settings, sectors and clients; (ii) if approaches that are ineffective are not be repeated; and (iii) if evaluation can feed into developing a stronger evidence base within health promotion.

In summary, all forms of high-quality, robust data can be used as evidence and form the spine of developing stronger evaluative culture. There are methodological strengths of each design and method if they are applied correctly to stated evidence and research questions. There are challenges facing practitioners when undertaking evidence-based decision making, but progress has been made addressing many of these. It is important to state that generating and implementing evidence is not a perfect process. A realistic goal is stated by Muir Gray (1997, p. 48): 'The absence of excellent evidence does not make evidence-based decision making impossible: what is required is the best evidence available, not the best evidence possible.'

The additional abilities and competencies of health promotion practitioners are addressed later in this chapter, but first we turn to thinking about practising ethically.

Working Ethically

This is not the only place in the book where 'ethics' are considered, as clearly we have a strand throughout the book of considering the values base, moral issues and ethics of what we do. Here however, we present some of the 'nitty-gritty' issues facing practitioners. Seedhouse (1997) has considered at length ethics in health promotion, producing an 'ethical grid' to aid decision making. He laments the lack of attention to ethics in health promotion training and in the health promotion literature (Seedhouse, 2001a). New (1999) has produced a useful report on values in public health, which is useful general reading and also picks up on those aspects that come more firmly under a public health remit such as immunization and screening, as well as behavioural modification and health education. Peter Duncan and Alan Cribb have written a number of articles and books on ethics in health promotion (e.g. Duncan and Cribb, 1996; Cribb and Duncan, 2002) and McKee et al. (2005) provide an overview of ethics in public health. Sindall (2002) has argued that 'Health promotion can no longer take its own moral credentials for granted'. He calls for debate about whether health promotion needs its own set of ethics in the same way that public health or medicine has, and for the development of a coherent ethical framework upon which to base health promotion practice. Clearly, with macro-level issues such as privacy, the right to interfere in people's lives, 'social engineering', the use of persuasion or coercion, 'nudging' and a whole raft of other ethical dilemmas, health promotion needs to engage with such a debate, in the interests of developing the profession.

Discussion of ethics in public health work often takes as its point of departure the tenets of health *care* ethics, and it is worth looking at these first. Indeed, many workers enter health promotion by first having worked in health care. Health care is usually concerned with patients or clients and thus the power differentials between them and the professionals who are caring for them raise ethical issues. Abuses of power are an obvious hazard, and a system of ethics has developed, which aims to protect the relatively vulnerable. Thus the principles of autonomy (not doing anything that goes against a person's wishes), non-maleficence (not doing harm), beneficence (doing good) and justice (treating people equally and with respect) provide a foundation for the doctor–patient relationship. These key principles apply to health promotion work too, but there are key differences between health promotion and health care work, and additional issues to consider. As we are dealing with healthy populations, and not necessarily with those who have identified themselves as in need of help, different kinds of 'contracts' between professionals and the community apply.

As health promotion is tacitly concerned with creating a 'good' global society, with positive ramifications for health, it is inevitably bound up with ethical and moral questions. We *are* making judgments about what kind of society we want to live in. Cribb and Duncan (2002) make a distinction between customary ethics and reflective ethics. The former refers to those aspects of everyday life that we hold to be part of custom or normative practice and are expected patterns of good behaviour; an example they give is that everyone 'knows' it is wrong to steal from a host, or to turn up very late for an event. However, 'Nothing can be accepted simply on the basis that it is customary. We have to be able to critically reflect on, and challenge, customary ethics' (Cribb and Duncan, 2002, p. 155). Otherwise, societies would be static with no room for change. Clearly, certain 'customary practices' that *have* been challenged as unethical – forced sex within marriage, female genital mutilation and beating of children, to name a few – had been seen as 'normal' aspects of life until challenged. Each of these issues has been taken up by health promoters and other social reformers, and many have been made illegal. The relationship between legality and morality is a complex one, and one that changes over time. Aspects of sexuality, for example, have variously been seen as legal and illegal, moral and immoral in different historical times and in different cultures. Whereas we view being gay, lesbian, bisexual or transgendered as needing to be legal and being moral, this would not be the case in those countries where gay people are persecuted with impunity, or where homosexuality is illegal. Some countries such as Uganda have recently not only discussed making homosexuality illegal, but making it a criminal offence not to report to the authorities if someone knows someone who is gay. The murder of the gay rights activist David Kato shows how much a matter of life and death this is. If health promoters are to work with sensitive areas such as sexuality, HIV/AIDS and reproductive health, then they must sort out their own ideas and understand their own moral codes!

Not Doing Harm

Arguably, the most important ethical principle is to do no harm. Some examples will be provided here from the area of weight and obesity. O'Hara and Gregg (2006) provide an interesting example of a discussion about the harm that programmes focusing on obesity can cause. Arguing that the weight-centred paradigm has stigmatized overweight and obese people, and that interventions to promote weight loss are not particularly effective and can produce psychological distress, they espouse instead a 'Health at every size' model as an alternative. There *has* been an increase in the stigma faced by obese children (Latner and Stunkard, 2003). However, whilst we would agree that the obsession with weight in Western countries is unhealthy, it is also the case that obesity *does* have health consequences, and many children and adults are unhappy when obese or overweight (Dixey, 1999b; McElhone *et al.*, 2005). Not to act in the face of expressed health needs would also be unethical. At least, obesity prevention programmes need to ensure that they build in measures to ensure that they do not cause harm, such as measures of self-esteem over the life of the project.

Dixey (1998a, b) has speculated on whether the focus on not being too fat has resulted in disordered eating, and also whether tackling one issue (child pedestrian accidents) has led to another – that of children becoming overweight due to lack of exercise and a rise in sedentary activities within the home, and to increased parental distress.

Voluntarism, Autonomy and Informed Choice

It goes without saying that it is unethical to coerce people. Rohinton Mistry's novel *A Fine Balance* (1996) graphically describes the rounding up of poor men, street dwellers and those with no power to resist during India's forced sterilization campaigns. This shameful period in the mid-1970s saw a policy of population control targeting men who already had two or more children, for compulsory vasectomies, but in the process and to meet quotas, other powerless men were also forced to have the operation. The other example that is often raised when discussing voluntarism is China's one-child policy. These examples are extreme, and are likely to occur in only a small number of countries. However, other issues do affect very large numbers of people, and another obvious example is of female genital mutilation and other traditional practices harmful to women. Where female genital mutilation is performed on girls, there is clearly no consent, and where it is performed on young women, there cannot be said to be consent given the strength of the cultural norms sanctioning the practice. Health promoters have made huge efforts to work on this issue but it is very persistent.

Health promotion works with the whole community, not only those 'at risk' or identified as in need. People thus do not necessarily ask for, or want, health communications or public service type broadcasts. They might not be able to avoid them, even if they wanted to, in the same way that commercial advertising is hard to escape. They do not sign consent forms, as patients are expected to. 'Voluntarism' is thus difficult to estimate, especially when health educators and promoters are trained in how to develop 'persuasive messages'. Commercial advertisers too, are adept at the art of persuasion, using emotional appeals with impunity. Is there really any such thing as 'free choice'? Or are we fooling ourselves that our actions are not influenced by significant others, by our socialization and by persuasive arguments?

Where there are democratic systems of decision making in place, decisions are easier to assess in terms of ethics. Adding fluoride or chlorine to water supplies usually raises its head in such cases; it is not possible to provide each person in a region with the means to consent. If a whole region makes the democratic decisions to add fluoride, then the consequences are easier to take than if a despot made that decision. Likewise, if decisions are made in democratic fora, they are easier to 'swallow', even if some people feel that their autonomy is compromised. Also, if actions compromise autonomy but save lives, it could be argued that those people saved have increased their ability to live autonomous lives in the future (as otherwise they would have been dead).

Surprisingly often in the health promotion literature, reference is made to 'captive audiences', and whilst most writers mean nothing sinister by this, it runs contrary to the ethos of voluntarism, and does need to be deconstructed!

Imposing Health Values

Downie *et al.* (1990) seem to overcome the moral dilemma of health promoters imposing their own values by taking a fundamentalist position, asserting that health is to be valued above all other values; health promotion 'endeavours to persuade people to adopt certain lifestyles, and is committed to furthering certain values'. This view is perhaps the honest one – health promoters often *do* believe that a healthy life is one where people prioritize health rather than hedonism or seeming recklessness. They would rather that people make the 'right' choices after hearing the evidence, rather than deciding to carry on with their 'unhealthy' behaviours. Ewles and Simnett (1985), in a 'whose life is it anyway?' fashion, question the 'ethical justification' for the imposition of these 'healthist' values, and seem to say that one set of values is just as good as another – for example, if some people prefer to live a sedentary life of enjoyment involving alcohol and tobacco, who are we to say that this is 'wrong'? Dixey (1999b) has raised similar concerns regarding beliefs in settings where religious ideas may be more culturally important than 'scientific' worldviews; in seeing it as important to wear a helmet on a motorcycle, a whole range of cultural issues were uncovered in Nigeria:

> The dominant discourse of contemporary health promotion tends to see fatalism as atavistic and unhelpful. However, 'fatalism' may be a rational perspective in the social and economic circumstances, and who can judge whether there are gods or a God who predetermine people's fate? Health promotion needs to recognise its secular, modernist, individualist biases, and its preoccupation with control and empowerment.
>
> (Dixey, 1999b, p. 206)

The Right to Intervene

We have agreed that states have a moral obligation to create the conditions in which people can be healthy. It also has a role in those cases where people are particularly vulnerable, such as with children, frail elderly, with learning disabilities or who are otherwise compromised. States in short, have a stewardship role (Calman, 2009). Most citizens accept that the state has a right to curtail certain freedoms in the public interest, but the whole issue of the relationship between the authority of the state and the individual is a complex one, and varies between societies. To a European, for example, the importance of the right for individuals to 'bear arms' (carry guns), so much a part of American culture, is baffling. This libertarian approach, which privileges the rights of individuals over the collective, runs counter to the 'social contract' assumed in many parts of the world. Those societies find it easier to accept John Stuart Mill's principle, that the state has the right to intervene when one person's actions harm other people. Thus banning smoking in cars where children are present is acceptable. Banning an individual smoking in the privacy of their own car is more contentious, as seen recently by reaction to the BMA's call to legislate against this.

Rationing – Deciding Who to Work With

Canada's Saskatchewan province's (Saskatchewan Health, 2002) guide to health promotion suggests that in deciding how best to use resources, decisions have to be made as follows:

Using the best available data and evidence on population health issues and effectiveness of interventions, weigh each possible issue in terms of:

- the degree of impact on population health status (as measured by mortality, morbidity, quality of life);

- the availability and effectiveness of interventions to address the issue;
- the cost to the community of pertinent health or social conditions and their treatment and prevention; and
- the potential to reduce health inequities.

(Saskatchewan Health, 2002, p. 20)

Not Acting – Doing Nothing

When we do nothing, we are supporting the status quo, which is itself a political act. Further, as Edmund Burke is reputed to have said, 'the only thing necessary for the triumph of evil is for good people to do nothing'. Doing nothing is one of the options available in the 'intervention ladder' (Box 5.5). Each of the options presents ethical challenges.

Whilst it would be unethical to act not knowing whether a course of action was going to be effective, if we waited until all the evidence was watertight, no action might take place at all. The importance of evidence-based practice will be taken up later in this chapter, but here we want to stress this as an ethical issue. When to invoke the precautionary principle was mentioned in Chapter 3, and there are many examples where thousands of lives would have been saved if that principle had been invoked. That asbestos could be a potential

---

Box 5.5. The intervention ladder.

The ladder of possible government actions is as follows:

- **Do nothing** or simply monitor the current situation.
- **Provide information.** Inform and educate the public, for example as part of campaigns to encourage people to walk more or eat five portions of fruit and vegetables per day.
- **Enable choice.** Enable individuals to change their behaviours, for example by offering participation in an NHS 'stop smoking' programme, building cycle lanes, or providing free fruit in schools.
- **Guide choices through changing the default policy.** For example, in a restaurant, instead of providing chips as a standard side dish (with healthier options available), menus could be changed to provide a healthier option as standard (with chips as an option available).

- **Guide choices through incentives.** Regulations can be offered that guide choices by fiscal and other incentives, for example offering tax-breaks for the purchase of bicycles that are used as a means of travelling to work.
- **Guide choice through disincentives.** Fiscal and other disincentives can be put in place to influence people not to pursue certain activities, for example through taxes on cigarettes, or by discouraging the use of cars in inner cities through charging schemes or limitations of parking spaces.
- **Restrict choice.** Regulate in such a way as to restrict the options available to people with the aim of protecting them, for example removing unhealthy ingredients from foods, or unhealthy foods from shops or restaurants.

(From: http://www.nuffieldbioethics.org/fileLibrary/pdf/Public_health_-_ethical_issues.pdf)

---

hazard to health was noted in the last years of the 19th century, but it was not banned until 100 years later, by which time it had caused thousands of deaths in Europe (European Environment Agency, 2002). As their report states,

> Preventive and precautionary public action ... requires a minimum measure of agreement between governments and stakeholders about the approach to causality under conditions of uncertainty, ignorance, disputed values and the high stakes of 'being wrong' in both directions, i.e. failing to reduce harmful exposures; or taking precautionary measures that turn out to be unnecessary.
>
> (European Environment Agency, 2002, p. 3)

Manipulating Behaviour

Health promoters potentially tread a thin line between educating, persuading and manipulating behaviour. 'Behaviour change' paradigms do not seem to see any problems with persuading or with 'persuasive interventions'. 'Nudging' was mentioned in Chapter 4. There has been much debate in the health promotion literature about the use of shock tactics as a means to change behaviour. The idea is to use the fear of consequences in order to shock people into doing something about their health. Ethical questions aside, evidence on the effectiveness of shock tactics is inconclusive. A very early study by Janis and Fresbach (1953) on persuading people to brush their teeth regularly found that approaches using high levels of fear resulted in them being less likely to brush their teeth. It seems that when fear increases, compliance in following the solution decreases. However, other studies have showed that fear appeals can have positive effects (Boster and Mongeau, 1984). Protection Motivation Theory (Rogers, 1983) helps to explain how using shock tactics might work: the motivation to take action is based on the individual's appraisal of the health threat and its solution, and the ability of the individual to take a particular action in dealing with the threat is important. Witte and Allen (2000) believe that fear can motivate an individual to take action as long as s/he believes they are able to protect themselves. An example of a fear approach is given by Hale and Dillard (1995, p. 65), who describe a 'well known fear appeal' campaign to reduce illegal drug use: 'The commercial shows an egg, a frying pan and then the egg frying. The voice-over says: "This is your brain. This is your brain on drugs. Any questions?" The intent of the message is to demonstrate that drug use kills brain cells.'

Curtis *et al.*'s (2011) work on the role of disgust in people's aversion to dirt and disease suggests that one of the most effective ways to get people to wash their hands after using public toilets is to put up a sign saying 'Is the person next to you washing their hands?', shaming them into washing their own hands. The Community-Led Total Sanitation movement in Nepal and Sierra Leone goes one step further and makes no apologies for using name and shame approaches.

The example of naming and shaming raises the question of whether the means justifies the ends – if serious causes of mortality such as childhood diarrhoea in poor countries are caused by some community members' poor hygiene, why should they not be called to account? This consequentialist or utilitarian argument would assert that if the greatest happiness of the greatest number is served by a certain course of action, then that course is justified. In our Community-Led Total Sanitation example, if a few people feel humiliated, then that is the price a few must pay for the greater good. The utilitarian standpoint is usually contrasted with the deontological or rules-based approach, where it is argued that if a rule exists (e.g. that people should never be deliberately humiliated) then this should hold, whatever the consequences.

Hale and Dillard (1995, p. 78) end their chapter on fear appeal by saying that

> Fear appeals have enormous persuasive potential and can promote better health. The effectiveness depends in large part on the structure of the message. At the least, an effective fear appeal must include a severe threat, evidence suggesting the target is especially vulnerable to the threat, and solutions that are both easy to perform and effective.

We would say that severe threats are unethical; interestingly, Hale and Dillard do not discuss ethical dilemmas. This area remains contentious, as often people only do recognize the need to change actions and practices when their concerns are raised, and when they experience a degree of cognitive dissonance (which health promoters deliberately try to raise). Perhaps at least Hale and Dillard's subtitle – 'Too much, too little or just right?' – is helpful when considering what degree of concern, interest and attention (but not fear!) to raise with people and communities.

We cannot do justice here to the very large number of ethical issues facing the practice of health promotion and readers will need to follow this up elsewhere. We now turn to thinking about new ways of working with people in the 21st century and specifically we consider new citizenship roles.

Active Citizenship – a New Role for Empowered People?

An implicit theme in this book concerns the relative roles of government, the private or commercial sector, the non-governmental sector and the community. Community participation was discussed in Chapter 2. In this chapter, we expand on what we could call civil society. We have stressed the importance of empowered people able to take control of the factors that determine their health, and thus to take control of their own lives. Citizenship is a progression from being a 'community member' as it implies an active, engaged and fully participating citizenship in order to bring about the 'good society'. How should health promoters work alongside these empowered citizens? The idea of people taking a more active citizenship role has been adopted by both left and right politicians, and is encapsulated in the notion of the 'Big Society'. This idea can be taken to mean that rather than 'big government', where government reaches into every aspect of life in passive communities, people should have a greater say in the running of their country's affairs.

We have also argued that it is the role of governments to ensure the health and safety of their populations. The commercial or business sector is often seen as developing products and ways of operating that harm health – either through employment practices that do not prioritize worker health, such as in poor factory conditions, or sweat shops, or by selling products that are clearly harmful, such as tobacco or 'junk' food. Private medicine and the pharmaceutical industry too have been accused of distorting health care, in promoting those areas that can be profitable (Bodenheimer, 1985; Eyer, 1985), and turning health into a commodity. This is obviously a simplified picture, and the private sector can obviously play a positive and constructive role in society, not least because it provides jobs and creates incomes. What is of interest here, however, is first how the political and policy landscapes have shifted such that the boundaries between these sectors have become blurred (Walt,

1994), secondly, how the non-governmental sector (NGOs) have emerged as key players, and thirdly, how empowered, active citizens can play a role in counteracting the agenda of the other sectors. The latter has been shown very visibly in the history of 2011. First there was the Arab spring, where across the Middle East ordinary people took it upon themselves to act against the governments that ruled them for so long. Secondly, we have witnessed the 'Occupy' movements, where across major cities in Europe and the USA people have occupied spaces near the financial centres of those cities in order to question the relationship between governments and the major financial institutions, and to question what is seen as the systemic failure of the international financial system to bring about economic stability and prosperity for ordinary people. The occupiers in London, organizing themselves under the name of OccupyLSX, say they want to reinstate the idea of the 'assembly' and ask people to stop seeing themselves as consumers and start seeing themselves as participants:

> … take back the initiative – because we've seen what happens when we let politicians take sole responsibility for how we organize our society: it's resulted in profound economic failure and material hardship. Change is possible if you want it – this is what we're trying to show people.
> (Colvin and Wargalla, 2011, p. 28)

The 21st century tacitly questions what it means to be a citizen – an active, engaged citizen:

> Upon what is citizenship based? In discussions about rights and responsibilities, obligations and entitlements, belonging and participation, a set of questions keeps insisting: how does one imagine oneself in connection with a community, a culture or a nation?
> (Frosh, 2001, p. 62)

There is also an implicit assumption that the

> … citizen in the information age requires a different range of skills and taken-for-granted knowledge to his/her predecessor and those skills and assumptions are constantly shifting. Without these skills individuals cannot properly perform their citizenship role. They lack the knowledge which would allow them to choose and argue on public-political issues and are therefore excluded from full citizenship.
> (N. Crossley, 2001, p. 40).

According to Kubow *et al.* (2000, p. 134), 'effective citizenship first requires the internalisation of a set of civic ethics or values'; a good person and a good citizen can be distinguished by the latter's engagement with civic society, contributing in some way to the public good. It is virtuous to be involved in community action, and it transcends self-interest. This participative citizenship, according to Kymlicka and Norman (1995, p. 293), holds the 'intrinsic value of political participation for the participants themselves'.

This implies that people participate in civil society for intrinsic rewards. It contrasts with the 'instrumental' motivation in theories of participation, where it is assumed that people are motivated by extrinsic rewards, such as gaining work experience, gaining new social contacts and so on. Parry *et al.* (1992) propose three other categories of motivation: the communitarian, educative and expressive. In practice, the boundaries between these motivations are blurred for people, and people may be motivated by a wish to express themselves, be educated and to identify with their communities, plus getting something out of the experience, which furthers their career or simply makes their life more meaningful and enjoyable. A communitarian model, however, suggests that where people strongly identify with their community, they are more likely to increase their participation, and in turn increased participation leads to greater identification with the community. By being more involved, people enhance their sense of belonging, are able to express themselves and somehow earn a sense of validation. Archer (2007, p. 7) suggests that we act as citizens 'to promote our concerns ... to advance or protect what we care about most'. But why are some people more willing (and able) to cooperate with others (Karsten *et al.*, 2000)? Clearly, those with some power already, and with skills and confidence, will be more likely to 'get involved'. Thus community assemblies, local councillors and lay involvement generally tend to over-represent the middle classes, the better educated and those with time and other resources to spare. However, as South *et al.* (2011) show, there are ways in which professionals can support people in civic engagement, such as in contributing to public health. Singapore is at the moment attempting to recruit 10,000 'health ambassadors', community members who can enthuse others, and in England community health champions are spearheading new ways for people to get involved.

Community health champions are a new way of describing lay health workers, those who formally or informally volunteer to promote health in their communities. The National Institute for Clinical

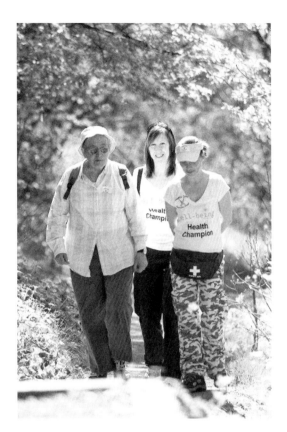

Health champions, encouraging others to be more active, England.

Excellence (NICE) Guidance on Community Engagement recommended recruiting community members to plan and deliver health promotion, which addressed the social determinants of health. The Altogether Better programme therefore aimed to recruit 13,500 community health champions by 2012. A comprehensive evidence review of the community health champions schemes (South *et al.*, 2010b) showed that there is a sufficiently strong evidence base on the positive impact of champions to justify their continued use, and that they can be a key resource for health. A further piece of research (White *et al.*, 2010c), in which key stakeholders and community health champions were interviewed, concluded that they have a very valuable role to play in creating better health in the civic landscape of the current century. Health champions are just one example of lay people getting involved in public health roles, as highlighted by South *et al.* (2010a) in the 'People in Public Health' project.

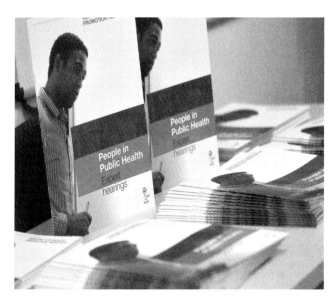

People in Public Health – lay people getting involved.

The changing relationships between the private, governmental and community levels can also be illustrated by taking a look at solid waste management. Management of waste produced by everyday life is a major problem to be solved by all societies. In countries such as England, there have been attempts to create more upstream solutions – to use less packaging, to recycle and to reduce waste – rather than expect a local council to collect waste from households and take it to landfill sites. This has resulted in a changed relationship between municipal authorities and citizens – the 'good' citizen sorts waste for recycling at the household level, takes climate change seriously and, in short, takes responsibility for some of his/her actions around waste creation. In poorer countries where there are less well-developed systems of local government and a low tax base to pay for services, different solutions have been found. In Kenya, Uganda, Tanzania and Zambia, the municipal authorities have franchised the collection of waste to community-based organizations, community-based enterprises and small and medium enterprises, so that they generate income for themselves and also provide a valuable public service (Tukahirwa, 2011). At Leeds Met, we have been involved for over a decade in providing support for aspects of these initiatives in Tanzania and Zambia, and have seen how they can empower women by providing income and social support (especially in the women-only or women-run organizations; Foster *et al.*, 2012).

Arguably, adults and young people gain experiences earlier in life, which lead to civic responsibility – or not. Clearly, children do have agency, and it is important to foster this in terms of them becoming active citizens as young people and also later in life. Where children are asked, they are 'very interested in their communities and, if given the opportunity, are willing to become involved in changing community conditions to promote their own well-being' (Kalnins *et al.*, 2002, p. 231). The Child-to-Child initiative (Pridmore, 1999) has been successful in encouraging children's involvement, and fostering the development of social responsibility, partially through its apprenticeship approach (Rogoff, 1993). It asserted that children could be partners with adults to improve health, though at times it has had to challenge the allegation that it 'uses' children as health educators. It has been shown to develop children's full participation and potential, and to make significant positive differences in adulthood (Serpell *et al.*, 2011). The Child-to-Child initiative has been evaluated latterly and shown to have had a role in developing civic responsibility in Zambia. An empowerment approach was developed in a rural primary school, using Child-to-Child approaches. It fostered cooperative learning, democracy in the classroom, and social responsibility.

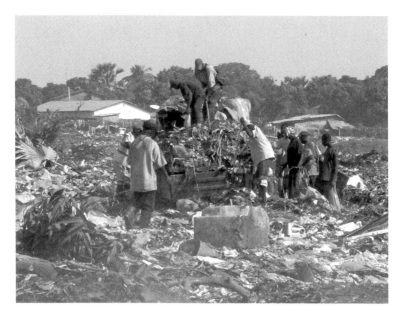

The problem of solid waste management.

In following up pupils, now adults, the evaluation showed that they had a sense of personal agency conducive to being active citizens in their current lives (Serpell *et al.*, 2011).

The Non-governmental or 'Third Sector'

The discussion so far has suggested that new forms of relationships are being created between the state, its citizenry, the private sector and what is increasingly being called the third sector. Pearce (2006) provides an overview of the key debates in the development discourse, as one of a collection of useful chapters in the book edited by Eade (2006). During the 1990s in particular, there was something of an 'explosion' of NGOs (Fisher, 1997). Salamon (1993, p. 1) has gone so far as to suggest that this explosion, at least in the 'third world' may 'prove to be as significant to the latter twentieth century as the rise of the nation-state was to the latter nineteenth century'. NGOs cover a range of types and scales of organizations, from large bodies with millions of dollars at their disposal to those run by one or two individuals from their own homes. The term 'NGO' covers community-based organizations, grass-roots organizations and people's organizations as well as the more familiar international NGOs such as Oxfam. These groups are creating new

opportunities for citizen engagement through coming together to form organizations. Some have become very powerful players, especially where they deliver services traditionally offered by government. The development of the third sector further blurs the boundaries between the four sectors, whilst Fisher (1997, p. 440) comments that 'political scientists are re-evaluating the role of voluntary associations in building vibrant civil societies and their impact on the relationship between society and the state'. What is interesting is the process by which activists have found ways of challenging established structures, changing the rules of engagement; NGOs represent new forms of associations, can manoeuvre themselves into political spaces and can tackle issues not high on government agendas. The emphasis on processes has led one commentator to suggest: 'NGOs are not things, but processes, and instead of asking what an NGO is, the more appropriate question then becomes how "NGO-ing" is *done*' (Hilhorst, 2003, p. 5).

This sector is seen optimistically by some, who see it as an expansion of civil society, and as a means for people to bring about the kind of society they want to live in – as many NGOs are fuelled by moral concerns, faith or politics. The sector asserts that there is more to it than 'being not for profit'; the values of the third sector are distinctive, have meaning to the sector and have been encapsulated as:

- empowering people;
- pursuing equality;
- making voices heard;
- transforming lives;
- being responsible;
- finding fulfilment;
- doing a good job; and
- generating public wealth (Blake *et al.*, 2006).

There are thousands of NGOs doing health promotion work. The duplication of efforts has been criticized – there are many hundreds of NGOS working in the HIV/AIDS field, for example – but Fisher suggests that whereas the impermanence and fluidity of these organizations and associations could be a weakness, 'the space created in their passing may contribute to new activism that builds up after them' (Fisher, 1997, p. 459). In other words, the political landscape has been permanently changed and there are now four sectors, with permeable boundaries, as suggested in Box 5.6.

Here we have called the citizen sector the fourth sector. It is not clear where a major, wealthy philanthropic foundation might sit, with more money to spend on health than many governments, and run by a businessman; or which sector might accommodate one of the women's community-based organizations mentioned above, which is a members' organization but run for profit, delivering a service that in another country might be run by a local council. The injunction to participate, get involved, be active, *will* lead to new groupings.

Osaghae (1995, p. 194) warns of using Western models to analyse civil society, as they fail to appreciate the role of rural, kinship and ethnic-based associations – 'there is a clear misrepresentation of the Western connotation of civil society to the African situation'. He chastises the Western preoccupation with the role of civil society organizations in challenging the power of the state and argues

that there is a need to focus more on the 'traditional' self-preservationist functions of civil society in Africa (Osaghae, 1995, p. 195). He argues that these associations have functioned more as 'shadow states', providing social welfare for groups and individuals when these have not been provided by the state. Box 5.7 provides a case study of a seemingly successful association in India.

These forms of voluntary associations and ways of people coming together to take action raise what in health promotion circles is called the bottom-up/top-down dilemma.

Resolving the Top-down/Bottom-up Conundrum

A central tension exists in health promotion as to how to resolve the problem of connecting bottom-up problem solving with top-down policy making and top-down programmatic interventions. In certain instances, anti-social behaviour clearly needs to be restrained, and also we would argue that in *every* area of discrimination, legislation is needed to change institutional culture and behaviour. In relation to people with disabilities for example, Barrett *et al.* (2003, p. 229) suggest that:

> It is agreed that policies which focus on awareness raising may alter attitudes to some extent, but will not change structural, institutional behaviour and this will not reduce inequality. Legislation is required to change institutional behavior rather than relying on persuasion.

Legislation is conventionally thought of as the singular example of top-down activity but what matters is the *process* of policy making, and that it is inclusive, participatory and ultimately democratic. The predominant discourse of the Ottawa Charter and subsequent iterations of health promotion methods is of community development; in practice, however, many health promotion textbooks espouse planning models and typical programme cycles where a scoping study or needs assessment is

Box 5.6. The four sectors of communal life.	
Public sector	Government, local authorities, public bodies, public sector workers
Private sector	Businesses, industry
Third sector	NGOs, charities, foundations, formal civil society groups, associations
Fourth sector	Citizens, people, communities, volunteers, user groups, self-help groups

carried out, an intervention is designed, appraised, approved, implemented, managed to fruition and evaluated – all with varying degrees of community 'consultation' or 'participation' but the control stays with the funders and professionals. The latter's priorities may be accountability to funders, cost effectiveness and reaching targets for coverage, number of people included and so on. The well-known North Karelia Project on coronary heart disease was an early example of a massive intervention, which does appear to have had some success (Tones and Tilford, 2001). In contrast, consider the Multiple Risk Factors Intervention trial (MRFIT),

which, in 1971, surveyed 400,000 men in the USA before randomly selecting 6000 for the intervention and 6000 for the control group. After 6 years, the trial showed no difference in mortality between the control and intervention group. Similarly, the COMMIT programme (Community Intervention Trials for Smoking Cessation), involved 11,000 smokers in 11 cities with a matched control group. At the end of the trial, a very modest difference was found between the two groups despite an expenditure of millions of US dollars (Smedley and Syme, 2000). In the present century, the mood seems to have swung against these large-scale projects and towards 'local solutions for local problems', which not only keys into the zeitgeist, but also the funding landscape.

Beattie's model (Fig 5.3) has become a mainstay of health promotion textbooks, offering a way of seeing relationships between more negotiated ways of taking action in relation to more authoritative or top-down methods, and at both individual and collective levels. The model is useful in terms of helping individual workers to see where they fit in the spectrum, and in making the point that on many issues, a full range of actions (i.e. actions in each quadrant of the diagram) is required. Table 5.4 takes this discussion further by outlining the characteristics of top-down and bottom-up approaches.

For some issues, a top-down, authoritative approach is needed because it is a matter of public safety – for example, many countries have laws protecting the public in terms of regulations surrounding food handling by retailers (to avoid food poisoning), or laws on speeding, driving after consuming alcohol and car maintenance. There are areas of public safety that are so important that they cannot be left to personal choice. The limits to top-down approaches and the use of law were discussed above in the section on ethics.

What we wish to discuss here is not so much these areas where the law or tough regulation is necessary, but rather, approaches to health promotion when working with communities or in health education, and more broadly, in developing healthy public policy or organizational change. Many health initiatives adopt a 'public address system' approach where messages are simply transmitted by an outside agent in a diffusionist model. That

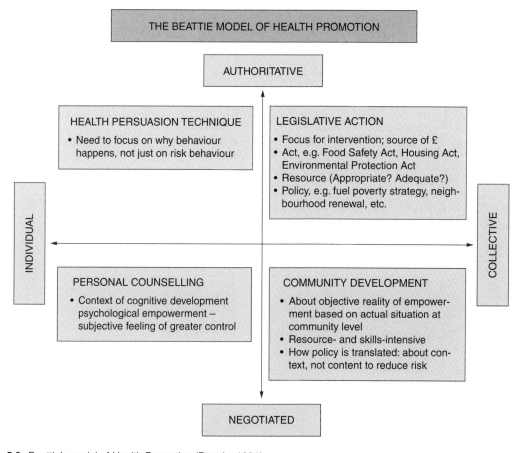

Fig. 5.3. Beattie's model of Health Promotion (Beattie, 1991).

Table 5.4. The different characteristics of top-down and bottom-up approaches (adapted from Laverack and Labonte, 2000).

Characteristic	Top-down approaches	Bottom-up approaches
Role of agents	Outside agents define the issue, develop strategies to resolve the issue, involve the community to assist with solving the issue.	Outside agents act to support the community in the identification of issues which are important and relevant to their lives and enable them to develop strategies to resolve these issues.
Power relationships	Power-over by the outside agent.	Power with and power from within. Outside agent surrenders some of their control.
Design	Defined short to medium-term time frame, fixed budget and large scale.	Long-term without a fixed time frame or design. Uses participatory approach and small scale.
Objectives	Objectives are determined by outside agent and are usually concerned with changing specific behaviours to reduce disease and improve health.	Community identifies objectives, which are negotiated with outside agent. These may be concerned with disease and behaviours, but also with community empowerment outcomes and political and social changes.
Implementation	Decisions over budget, strategy, administration, etc. essentially rests with outside agent.	Decisions are constantly being negotiated between the outside agent and the community.
Evaluation	Evaluation concerned with targets and outcomes often determined by the outside agents.	Evaluation concerned with process and outcomes, and inclusion of the participants.

'agent' is seen as having superior insight into the needs of the 'recipient' community and has produced an idea that it is believed will benefit that community. Paolo Freire describes in a stark way how well-meaning professionals actually commit acts of 'cultural invasion' in their belief that they have the answers to other people's problems (Freire, 1972). Central to health promotion thinking and values is that change occurs from below – impositions from the top and without clear and supportive frameworks for implementation are unlikely to produce change. As far back as 1976, Rogers (1976) was calling for a new paradigm arguing that this approach doesn't work. Community-led approaches with full ownership of stakeholders and strong partnerships are more likely to bring about sustainable change. Moreover, Walker (quoted in Attwood *et al.*, 2003, p. 4) suggests, 'Bright ideas dreamt up at the centre sink time and time again … [due to] … the absence of a grassroots delivery system that is both accountable and effective'. Attwood *et al.* (2003, p. 5) write about 'Mad Management Virus', which believes that 'Programmatic top-down approaches always work', and 'The more inspection and control, the better the outcome'. The Mad Management Virus sets targets and believes that these will produce specified results; it also believes

that these methods have no harmful effects on people's morale, levels of trust or engagement. In contrast,

'Positive and successful paradigms of change put users and communities at the centre, taking the view that effective lateral cooperation around action and learning can transform communities of place, interest, practice or influence.

(Attwood *et al.*, 2003, p. 7)

The aid sector, development and health promotion abound with examples where programmatic, top-down initiatives were ineffective and resulted in both rejection by the community and unsustainable interventions. As an example from the sphere of schooling, Wrigley (2000) argues that to bring about school improvement, top-down initiatives fail and only an empowerment approach will work. Attwood *et al.* (2003, p. 11) suggest a whole systems approach: 'Innovators employing whole systems methodologies seek to work in the uncomfortable spaces where the top-down collides with the horizontal and networked world of implementation. Restraining the top-down impulse in order to create virtuous cycles of hope, collective innovation and pride of purpose is what this book is all about.' The book is recommended as very useful further reading.

That people have to come up with their own solutions was recognized by the seminal work of Everett Rogers on the diffusion of innovations, whilst both Carl Rogers and Paolo Freire believed that all people have within them the ability to come up with their own solutions, as we discussed in Chapter 4. E. Rogers was interested in why some farmers adopted innovations (such as new types of seed) more readily than others. In summarizing a large body of evidence on effective adoption of new ideas by communities (Rogers and Shoemaker, 1971), they developed a matrix, which showed that where people identified both the need for change, and came up with their own solutions, change was more likely to be implemented and long-lasting, than where these were identified by outsiders. It could be hypothesized that the greater the level of outside 'intervention', as in a 'public address system' approach, the less participation there will be and the less conscientization will occur.

These questions raise important dilemmas for health promotion professionals in terms of how to work with communities and organizations. Laverack and Labonte (2000) have proposed a 'middle-out' way of working, which provides a role for workers to liaise with those above (the policy makers and so on), and the communities on the ground or 'below' – not that we like this sense of a hierarchy, but the terminology is what has become custom and practice. They also show how a 'parallel track' approach could keep a programme on track whilst also meeting empowerment objectives and methods (Fig. 5.4).

This still raises issues for the ways in which those with expertise can work with communities. Many people have skills that they have taken years to acquire, are motivated to work with communities in need and sometimes themselves come from backgrounds that are not that dissimilar from the communities in question. How can this expertise be harnessed and used appropriately, avoiding 'cultural invasion', insensitive top-down programme planning and taking into account the skills and knowledge of the community members? An example might be that a dietician with a commitment to working with parents in a poor housing area in Leeds would see it as obvious to offer nutrition and 'healthy eating on a budget' classes in local Children's Centres. The class would be advertised and take-up, typically, would be low. Those parents might not see this as a priority, or might want to tackle a more pressing issue such as the poor quality of the local

green spaces and children's play areas. If a health promoter worked with these parents, who gained knowledge and confidence in tackling the local council about their issues, they might in the future identify other issues on which they wanted some input. One of these could be thinking about how to grow more of their own food, to develop a food cooperative, and also to learn about cooking ... in which case they might approach the dieticians and invite them to work alongside them.

One initiative in which we were involved was a project with ten primary schools in Leeds to consider how they could promote more exercise and healthier eating with the longer-term goal of preventing obesity. The medically trained on the team assumed that we go into the schools with a prescription for what they needed to do in order to achieve reductions in children's body mass indexes (BMIs). The health promoters on the team were seeing the process very differently – that we would approach the school staff and ask them if they wanted to develop their own action plan for setting about the objectives. In this way, each school had a different plan, but they were all geared towards making the school a healthier place in terms of eating and exercise. The staff 'owned' the ideas and thus had an investment in bringing them to fruition. The process evaluation showed that the schools had changed in terms of their thinking and organizational cultures, but the measures such as BMI did not show any changes. If the latter was the yardstick for success, it would have been said that the project was a failure; in fact, significant differences had occurred in the schools. The point of relating this experience here is that organizational change needs to put the people in that organization at the heart of the imitative.

Skills of Health Promoters

What does all this indicate for the development of health promoters as professionals? A compounding factor is that it appears from some of the discussion above and from a number of studies (Carter *et al.*, 2009; South *et al.*, 2011) that training lay people to perform health promotion work can be as effective, if not more so, than when professionals do that work. Carter *et al.* (2009) have shown how lay people are more effective at taking accurate blood pressures (and people do not get as stressed) than physicians. The 'Watch it!' weight management

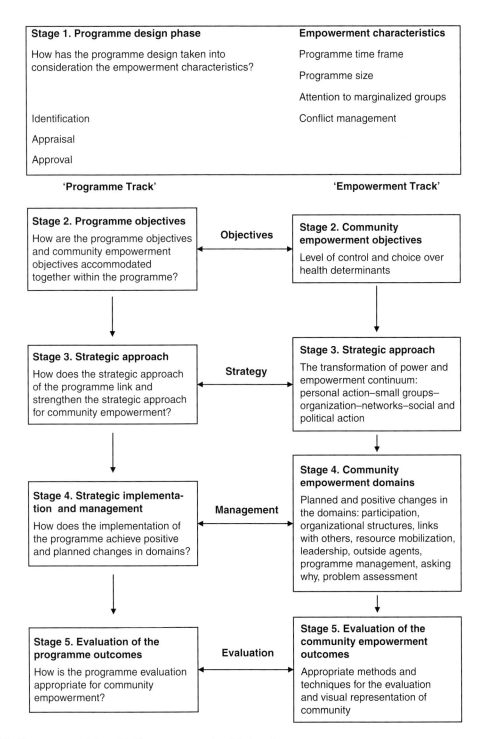

Stage 1. Programme design phase	Empowerment characteristics
How has the programme design taken into consideration the empowerment characteristics?	Programme time frame
	Programme size
	Attention to marginalized groups
Identification	Conflict management
Appraisal	
Approval	

'Programme Track' — 'Empowerment Track'

Stage 2. Programme objectives
How are the programme objectives and community empowerment objectives accommodated together within the programme?

Objectives

Stage 2. Community empowerment objectives
Level of control and choice over health determinants

Stage 3. Strategic approach
How does the strategic approach of the programme link and strengthen the strategic approach for community empowerment?

Strategy

Stage 3. Strategic approach
The transformation of power and empowerment continuum: personal action–small groups–organization–networks–social and political action

Stage 4. Strategic implementation and management
How does the implementation of the programme achieve positive and planned changes in domains?

Management

Stage 4. Community empowerment domains
Planned and positive changes in the domains: participation, organizational structures, links with others, resource mobilization, leadership, outside agents, programme management, asking why, problem assessment

Stage 5. Evaluation of the programme outcomes
How is the programme evaluation appropriate for community empowerment?

Evaluation

Stage 5. Evaluation of the community empowerment outcomes
Appropriate methods and techniques for the evaluation and visual representation of community

Fig. 5.4. The accommodation of bottom-up approaches into top-down programmes.

programme deliberately recruited people who had not previously trained in a health field (Dixey *et al.*, 2006) and 'health trainers' are another cadre of workers in the UK contributing to health promotion but without having gone through conventional medical training. Village health workers, working on a voluntary basis have a long history in many countries (Campbell and Scott, 2011). Labonte and Laverack (2010) provide a critical commentary on the whole debate about developing community capacity for health promotion. All this has implications for the notion of professionalism, professionalization and how professionals work alongside both communities and lay workers. Evans (2008, p. 23) has attempted to define 'professional' – it is an 'articulated perception of what lies within the parameters of a profession's collective remit and responsibilities', but as Holroyd (2000, p. 39) points out, 'Professionalism is not some social-scientific absolute, but a historically changing and socially constructed concept in-use'. There is agreement that professional work incorporates a body of knowledge, a set of ethics, often a professional body, which regulates its members, and also, a commitment to learning, professional updating and continuous professional development. It is not at all clear what the 'profession' of health promotion is, or what the health promotion professional would look like. One attempt to clarify this has been the discussions that led to the Galway Consensus, which as the name signifies, is a global consensus on the competencies for the specialist health promoter.

The Galway Consensus

A team of academics and practitioners, including John Allegrante, Collins Airhihenbuwa, Maurice Mittelmark and Margaret Barry have been instrumental in developing the Galway consensus, arguing (Allegrante *et al.*, 2009; Barry *et al.*, 2009) the critical need to consider what skills and competencies are required by health promoters in addressing current health challenges, such as tackling health inequities and social determinants of health, promoting healthy ageing and positive mental health. The MDGs and the report of the WHO Commission on Social Determinants of health, call for actions that require a complex mix of technical skills, expertise and leadership. Once identified, these need to inform the basis of education and training development of health promoters, so there are

important implications for colleges and universities.

The eight domains identified are:

1. **Catalysing change** – Enabling change and empowering individuals and communities to improve their health.
2. **Leadership** – Providing strategic direction and opportunities for participation in developing healthy public policy, mobilizing and managing resources for health promotion, and building capacity.
3. **Assessment** – Conducting assessment of needs and assets in communities and systems that leads to the identification and analysis of the behavioural, cultural, social, environmental and organizational determinants that promote or compromise health.
4. **Planning** – Developing measurable goals and objectives in response to assessment of needs and assets, and identifying strategies that are based on knowledge derived from theory, evidence and practice.
5. **Implementation** – Carrying out effective and efficient, culturally sensitive and ethical strategies to ensure the greatest possible improvements in health, including management of human and material resources.
6. **Evaluation** – Determining the reach, effectiveness, and impact of health promotion programmes and policies. This includes utilizing appropriate evaluation and research methods to support programme improvements, sustainability and dissemination.
7. **Advocacy** – Advocating with and on behalf of individuals and communities to improve their health and well-being and building their capacity for undertaking actions that can both improve health and strengthen community assets.
8. **Partnerships** – Working collaboratively across disciplines, sectors and partners to enhance the impact and sustainability of health promotion programmes and policies.

The Galway meetings have had representation from all parts of the globe and it is felt that the skills outlined apply to people practising anywhere in the world. Prior to the Consensus, a number of attempts had been made by the professional associations representing health promotion, to outline the core skills, and to differentiate these from public health skills. Health Scotland, for example, produced an extraordinarily detailed 112-page report listing the competencies of health promotion practitioners in 2005 (Health Scotland, 2005). The Society for Health Education and promotion Specialists in England had previously described the skills base (SHEPS, no date).

The competency approach has been criticized by some; Eraut (2004, p. 264) for example notes that 'from a learning viewpoint, competence is a moving target'. Professional learning is an ongoing process through practice (Eraut, 2001), and it is difficult to measure professional competence and professional learning (Daley, 2001) and to provide assurance of competence, particularly relating to informal learning such as in reflective practice (Friedman and Philips, 2004). Often competencies are measured against professional and occupational standards, but their rigidity can lead to a mechanical assessment of professional competence, which is not suited to the dynamism and complexity of the current public health environment (Cole, 2000). In relation to health promotion, Naidoo and Wills (2005, p. 10) have argued:

> The concept of competence has aroused much controversy. It can be seen as narrow and mechanistic, focusing on tasks and not enabling practitioners to acquire the value base essential for critical practice. All practitioners need to be not just technicians but reflective practitioners with a professional literacy. Competencies cannot cover all types of activities nor the personal processes entailed in health improvement. In specifying a range of activities in which the practitioner must perform, the role of theory and understanding is diminished. 'Knowing' becomes merely preparation for 'doing' with no requirement to reflect on theoretical bases or make sense of working practice.

The debate about a competence-based approach notwithstanding, recent decades have seen a twin track of developing the competencies for health promotion specialists and of encouraging those who could who do some health promotion as part of their main role, to develop health promotion (or at least health education) skills. The latter has usually been linked with the Ottawa Charter's call to reorient health services. We can perhaps identify *three* levels:

1. Specialist health promoters: those who have health promotion (or an equivalent) in their job title and who work for all of their time in health promotion activity; these might be health trainers, health improvement officers, etc.
2. A range of workers who have a health promotion function as part of their role, such as housing officers, social workers, community workers, nurses, doctors, clinical officers, midwives, teachers, youth workers, play workers, dieticians, pharmacists, counsellors; these workers need to have skills to enable them to do health promotion.
3. Workers who need to have a health promotion awareness, such as transport planners, architects, leisure and hospitality management workers, education officers, politicians, policy makers, etc.; these workers need to be aware of how their actions impact on health and to be aware of how they can contribute to health-promoting settings.

The Galway Consensus perhaps relates most to the first of these groups. For the second and third groups, if more preventive and upstream ways of working are to be adopted, there are implications for the kinds of skills required by *all* those who can contribute to public health – whether currently working within the health (care) service, such as nurses, physiotherapists, occupational therapists, dentists, pharmacists, or outside of it, as planners, community workers, environmental health officers, housing officers, teachers … and many more. In the UK, there has been a plethora of discussion papers about the development of the public health workforce to make sure it is 'fit for purpose' for the 21st century (DOH, 2005) and the Royal Society for Public Health hosts a 'Shaping the Future of Health' promotion website (http://www.rsph.org.uk/en/health-promotion/). Much of this discussion however, has been restricted to those working within the National Health Service (NHS) and there have been similar discussions in other countries about how health workers can contribute to broader public health goals. This picks up on the relatively neglected aspect of the Ottawa Charter, of reorienting health services.

A lot is known about the roles of various cadres of health workers in effective health communication, and behaviour change in terms of source credibility. Health visitors for example are seen as respected and credible educators by new mothers (Weeks *et al.*, 2005). Dieticians have a mixed response in terms of perceptions of their effectiveness in giving health messages (Hancock *et al.*, 2011). Much could be gained by training health workers in health promotion skills and recent years have seen interest in the role of pharmacists, and also in the role of other workers who have contact with the public, including barbers and hairdressers (Linnan and Ferguson, 2007). One of the areas of development has been in helping people to make appropriate and timely use of health care services, which is an important aspect of health education. Late presentation (for example of cancers) tends to be associated with lower socio-economic status in the UK and other developed countries. Health workers can also play a large role in encouraging parents to present children for the full range of vaccinations and in encouraging women to present early for antenatal care. Research shows that poor attitudes of health care workers is one determinant of under-utilization of services in India (Navaneetham and Dharmalingam, 2002), Jordan (Obermeyer and Potter, 1991), Pakistan (Stephenson and Hennink, 2004), Mali (Gage, 2007) and Ethiopia (Mekonnen and Mekonnen, 2003), and improvements in perceived quality of service have led to greater utilization in Bangladesh (Koenig *et al.*, 1997). These 'poor attitudes' are perhaps not surprising given the conditions many workers find themselves in. Health workers in Asia and Africa are often underpaid, lack opportunities for professional development, have high workloads and poor morale, and work in health services with poor infrastructure. Insufficient supply of health workers due to low numbers being trained in the first place is also a major factor, related to the low level of capacity of higher education institutions, particularly in many African countries (Dovlo, 2005; Dixey and Green, 2009). (This issue is explored further in Chapter 6.)

Many working in health promotion take on a training role, especially training others in health promotion skills. This is not mentioned in the eight domains of the Galway Consensus, but it is an important aspect, and some health promotion workers have an exclusive training role. There is a surprising lack of literature on the qualities that are held by highly skilled and effective trainers and how to measure these. Another relatively neglected area of work in the literature on skills is that of handling information, running public resource centres and the sorts of skills held by librarians, IT specialists, journalists and media personnel.

Developing the public health workforce is an explicit part of the UK government's strategy to improve health outcomes. *Choosing Health* (DOH, 2004) and the Darzi Report (2008) both identified the need of the health workforce to respond better in terms of promoting health. The Public Health Skills and Career Framework was published in 2008 (Public Health Resource Unit, 2008), as a

tool for describing the kinds of skills needed across the entire public health workforce, and was intended to recognize everyone's contribution to improving health, even if not in posts traditionally seen as 'health work' and those for whom 'health work' is a part of their job alongside other responsibilities. The framework provides an outline of which skills are required, which can then be used to commission a range of education and training opportunities that might provide those skills. A range of providers have responded, and offer education and training across the various levels of the framework; the concept of a skills escalator has also developed, whereby staff, once on the 'escalator', can progress. The framework has given impetus to the discussion about what kinds of skills are needed by any workers who come into contact with the public and who thus might have opportunities to carry out opportunistic or more structured health promotion activities. Naidoo *et al.* (2003) have discussed the framework's role in developing the public health workforce and described how it might work in relation to working with asylum seekers in England. Latterly, 'health trainers' have emerged as the newest addition to the public health workforce as an innovative means of tackling inequalities and helping individuals to think about their health and lifestyle.

Leadership

Arguably the chief task of specialist health promoters is to play a leadership role, and other competencies fall under this. As change agents and advocates, partnership builders and planners, such workers are expected to *lead* health promotion into the 21st century. St Leger (2001) has commented on the need for the next generation of health promotion leaders who are not only technically competent, but who are also able to lead theoretical developments, to reflect on the purpose of health promotion and to relate health promotion to broader social issues. As specialist health promoters are involved in working with communities and increasingly, with organized, active citizens, in developing healthy public policy, and working with governments, civil servants, with the complex NGO scene, developing health communication strategies, working with media organizations and negotiating the complex world of PR and public messaging, leading on organizational change to create healthy settings and raise positive health awareness across all sectors, there is a need to develop clear leadership skills. There is not the scope in this book to elaborate on leadership, and whole books are available on this. What we would say is important is that leadership remains true to health promotion principles. This requires adoption of the new thinking about leadership, as Attwood *et al.* (2003, p. 17) comment: 'The new leadership "game" is engagement and involvement, not hierarchical domination, and effective leadership involves the many rather than the few.' They quote Drath and Palus (1994, in Attwood, 2003, p. 17), who liken ideas of 'the powerful individual taking charge' to the 'white-caps on the sea – prominent and captivating', but with no recognition of the 'far vaster and more profound phenomenon out of which such waves arise'. In opposition to this 'heroic form of leadership', Attwood *et al.* (2003) argue that leaders should provide coherent frameworks within which others have space to think, to decide things for themselves, and to decide what needs changing and what does not. Thus, effective leaders develop 'holding frameworks':

> ... the job of leadership is both to set in motion the processes by which the container or framework is established, and to ensure that it operates like a membrane so that those involved (stakeholders in the issues concerned) are affected by the uncertainties of the external environment in ways that support rather than stultify their sense-making and learning.
>
> (Attwood, 2003, pp. 61–62)

The notion of holding frameworks derives from psychotherapy, where, as it can be imagined, the therapist provides a space in which to facilitate a client to work out solutions. If there is real belief that people have within them the capability of producing solutions to their own problems, and are not powerless (which we have said is central to health promotion values), then in one way the task of leadership is straightforward – it is simply to get everyone in the same space, and to have the facilitation skills to manage the engagement, resolve potential conflict and move to resolutions. (In practice, it is more complicated!) The framework can provide a set of values, purpose and strategic direction; the leader also needs to understand the 'big picture' and keep this in focus. In bringing about significant change, for example developing a Healthy City initiative, there would be considerable complexity, multiple stakeholders and a very

long-term vision. Thus, leaders in health promotion often find themselves managing networks, or even networks of networks. Networking is a skill in its own right and although linked to partnership building, it is distinct from that. The importance of networks in organizational learning and knowledge transfer and management was discussed above.

If health promoters are to get health promotion onto agendas, and mobilize organizations and communities, they need to be able to play leadership roles in networks. Part of this role involves 'knowledge renewal' (Ballantyne, 2000) or knowledge exchange. The leadership roles include: energizing and encouraging people to share experiences; 'code breaking' or helping people break into each others' worlds and language; diffusing knowledge, letting it circulate, be tested, tried out and incorporated into new practices (Senge, 1994; Horsman, 2004). Working with networks throws up a number of issues, as identified by Attwood *et al.* (2003, p. 154):

- How are the effectiveness, quality and success of networks to be defined and evaluated, and how would these be agreed?
- How can networks be effectively led?
- How are they to be governed – who is eligible to join, how should behaviour be regulated and conflicts resolved?
- Where does accountability rest – in the participating organizations or within the network, or somewhere else?
- How can the network be supported in terms of overheads, infrastructure and so on, and how are these to be managed?

Summary

This chapter has attempted to discuss some challenges in the practice of health promotion, ending on the challenges in terms of the skills required to do health promotion work. Some of these challenges reoccur in the next chapter, particularly when discussing capacity building for health promotion at a societal level rather than the individual level, as we have done here. Working ethically, developing evaluation skills and evidence-based practice are contentious areas and we do not pretend to have produced all the answers here. It remains to be seen whether settings approaches will really 'deliver'. Many factors run counter to organizations wishing to become healthier settings, not least the imperative in some sectors to be profitable or show 'value for money'. However, as we suggest in the next chapter, health promotion is an optimistic profession, and the future development of health promotion will be explored next.

Further Reading

Barnes, M. and Prior, D. (2009) *Subversive Citizens. Power, Agency and Resistance in Public Services.* The Policy Press, London.

Douglas, J., Earle, S., Handsley, S., Jones, L., Lloyd, C.E. and Spurr, S. (2010) *A Reader in Promoting Public Health: Challenge and Controversy*, 2nd edition. Sage, London.

Green, J. and South, J. (2006) *Evaluation.* Open University Press, Maidenhead, UK.

Green, J. and Tones, K. (2010) *Health Promotion: Planning and Strategies*, 2nd edition. Sage, London.

Scriven, A. and Hodgins, M. (2012) *Health Promotion Settings: Principles and Practice.* Sage, London.

6 Towards the Future of Health Promotion

RACHAEL DIXEY

This chapter aims to:

- explore the role of the epistemic and academic community of health promoters;
- suggest that there are new and emerging public health problems to take into account;
- reinforce the need to defend the radical intent of the Ottawa Charter and to develop further anti-oppressive practice;
- describe how the health promotion discourse is changing, and moving into new realms of well-being;
- reinforce the importance of hearing lay voices and understanding 'healthworlds'; and
- present some ideas for moving forward the value base of health promotion.

Introduction

This chapter has the task of reflecting on the state of health promotion in the 21st century. It would perhaps require another book to consider fully where health promotion is going, its potential as a social movement to bring about a fairer, more just world in which everyone has good health and can achieve their potential, and whether contemporary health promotion has the answers to the issues of the 21st century and its concomitant threats to health. This begs the question of what characterizes the 21st century; we suggest that globalization and climate change are two of the defining features, amongst others. What this chapter does is start to address some of these questions and suggest what the academic community can offer.

The opening chapter mentioned the existence of a number of implementation gaps, including the failure to close the gap between intentions (such as in HFA2000, the MDGs or the original aims of the Ottawa Charter) and progress on the ground, as measured by inequalities in health. This chapter considers the slow, uneven progress towards developing health promotion globally by considering its tardy implementation in the continent of Africa. The politically fraught nature of developing health promotion will be exemplified by charting its fortunes in England, where currently health promotion is in a major decline. The chapter illustrates

how language reflects power, and that the discourse around public health in England has quietly dropped 'health promotion'. This reminds us that discourse not only reflects reality, but it helps to construct it, and as that construction can shut off other ways of seeing, it is very powerful.

The epistemic health promotion community has drawn attention to the ways in which the radical intent of the initial key documents and conferences, which brought paradigm shifts in thinking and which are essential milestones in our history, has been diluted by the political forces that have no interest in prioritizing social justice in health. Hall and Taylor (2003) suggest that as soon as the Alma-Ata conference was over, primary health care came under attack and papers abound with the notion of a retreat from Alma-Ata, such as Campbell and Scott (2011). The health promotion community has been vocal in defending the legacy of Ottawa and Alma-Ata but as *health promotion* remains a contested concept, there has been disagreement amongst that community too. Our view is that the original radicalism *has* indeed been diluted, though the high-level activities on social determinants have restored some of this.

Leadership in health promotion for the 21st century has never been more essential. What has been already won needs be guarded and energy is required to stay involved in the politics of implementing the vision. Health promotion is an intellectual activity applied practically. Academic health promotion plays an essential role in developing the theory behind practice; it also plays a crucial role in defending health promotion, developing the evidence base to show whether and how it works. By academic, we do not merely mean those who work in universities or other higher education institutions (HEIs), but all those who contribute to the literature on health promotion, to theory-building, evaluation studies and so on. They could be working in para-statal bodies, NGOs, government or as freelancers, as well as in HEIs.

The academic community, in our view, has a fivefold role:

1. To maintain a watch on the implementation of the vision, to ensure that health promotion ideas remain radical and do not become distorted and diluted, and thus to carry out analysis, such as discourse analysis, to ensure this.
2. To continually refresh the theoretical base, move across disciplinary boundaries, and draw on relevant ideas which can enrich understanding and thus inform practice.
3. To challenge health inequities and oppressive practice and to present critiques of systems of stratification or divisions which mean that people cannot reach their full potential.
4. To suggest ways of theorizing and understanding key challenges of the 21st century – among them, globalization, climate change, engaging with communities and the 'search for meaning'.
5. To take seriously the need to develop the evidence base for health promotion, publishing both what works and what doesn't, whilst also defending the value base, and bearing in mind that 'what really counts can't always be counted'.

These five dimensions are not in any particular order – they are all important.

It goes without saying, too, that the academic community needs to publish, but more than that, needs to dialogue and engage with policy makers and others in power. In addition, we would argue that HEIs, including universities such as our own, have a fourfold role:

1. To carry out high-quality research that makes a difference on the ground.
2. To develop capacity in health promotion, thus developing the health promotion workforce and adding to human resources for health.

3. To engage with communities.
4. To model a settings approach by becoming health-promoting universities.

Implementing the Vision of Health Promotion

The changing discourse of health promotion

Academics and practitioners have questioned whether health promotion has strayed from its radical roots based in the Alma-Ata Declaration and the Ottawa Charter, and also whether progress has been made on primary health care or on Ottawa's five action areas (Baum and Sanders, 1995; Hall and Taylor, 2003). Arguably, much progress has been made in building public policy, though Sparks (2011) warns against the 'misdirection' generated by opponents of healthy public policy. Developing healthy public policy has been key to the modern health promotion movement but has more recently come under attack by those who wish to 'roll back the state' in the current neoliberal climate. Despite the clear evidence that using public policy to tackle, for example, tobacco control or road safety, and that it is nearly impossible to do so without regulatory support from above, those on the political right use the arguments about individual freedom and the 'nanny state' to dispense with those regulatory, policy frameworks and legislation that promotes health. Sparks' response to this threat is to suggest that we need to build persuasive arguments and a firmer evidence base of what works in terms of the role of healthy public policy – 'The impending 25th anniversary of the Ottawa Charter is a fitting occasion to rekindle our efforts' (Sparks, 2011, p. 262). The special edition of *Health Promotion International*, mentioned in Chapter 1, contains a detailed investigation of the impact of the Ottawa Charter and its continuing relevance.

Other areas of the Ottawa Charter have not fared as well: whilst the environmental movement has given attention to the emphasis on supportive environments, and the application of newer concepts such as social capital has led impetus to the creation of strong communities, the development of personal skills has been lower on the agenda. Nutbeam (2008, p. 439) argues that, 'the Ottawa Charter led to relative neglect of health education as a tool for health promotion'. He suggests that the development of concepts such as health literacy has given renewed energy to the importance of health education, and we would assert too, that this is a key aspect of health promotion. (Health education was considered in Chapter 4.) The newer cadres of health workers such as health trainers, mentioned in Chapter 5, are increasingly contributing to the development of personal skills, confidence and health literacy. In the USA, given its more individualistic orientation in health promotion and its emphasis on health education, has perhaps led to greater theoretical development here than in the rest of the world (Lightsey *et al.*, 2005).

The final area of action, reorienting health services has perhaps been the most disappointing and most difficult to see progress in. Not only has the radical vision of Alma-Ata failed to materialize in bringing primary care to developing countries, but in those 'industrialized countries' represented in Ottawa, there has been a corresponding lack of a shift in emphasis towards prevention, primary (rather than tertiary) care, or increased funding for health promotion within health care. The importance of health care services, whilst recognized in 'developed' countries, is perhaps underplayed in countries where good quality health care, and free access to it, is taken for granted (except in countries such as the USA where millions do not have free health care), but the disease burden in parts of the world is not only high, but access to health care

is highly problematic. This aspect of promoting health needs not to be neglected. Possibly one reason for the failure is a lack of interest in 'healthy' people by those who have been motivated to train to 'help sick people'.

Secondly, however, there is a lack of incorporation of what is known about people's health-seeking behaviours into service planning. There are many studies about people's behaviours in relation to health and illness, from uptake of services such as immunization and screening to illness behaviours and seeking medical help. For instance Chen *et al.*'s (2006) work on lay beliefs about hepatitis among North American Chinese shows why they do not seek health care in the form of vaccinations – because they saw hepatitis as caused by harmful food, alcohol, stress and lack of adequate rest, as much as infection, and strategies to prevent it were more likely to involve tackling stress and getting rest. Similarly, de-Graft Aikins *et al.* (2010) explored ideas about chronic illness in Ghana and Cameroon, and found that the complex ideas about the causes of, for example, diabetes, led to people engaging in 'medical pluralism' – that is not only using biomedical help but also ethnomedical and faith healing systems. In relation to the choice of health systems, Siahpush (2000) explored studies on people's use of alternative or complementary therapies. Much is known about men's health-seeking behaviours,

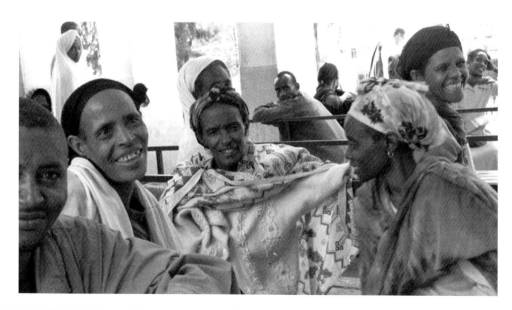

Women attending a primary health care clinic, Jima, Ethiopia.

but this is not reflected in any major way in finding alternative means of gendering service provision. Thus, for instance, White and Johnson (2000) explore men's delay in seeking help for chest pain, Buckley and O Tuama (2010) Irish men's behaviours as health consumers and Matthewson (2009) young men's health-related behaviours in Senegal. According to Saltonstall (1993), health becomes a way of 'doing gender', and so men's actions are very much linked to hegemonic concepts of masculinity. These need to be understood if health services are to be effectively reoriented. There was also some discussion of the role of health workers' attitudes in Chapter 5 in terms of reorienting services.

Relatively recently, discourse analysis has been used to dissect the texts which have enshrined the basic principles and goals of the modern health promotion movement. Discourse analysis of this kind helps to illustrate how 'social movement frames gain wide appeal but over time lose their progressive formulation that incited their production or, more are used to counter progressive goals' (Naples, 2003, p. 89). In other words, the radical nature behind the original movement becomes diluted and subverted by the 'powers that be'. Discussion of discourse usually begins with Foucault's understanding of the term, as

> ... systems of thoughts composed of ideas, beliefs and practices that systematically construct the subjects and the words of which they speak. He traces the role of discourses in wider social processes of legitimation and power, emphasising the constitution of current truths, how they are maintained and what power relations they carry with them.
>
> (Lessa, 2006, p. 285)

Discourse analysis starts with the premise that language is central to the creation of discourse/s and therefore that language is central in reflecting and perpetuating power structures (Lupton, 1992). Discourses thus create 'regimes of truth' (Lessa, 2006, p. 285), which come to be 'hegemonic', i.e. those regimes of truth come to be accepted as the norm, keeping in place the status quo in terms of power structures. Scott-Samuel and Springett (2007) put this clearly when they write:

> Gramsci, Foucault and Bourdieu have all pointed to the relationship between discourse (that is, knowledge associated with a particular theme – such as public health) and power. Their mutual nature ensures that as a particular discourse becomes more prominent, the power of the groups whose interests it represents

increases. Just as discourse shapes relations of power, the latter in turn shape how and by whom discourse is influenced over time.

Their perspective on how the discourse has changed in England, resulting in a dramatic decline in the fortunes of health promotion, is discussed below. Particular groups, through their ability to influence and sponsor the dominant discourse, are able to promote their own interests; they have a 'voice'.

Porter (2006), in a useful paper, compared the Ottawa Charter and the Bangkok Charter using critical discourse theory to analyse how the health promotion discourse has changed in highly significant ways from 1986 to 2005. She argues that the language of the Bangkok Charter has become far more timid; whereas the Ottawa Charter *directed* and said 'we must', Bangkok merely makes suggestions and calls for certain actions to take place. Whilst Ottawa was framed in terms of a 'new social movement' discourse (emphasizing empowerment, action on social determinants, community participation), Bangkok replaces this with a 'new capitalism' discourse, where adjustments to health status are made by changes to the economy. Whereas sociology and ecology framed Ottawa, resulting in a stress on a 'socio-ecological' approach, Bangkok privileges economics – 'Discursively, this proposes cleaning up messes of new capitalism, but not questioning their sources' (p. 77). Porter sees a move from 'participatory democracy' to 'global technocracy': 'Ottawa foregrounds people, whereas Bangkok emphasizes policy and functions ... Ottawa explicitly constructs people as diverse and complex', whereas Bangkok emphasizes global governance with little mention of local action (Porter, 2006, p. 76). The social justice agenda of Ottawa is replaced by a concern to improve health opportunities rather than suggesting that these need to be equitable. She argues that the discourse analysis suggests that the holistic view of health of Ottawa has been lost, people have become consumers, and there is a shift from workers and their needs to employers' roles.

Raphael (2003) has shown how the health promotion discourse in Canada shifted through the adoption of the term 'population health', which has served to depoliticize health promotion; moreover, despite being a world leader (Pederson *et al.*, 2005) in the development of health promotion, Raphael argues that the approach in reality in Canada is still very downstream and medically oriented. More recently his discourse analysis (Raphael, 2011) of the social determinants of health (SDH) shows how varied are the responses to the SDH agenda. He identifies seven discourses, ranging from conservative to radical; at one end, SDH is seen merely as being concerned with identifying those in need of health and social services, a problem that will be solved by extending service provision to those groups. At the other extreme are discourses that see SDH resulting from economic and political structures and their justifying ideologies, and as centring on identifying those classes and interests that benefit from social and health inequalities. The more conservative discourse is capable of derailing the original intent of the Marmot review of the SDH.

This next section considers the challenges facing the development of health promotion in sub-Saharan Africa. It later goes on to discuss how 'health promotion' has lost its place in England. In some European countries, health promotion appears to be on the ascendency (Ziglio *et al.*, 2005); Poland, for example, in its period of political–economic transformation, can be seen to be developing its Ottawa Charter credentials (Tobiasz-Adamczyk *et al.*, 2009), and health promotion seems alive and well in the Scandinavian countries. Whereas the Ottawa Charter was principally concerned with the health of 'industrialized nations', and the Lalonde report with developing new approaches to the ill health of an affluent society, the Alma-Ata Declaration in 1978 was a more relevant cornerstone on which to reorient health and health care in resource-poor countries, and it was only really the Jakarta Declaration that made prominent the needs of the 'developing' world. Indeed, the conference in Indonesia helped to infuse energy into health promotion there, although the state of Indonesian health promotion remains patchy (Chu, 2003). Another middle-level-income country, Brazil, has developed health promotion along the lines of Ottawa (Carvalho *et al.*, 2005; Tavares *et al.*, 2005), although the challenges facing Latin America remain huge. It has been described as the most inequitable continent with enormous epidemiological complexity (Arroyo, 2005). The relatively wealthy and middle income countries of South-east Asia have developed 'Boards' to organize their central agencies for health promotion, such as the Singapore Health Promotion Board, or the Thailand Health Promotion Board and that in Malaysia; Korea meanwhile has a Health Promotion

Foundation, as does China. Russia has struggled to build health promotion into its emerging reformed healthy systems (Tillinghast and Tchernjavskii, 1996) and the former Soviet Union generally is faced with many public health problems (Godhino, 2005). After Jakarta, subsequent international conferences, particularly Mexico, addressed the glaring equity gaps between the richest and poorest countries. This is not to say that the Ottawa Charter is inappropriate for resource-poor countries, but countries that have not gone through epidemiological or demographic transitions have a range of health issues not faced by wealthy, industrialized countries. Health promotion in resource-poor countries tends not to be principally concerned with tackling the determinants of health, but with Information, Education and Communication (IEC) activities, encouraging people to make better and more timely use of health services, and encouraging community mobilization.

Bringing health promotion about in sub-Saharan Africa

Africa is a huge continent and generalizations about it are usually not a good idea. It is essential to counter the negative view and misperceptions of Africa held by the West. For example, whereas Africa is seen as famine-ridden, only one of the 20 largest famines (in terms of lives lost) during the 20th century occurred in Africa (Keneally, 2011). Several African economies are growing at rates higher than those in Europe. However, it is generally understood that Africa remains the least 'developed' continent, characterized by a high disease burden, large number of wars and civilian conflicts, and high dependency on overseas aid. Collier (2007) has gone so far as to adopt the term 'Africa+' to describe the 'bottom billion' – those poorest countries including the poorest in the continent of Africa, plus Haiti, Bolivia and the Central Asian countries Laos, Cambodia, Yemen, Burma and North Korea. Whilst this use of 'Africa' as a pseudonym for poverty, corruption, conflict and marginalization is to be resisted, there do remain important questions about why many African countries contain a disproportionate amount of health and development problems.

Health promotion in Africa is generally recognized as being in a poor state (Sanders *et al.*, 2008; Amunyunzu-Nyamongo and Nyamwaya, 2009).

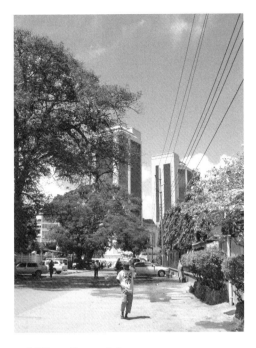

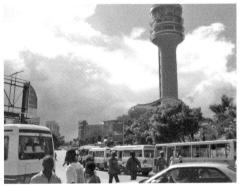

Images of Africa – Dar-es-Salaam.

Loss of trained health care personnel in sub-Saharan Africa, due to migration, death and other factors is threatening the sustainability of health systems in many African states. The crisis of health care staff has been cited as one reason why sub-Saharan Africa will not meet the MDGs (Economic Commission on Africa, 2005). The 'health worker crisis' refers to the severe shortage of trained health staff – doctors, nurses, allied health professionals – that characterizes most African health care systems (WHO, 2006). The size, nature and causes of this crisis have been well explored elsewhere, with, for example, Dovlo's (2003, 2005) and Huddart and Picazo's (2003) descriptions of the 'brain drain' and its effect on retention of health professionals in Africa. The centre of the problem, according to Dovlo's analysis, is the 'huge demands emanating from the developed countries' (Dovlo, 2003, p. 1), where health workers are pulled towards better salaries, better conditions of service and opportunities for professional development.

The crisis facing health care systems raises a larger and more fundamental question of whether health care workforce planning based on 'Western' models are – or ever were – sustainable. The emphasis on expensive, curative care in poorer countries was challenged by the Declaration of Alma-Ata (WHO, 1978), which attempted to divert more funding into primary care, accessible to the majority, rather than into tertiary care in the urban centres. Universal primary care has been subverted and the original ideals diluted (Baum and Sanders, 1995). There remains a lack of emphasis within Ministries of Health on preventive public health, of 'upstream thinking' and of tackling the determinants of poor health. Ironically, the lack of trained health (read 'medical') staff *has* resulted in the need to rethink how health care is provided, resulting in cadres of village health workers, public health officers and clinical officers, all of which can be provided more cheaply than expensively trained doctors.

The Nairobi Conference was the first international health promotion conference organized in Africa, enabling more Africans than previously to participate. Catford's (2010), conference reflections describe Africa's opportunity 'to light the way' forward for health promotion, thus closing the obvious 'implementation gap' between the rhetoric and the reality. He commends the 'vitality, level-headedness and commitment' of African participants, despite the 'lack of resources and infrastructure' available for health promotion in their countries, and comments, 'We look in eager anticipation to see how Africa moves ahead in closing the implementation gap in health promotion' (Catford, 2010, p. 3). Is this feasible, given that many African nations face lack of access to safe water and sanitation, serious communicable diseases, so-called 'tropical' diseases such as malaria, and high rates of infant and maternal mortality? Globally, Africa experiences the highest rates of HIV, putting huge strains on already stretched health care services and on the fabric of those societies worst affected. Bartram and Cairncross (2010) suggest that diarrhoeal diseases claim more lives of children under the age of 5 in developing countries than does the combination of malaria, TB and HIV/AIDS; 75% of mortality in poorer counties is associated with poor hygiene, water and sanitation. Few households have water connected to their houses, leading to contamination before use. Poor roads, undeveloped transport systems, poor telecommunications and large distances between health facilities feature in many rural communities, affecting access to basic preventive and curative services (Mooney, 2000; Skinner *et al.*, 2005; Peltzer, 2007). Poor quality of care and negative attitudes of health care staff have been shown to affect use of services (Kebaabetswe, 2007). Front line health workers are often underpaid, lack continuing professional development opportunities, work in poor conditions with chronic understaffing and have low morale.

Two Africans writing about health promotion (Amunyunzu-Nyamongo and Nyamwaya, 2009) comment:

> The most confounding factor to health promotion development in Africa emanates from the fact that health promotion activities are in most cases, planned, managed and controlled exclusively by health staff, mostly from within the ministry of health. The main actors are health workers whose concept of health is based on the conventional public health model and whose focus is on interventions revolving around curative services.
>
> (p. 21)

Nyamwaya (2003, 2005) suggests that health promotion development *has* accelerated over the last 20 years, but there remains 'an undeclared war for supremacy among different practitioners … health education practitioners, medical doctors, nurses and professionals from areas such as social mobilization, behaviour change communication and social

marketing, who are jostling for niches' (Nyamwaya, 2003, p. 2). In terms of health promotion, Amunyunzu-Nyamongo *et al.* (2009, p. 185) comment that, 'the continent is characterized by a worrying disconnect between policy and implementation which remains one of the key challenges to the development of health promotion in the region.' Amunyunzu-Nyamongo *et al.* (2009) point to six areas that require attention if health promotion is to develop in Africa. These are: (i) to invest in health; (ii) to develop more robust health systems; (iii) to build capacity in health promotion; (iv) to work within traditional and new settings; (v) to cultivate political will; and (vi) to generate evidence of health promotion effectiveness. Sub-Saharan Africa, the world's poorest region, has the highest disease burden, least number of trained health personnel and least developed infrastructure for health promotion.

Although there is substantial 'health promotion' or health education type activity in Africa, it is not 'big picture health promotion', occurring at a policy level true to the Ottawa Charter – addressing the SDH or concerned with tackling inequalities, empowerment and with people taking control of their health. On the other hand, there *is* 'small picture' health promotion, which can be seen as an adjunct to the medical enterprise, concerned with health education, encouraging people to make better use of preventive health services and so on. Moving into more radical 'big picture' health promotion remains challenging. The 'implementation gap' continues.

If African colleagues are to take forward the health promotion agenda in Africa, the academic infrastructure needs strengthening. Outside South Africa, the academic infrastructure for health promotion is under-developed, and where health promotion *is* offered, it tends to be as part of a medically dominated university public health department. Onya (2009) describes the 'serious' lack of training capacity in African health promotion, related partly to the low level of capacity of higher education institutions in Africa. Before 1960, only 18 of the 48 sub-Saharan countries had a university (Sawyerr, 2002), despite which African universities are acknowledged to have performed well in terms of producing human resources to replace colonial officials (Ajayi *et al.*, 1996). However, in the interconnected global knowledge economy of the 21st century, and the marketization trajectory that universities in the global North have been on for some time, African universities face becoming marginalized (Sawyerr, 2002).

Understanding the Demise of 'Health Promotion' in England

The history of health promotion in England demonstrates the way in which the dominant ideology and the views of the government in power affects policy towards health and its determinants. Currently, there is a great deal of pessimism among the health promotion community in England; it has fared better in Wales and Scotland, but in England, Scott-Samuel and Wills (2007, p. 115) have gone as far as to say that health promotion 'may either be dead or just becalmed and waiting to be brought back to life'. Scott-Samuel and Springett (2007, p. 211) show how 'the words health promotion have been steadily disappearing from the public health discourse in England'. During the 1970s, the Labour government continued to emphasize health education and narrow lifestyle approaches; it did not appear to recognize the shifts being fostered by the Lalonde report. The arrival of the Thatcher government in 1979, and its suppression of the Black report into inequalities in health, did not presage a new dawn, but surprisingly, health promotion did 'develop and even flourish in the context of local government and the non-statutory sector' (Scott-Samuel and Springett, 2007, p. 212). Despite a government 'diametrically opposed to [a] social justice agenda' (Scott-Samuel and Wills, 2007, p. 116), the 1980s saw a period of health promotion activism, where the settings approach, strong Health Cities networks, the Health For All movement and fora provided by journals such as *Radical Community Medicine* and the pressure group Public Health Alliance, 'temporarily liberated health promotion from the distortions of biomedicine and placed it firmly in the hands of the local state' (Scott-Samuel and Springett, 2007, p. 213). Later, when the NHS was reorganized, public health came under the newly formed Primary Care Trusts, and health promoters were thus embedded within the health (sickness) service. Many of us would argue that placing health promotion and the wider public health within local government, which are inherently political bodies, is more helpful than placing them within the National Health Service, where officers have to exempt themselves from political activities. There is an irreconcilable contradiction here. (Incidentally, although there are further setbacks for health policy under the more conservative government elected in 2010, at least the proposed move back to local authorities is a welcome move.)

The New Labour government of 1997 appeared committed to tackling poverty, deprivation and health. Due to misguided attempts at strengthening public health (looking at it charitably), Scott-Samuel and Springett (2007, p. 213) suggest that it was over 5 years into their term of office that New Labour 'began to listen to the message about its destruction of health promotion'. Although it introduced a range of initiatives that were welcomed by the health promotion community – neighbourhood renewal, Sure Start (to provide pre-school children with a better start in life), the social exclusion unit – these social projects were not, according to Scott-Samuel and Wills (2007, p. 117), part of a 'coherent health-focussed strategy'. Health promotion has been subsumed into public health, which itself is still, despite re-branding itself from *public health medicine*, allied to a medical model. Health promotion specialist teams were disbanded and scattered throughout the NHS. The term 'health improvement' crept into the policy language; as Scott-Samuel and Springett (2007) comment, 'Health improvement is a target' – it does not signify the values and processes of health promotion, which is a coherent ideology with sets of principles and methods of working. The move away from 'health promotion' reflected, in part, a theme that 'health promotion has not worked'. French and Milner wrote in 1993, 'We have come to the conclusion that health education/promotion practice in this country, funded at current levels, cannot have any major impact on mortality or morbidity at the overall population level' (French and Milner, 1993, p. 98). They made a case for a new term, health development, and called for a more realistic approach to improving the health of the population, given funding levels. They outline this new way of working in their paper, which includes not working to produce structural change, but instead to focus on working at the personal and small group level. In a response to their ideas, Brown and Piper (1993) suggest that what French and Milner describe could equally be described as health promotion, but to abandon structural change would be to move in a more conservative direction than many health promoters would want to. Later, the term health improvement came to predominate, though *health development* is also present. Each iteration, it can be argued, waters down the progressive intent of the early health promoters.

Despite this gloomy picture, what is occurring on the ground might be more cheering. The 2011 Health

Promotion Awards in England, for example, awarded by the Royal Society for Public Health illustrated that 'In a changing public health landscape, health promotion still features as a mainstream approach to improve health and address the wider social determinants' (Araujo, 2011, p. 15). Moreover,

> This year's winners illustrate the importance of partnership working and the enduring relevance of the Ottawa Charter approach to improving and sustaining community health and well-being. The impact that each project has had on its local community shows that when it comes to improving health, a joined-up approach is key. This is a sentiment that Sir Michael Marmot, Director, UCL Institute of Health Equity, was keen to emphasize when he congratulated one of the winners ...
>
> (Araujo, 2011, p. 15)

Thus there remains the possibility for 'street level bureaucrats' and dedicated health promoters to carry on activities despite the lack of endorsement from government policy, but with the welcome support of key players such as Michael Marmot. In addition, documents such as Shircore (2009), which is a key government policy document, clearly demonstrates the role of health promotion.

These case studies of countries in Africa and of England illustrate that there remains an on-going battle to wrest control of health promotion from health *care* sectors and the dominance of the biomedical model. This resonates with Tobiasz-Adamczyk *et al.*'s (2009) account of the early failures of health promotion in Poland, because it was dominated by the biomedical model and its interventions not only reinforced, but in some cases, increased existing health inequalities. Many countries have made attempts to increase health promotion but, failing to appreciate the Ottawa Charter's central idea that the key sectors to promote health lie outside the health (care) sector, tend to send health (care) workers on courses. As an example, two of us from Leeds Met were asked to run a health promotion course for the Eastern Mediterranean Regional Office (EMRO) of the WHO. This 2-week course aimed to reorient health systems in the participating countries (mainly in the 'Middle East') towards a more health-promoting approach. All those sent on the course were medical doctors. Whilst there are medical doctors who have made massive contributions to health promotion (among them, Michael Marmot, David Sanders, David Werner, Alex Scott-Samuel), they have done so by moving away from a clinical, down-

stream place of working. Normally, doctors are not well placed from where they sit to undertake health promotive, upstream strategies. We will always need doctors to rescue the ill and diseased and it is vital that they are there. However, the failure to appreciate the social model of health seriously hampers the development of health promotion. It means that health promotion continues to be seen as an adjunct to the medical, health care enterprise.

Refreshing the Theory Base

There is no dispute that health promotion requires a robust theory base. McQueen *et al.* (2007) have arguably led the debates on developing appropriate theory bases for health promotion in the 21st century.

Mittelmark (2005) has expressed frustration that health promotion tends to be insular and is missing opportunities for theoretical development due to a lack of attention to the importance of communicating with other disciplines. He gives the example of community psychology as one where there are clear parallels between the two areas:

> With its longstanding emphases on person-environment fit in community settings, coping and social support, promotion of social competence, stimulation of citizen participation and empowerment, and organizing for community and social change, community psychology bears a striking resemblance to health promotion.
>
> (Mittelmark, 2005, p. 55)

Nelson and Prilleltensky's work (2010) in community psychology, where they see its mission as advancing the liberation and well-being of oppressed communities, would concur with this.

This statement suggests what Mittelmark, a key figure in contemporary health promotion, sees health promotion *as*. It also suggests that students of health promotion need to read in other disciplines, and to look critically at what disciplines health promotion *does* draw on. The usual starting point for considering the multidisciplinary nature of health promotion is Bunton and MacDonald's (1992) seminal book. They provide discussion of the contribution to health promotion of sociology, psychology, education, epidemiology, economics, social policy, marketing and communications. At the point they wrote that book, there was a concerted effort to move health promotion in the direction of a social model of health (as opposed to a medical model) and thus there is a discernible lack of attention to the disciplines of medicine, nursing or social work: knowledge areas based on a personal relationship between professionals and clients/patients have tended to be less favoured within the health promotion academic community in the attempt to move health promotion more towards social policy and strategic level development. These mentioned areas undoubtedly have made important contributions; social work, for example, was among the first to discuss empowerment (Gutierrez, 1991) and to develop a coherent value base for practice based on a changed power dynamic between professionals and clients (Dalyrymple and Burke, 2001).

Our overview of lay people's ideas about health and illness has continually made reference to the social and cultural context of such ideas. In this, sociological and anthropological accounts frequently differ from psychological accounts that usually stress theories of social learning and social cognition (Stainton-Rogers, 1991).

As a discipline that draws on other primary disciplines, health promotion is something of a 'hybrid' discipline, or as Seedhouse (1997) describes it, a 'magpie profession'. (A magpie is a European bird, which, like other members of the crow family, likes to collect objects at random and take them to its nest.) Thus health promotion has much in common with a range of areas with double-barrelled names: environmental psychology, political ecology, cultural epidemiology, social psychology, behavioural economics, which, according to Mittelmark (2005), would enrich health promotion. A further example of a secondary discipline that health promotion could draw on is leisure studies, which is essentially concerned with how people gain meaning in their lives through their non-work activities, the role of purposeful activity in mental and emotional health, and how people use their leisure time for pursuits that are health-enhancing. There has been a similar debate within leisure studies to that within health promotion, about whether it is truly a discipline in its own right. As an example of how interesting material can be found in a variety of academic journals, the *British Journal of Guidance and Counselling* has a whole edition devoted to the relationship between leisure and health, with eight papers on this theme (e.g. Trenberth, 2005).

The need for academic health promotion to extend beyond borders fits with all the thinking within the *practice* of health promotion that, as the determinants of health lie outside the health (sickness) service, there is a need to develop partnerships,

inter-professional and inter-sectoral collaboration, and to liaise with sectors such as transport, housing, employment, education, agriculture, architecture, urban design, media – in short, with those sectors where health *originates*. It makes sense, therefore, that health promotion as an academic discipline, needs to cross boundaries and to capitalize on the insights of any relevant disciplines. This leads to a discussion of whether health promotion is multi-disciplinary and/or interdisciplinary.

Health promotion describes itself as eclectic and multidisciplinary (McQueen, 2001). Multidisciplinarity is usually taken to mean that several disciplines have something to offer in understanding a phenomenon, such as the rise of gang violence; interdisciplinarity is taken to mean that disciplines borrow ideas from each other, in a transfer of insights. Given the complexity of the determinants of health in the complex world of the 21st century, there is a need perhaps to go further than this. Albrecht *et al.* (1998) call for a transdisciplinary paradigm in order to understand human health, where a unified conceptual framework can incorporate the diversity presented by different disciplines and thus help to understand the complexity of the world. How a transdisciplinary paradigm could be adopted in health promotion remains to be discussed and worked out. What is important is that health promotion does not occupy a liminal disciplinary space, being neither one thing nor another. Already, it is difficult for those outside health promotion to always grasp fully what it is about; this means it is more difficult for managers (such as in universities or health ministries) to appreciate what it is, especially in comparison to such well defined areas as nursing or physiotherapy, making it easy to marginalize it.

A further challenge for the development of the theory base of health promotion is to ensure that it does not remain Eurocentric. MacDonald (1998) espoused his view over a decade ago, that health promotion *is* a Eurocentric phenomenon and more recently, there have been calls to develop a critical public health in the global South (Colvin, 2011). Airhihenbuwa is one of the main critics who have pointed out how Western models of, for example, psychology, do not serve well those societies that do not derive their values from individualistic norms, and he also suggests that health promotion has been mishandled in Africa by emphasizing for example, individual empowerment, rather than understanding the collective and communitarian nature of those societies. He writes:

Theories based on the individual, which may be effective and meaningful in Western context, have lesser relevance in self-effacing cultures of Asia, Africa, Latin America, and the Caribbean. In these regions, family and community are more central to the construction of health and well-being than the individual, even though the individual is always recognized as an important part of the cultural context. In these cultures, individuals are less likely also to express themselves and less likely to articulate their level of well-being from the standpoint of 'ego' (the 'I'). It is the state of well-being of family and community that regulates how individuals measure their state of health. Moreover, theories and models based on measuring how the individual feels about himself or herself (e.g. 'I feel good about myself') could never capture the health locus of control in many societies because such control rests somewhere outside the self. Within this self-effacing construct, individuals are not always accustomed to expressing their attitudes and beliefs by using extreme descriptors often found on social science survey instruments such as 'strongly agree' or 'strongly disagree'. In fact, to do so within such a cultural context is considered disrespectful. Yet instruments designed to measure health behavior, for example, self-efficacy, often are presented on such a continuum of two extremes (strongly agree to strongly disagree) in cultures where such measures are not only irrelevant but could also be considered offensive. To capture the complexity of the context within which an individual is part, one needs a framework that underscores the component of context that features culture as a central and organizing theme (Sue, 1994; Airhihenbuwa, 2007). The professional and cultural partiality of the Westernized approach to the understanding of self renders problematic findings from much social and behavioral science research in Africa, Asia, Latin America, and the Caribbean.

(Airhihenbuwa and Obregon, 2000, pp. 10–11)

The privileging of Northern discourse is not unusual in academic circles, despite the postmodern questioning of what counts as legitimate knowledge (Best and Kellner, 1997; Sharp, 2008). This has implications for health promotion. Robins (2004) for example, argues that tackling the massive AIDS epidemic in South Africa will not be effective using 'Northern' approaches, without incorporating local interpretations of HIV and AIDS. The role of lay knowledge has been debated in health promotion: for instance, Popay *et al.* (1998, p. 619), in their exploration of the place of lay knowledge in theorizing about

health inequalities conclude: 'Lay knowledge therefore offers a vitally important but neglected perspective on the relationship between social context and the experience of health and illness at the individual and population level.'

In work on lay epidemiologies, the idea has been extended recently into notions of 'community epidemiologies', for example in the work of Salant and Gehlert (2008), on African Americans' ideas about breast cancer risk. The authors argue that, when discussing breast cancer risk, whether in nostalgic memories about traditional ways of life in the South, or references to competing health risks and the sense of being victimized by outside forces, community played 'a central conceptual role in participants' responses' (p. 612).

Others are more critical of this postmodern privileging of all accounts of health and illness, whether professional or not; Prior (2003), for example, acknowledges the experiential dimensions of lay knowledge, but points out the limitations of such knowledge and challenges the notion of lay 'expertise'. Allmark and Tod (2006) explore the ethical dilemmas for health professionals posed by a lay epidemiology that conflicts with medical advice, but conclude: 'engaging with lay epidemiology is likely to increase the effectiveness of public health work, as well as helping ensure that it is ethically sound' (Allmark and Tod, 2006, p. 463). That position is endorsed by Henderson (2010, p. 5), who suggests that if health professionals privilege scientific knowledge over lay knowledge this risks 'misunderstanding the manner in which the experiences and belief of their clients impact health-seeking behaviour', and this will undermine their practice.

Challenging Oppression

The third of the roles of academic health promotion outlined at the start of this chapter was to challenge health inequities and oppressive practice, and to present critiques of systems of stratification or divisions, which mean that people cannot reach their full potential. Academics have provided a sociology *of* health promotion (Bunton *et al.*, 1996) and also made use of critical theory to challenge orthodoxies in order to bring about transformational change. Health promoters need to be self-reflexive, reflective practitioners who do not get lost in theory, but who use theory to better understand the complexities of real life and thus come up with robust means of bringing real health and social justice to people on the ground. A key aspect of health promotion is to develop anti-oppressive practice and thus to challenge oppression wherever it is encountered. What does the academic community within health promotion have to say about ageism, sexism, racism and disability? Has it developed robust critiques?

Jenny Douglas has provided consistent critiques of health promotion from a black perspective (1995, 1997). She argues that the discourse of multiculturalism disguises the issues facing black and minority ethnic communities in Europe:

> A failure of the multicultural approach is the lack of acknowledgement of the material causes of ill health in black and minority ethnic communities in relation to poverty, discrimination, poor housing, poor working conditions, employment and racial harassment. All of these areas have been documented but have had little impact on the development of health promotion programmes ... It is almost as though by addressing the health promotion needs of black communities from a cultural perspective, issues of inequality were also being dealt with.
>
> (Douglas, 1995, p. 74)

She says that

> Nowhere in the literature accompanying and supporting the WHO's strategy [Health For All] is any reference made to black and minority ethnic communities and migrant communities in Europe. Thus although equity underlies the approach of Health for All, there is no recognition of this in relation to racial discrimination and racism.

Hylton (2010, pp. 336–338) argues that critical race theory (CRT) has emerged as an effective framework to challenge racism in his chosen area of study (sport) but also within society more generally:

> CRT is intrigued but suspicious of parts of any society that claim to be accessible and fair across racial and ethnic divides ... For CRT advocates the question is not *do we* live in a racist society? Rather it is a conclusion: *we do* live in a racist society and we need to do something about it.

This would be our conclusion too – that racist acts are not aberrational but are deeply embedded into global society; they are not simply acts of individual agency, but part and parcel of institutional life. It is therefore incumbent upon health promoters not only to examine 'whiteness' (especially for those who *are* white), in order to understand whiteness as a process and to see its role in upholding systems of power, but also to consider the institutional racism of their respective organizations and the structures of power within their national contexts.

Following these basic tenets of CRT, we also assert that the other forms of discrimination *do* exist; we do not feel we need to make a case to show that they do. Thus sexism, ageism, discrimination against people who are differently abled, who are gay, lesbian or transgendered, who are from particular classes, castes or ethnic groups, all flourish. There is also discrimination against people with particular health statuses, for example those who are obese, who have experienced mental ill health or other stigmatized illnesses, including HIV/AIDS.

Despite the presence of many in health promotion who would call themselves feminists, there is scanty critical feminist critique of health promotion, such as that provided by Lesley Doyal (1995) or Wilkinson and Kitzinger (1994) of health in general. A notable contribution in health promotion is Moore's (2010) excellent feminist critique of the 'new health paradigm' in which she suggests a 'new feminist critique of health promotion'. Furthermore, in their attempt to 'ignite an agenda for women and health promotion', Pedersen *et al.* (2010, p. 259) note,

> Despite the general acceptance of gender as a determinant of health and the inclusion of women and girls as important subpopulations in population health frameworks, health promotion has not articulated how to integrate gender into its vision and practice. Nor has the field addressed fully how its theories, methods and activities may sustain gendered forms of oppression that contribute to women's health inequities.

They go on to suggest a framework for women's health promotion. There *are* clear feminist voices within health promotion, who hold the view that patriarchy is a major obstacle to women achieving their full potential, as explored by Daykin and Naidoo (1995). The task is to keep high on the agenda those social issues that affect women's health and well-being, such as gender-based violence, traditions harmful to women (such as genital cutting), sexual harassment, forced marriage, as well as trying to gain more attention for those conditions that predominantly affect women. These include family planning, reproductive health and women's cancers. A strong case can be made, for example, that although breast cancer receives a disproportionate amount of attention (compared with other cancers), the causes of this cancer are under-researched and are relatively ignored. The reason for the rise in breast cancer across the developed world is not seen as worthy of investigation; some women argue that if a type of cancer affected one in nine men in the UK and USA (as breast cancer does women), then more action would have been taken to tackle the causes! Attempts to get the wider, environmental causes of breast cancer on to the policy agenda in the UK have been thwarted (Potts *et al.*, 2007, 2008), whilst these same attempts *have* been successful in the USA (Steingraber, 1997), highlighting the complex politics and ideologies of cancer (Potts, 2000). A number of issues affecting the health and well-being of women and stopping them realizing their potential are seen as 'cultural' issues. In this light, it can be argued that 'multiculturism' has not served women well.

There are also calls to recognize the role of gender, with a number of authors calling for more gendered epidemiology, and for gender mainstreaming in health promotion (Ostlin *et al.*, 2007; White and Richardson, 2011). Keleher (2004) draws attention to women:

> It is when we discuss gender and inequities as social experiences that key issues for health promotion arise; these are particularly issues for women's health. There is a responsibility for anyone, whether decision-makers or advocates, when talking about gender, not to use it selectively, i.e. to only mean biological or psychological differences, but to use it comprehensively – to recognize and take responsibility for the stereotypes, societal expectations, discriminations, power relationships and social and sexual norms that shape so much of women's experience, and the social, cultural and economic environment that shapes women's opportunities. Women's particular health issues, their social position, reduced income and long-term financial security, and their vulnerability to stereotypical attitudes and assumptions about their roles in society, are different to those of men, and are frequently disempowering. Indeed, the 1997 UNDP report … states that no society treats its women as well as its men. Key areas where inequities persist include women's financial security, reproductive and sexual health, emotional and mental health, violence, and caring.

(Keleher, 2004, pp. 277–278)

Meanwhile A. White *et al.* (2011) and EC (2011) draw attention to men's health and the need for particular attention to their poorer health status in key areas (White and Pettifer, 2007; Conrad and White, 2010) requiring health strategies designed specifically for men.

Children and young people too are often neglected in health promotion. This might seem a surprising assertion when they feature so strongly in health promotion interventions; in industrialized countries, many examples can be found of attempts to curb teen use of alcohol, reduce teen pregnancies, encourage healthy eating, more exercise or educate young people on how to become responsible, healthy adults. What we mean by neglect is that their voices are not heard and children and young people are seen as problematic, are pathologized and requiring to 'be educated'. Indeed young people *do* face health issues that are problematic. For example, in a sample of 1943 Australian adolescents (15–19 years and tracked to the ages of 25–29), 10% of girls and 6% of boys reported self-harming (self-cutting, burning, overdosing, poisoning and self-battery). The incidence of self-harming decreased as the young people became young adults (Moran *et al.*, 2011). Young people's mental health has only relatively recently been placed on the agenda. What is viewed as 'problematic' or 'troublesome' by health professionals (or 'experts') is not necessarily seen as such by young people themselves. A recent example of this disconnect highlights the importance of establishing the meaning that young people give to their behaviour. Research with young women into risk-taking and health found that taking risks served a function and purpose; a space to escape from the pressures of everyday life (Cross *et al.*, 2011). We need to take such things into account when designing interventions that aim to reduce so-called 'risky' behaviours. This highlights the importance of consultation with, and the participation of, young people in health promotion efforts.

Children are often seen as 'captive audiences' for health education, particularly if they are in institutional and instructional contexts such as schools. There are good examples where children and young people are consulted or are full participants in deciding when and how to tackle their health issues (e.g. MacGregor *et al.*, 1998; Alderson, 2000). In terms of methods to include young people, Noreen Whetton was a pioneer. She developed the draw and write technique to find out what really quite young children (in primary school) felt and needed in terms of health issues. Later, Berry Mayall (1994) produced extraordinary insights from children in her work in primary schools in

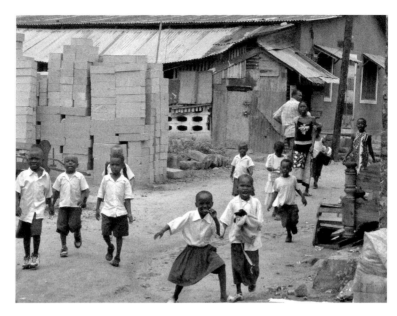

Children and young people – are their voices heard?

England. Some of our work with children (Dixey *et al.*, 2001a, b) has shown how focus groups can be used with primary school aged children, illustrating children's sophisticated understanding of healthy eating and weight issues. These young people negotiated the complex and contradictory messages received by living in contemporary media-driven and celebrity-obsessed society, showing that lack of education about healthy eating is not the only, or even the main issue. *Not* asking children and young people what they think and believe is common even in initiatives acclaimed as being 'bottom-up' and participative, but the methods *are* there *to* include them.

Although it is obviously essential to prepare children and young people for adult life, this is not the only reason for health promotion with young people – rather, they have the right to a happy and fulfilling childhood *now*. Therefore they have health promotion needs as children and young people *now* so that they can enjoy that childhood and process of growth into being healthy young people.

Health promotion is surprisingly quiet about some of the issues affecting children in resource-poor countries. The literature reflects the concerns of adults, focusing on child survival, diseases and conditions; these are clearly important but there is a relative neglect of issues such as children's mental

health, and 'social' issues such as abuse, lack of power, child rights, child labour and the use of children in conflicts.

At the other end of the age spectrum, the voices of the aged are also often invisible. As Billings and Hashem (2009, p. 7) point out,

> Studies that develop models of healthy ageing have mostly involved measuring clinical and functional aspects, and there are a few investigations into older peoples' own views of what the connections are between old age and a positive sense of well being and mental health. These studies are significant in revealing a number of components that can be seen as having salutogenic qualities, but are not captured by other models.

Cattan (2009a, 2010) has critiqued ageism within society and within health promotion; her work on loneliness and mental health among elderly people living in the UK is not just poignant – it is a damning indictment of the way in which elders are perceived and subsequently treated in highly industrialized, capitalist economies (Cattan *et al.*, 2005). As people live longer and poorer countries go through the demographic revolution, healthy ageing is likely to be a larger part of health promotion.

Vincente Navarro has perhaps been the most consistent voice writing from a neo-Marxist perspective

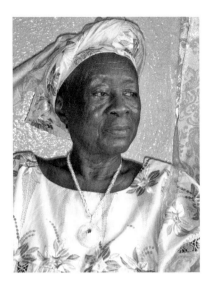
Ageing with dignity.

and thus highlighting the important role of class. This perspective has gone somewhat out of fashion amidst the rhetoric of new, 'classless' societies. He points out that 'race mortality differentials are large in the US, but class mortality differentials are even larger' (Navarro, 2009, p. 5). A young African American is 1.8 times more likely to die from a cardiovascular condition than a young white American, but a blue collar (i.e. working class) worker is 2.8 times more likely than a white collar businessman to die from a cardiovascular condition. The fact that 'class has almost disappeared from political and scientific discourse' (p. 7) being replaced by 'less conflictive categories' such as 'status', which are less threatening to the social order, disguises these inequities. He argues that ignoring the existence of class means that inequities within countries are glossed over, and there is a lack of recognition of the wealth of those at the 'top' of the poorest countries. 'The wealthiest classes in Brazil, for example, are as wealthy as the wealthiest classes in France' (p. 8), making nonsense of the idea of rich and poor countries. Bangladesh, heralded as the 'poorest country in the world' is not poor. 'It is a rich country. Yet the majority of its people are poor' (p. 9). He quotes an article about Bangladesh as saying:

> Bangladesh has enough land to provide an adequate diet for every man, woman and child in the country. The agricultural potential of this lush green land is

such that even the inevitable population growth of the next 20 years could be fed easily by the resources of Bangladesh alone. (p. 9)

The maldistribution of wealth and the class privileges embodied therein are drastically underestimated by the WHO, according to Navarro. In regard to the Commission of the Social Determinants of Health, he suggests that 'The Commission's studious avoidance of the category of power (class power as well as gender, race and national power) and how power is produced and reproduced in political institutions is the greatest weakness of the report'. Such class-blindness means that we see it that 'inequalities kill', whereas Navarro suggests that it is 'those who benefit from the inequalities that kill'. This standpoint conforms with Raphael's seventh SDH discourse described above, and if the analysis is located here, it has fundamentally different outcomes for how to address the SDH. This is not at all to suggest that Navarro is scathing of the report – he has suggested that its authors should receive the Nobel Peace Prize. *But* he feels that the report does not go far enough.

In keeping with our social model of health, it is unsurprising that we are critical of medical models of disability. That model has long been seen as insufficient to understand disability, and disabled writers, notably Oliver (1983, 1990), developed a social model of disability from the point of view of disabled people. This shifted the dominant paradigm away from individualized situations of impairment, towards disabling environments and systemic barriers to living fulfilling lives as disabled people.

> The social model of disability is underpinned by the view that economic and social barriers are so pervasive that disabled people are prevented from attaining for themselves a reasonable quality of life. Policy is more oppressive where institutional practices are geared towards care and control rather than empowerment and enablement, which means that the expert contribution of disabled people in preventing barriers is neither asked for nor understood.
> (Barrett *et al.*, 2003, p. 229)

Whereas the medical model assumes that disabled people have a 'problem', based on dependency, deviation from the norm, and that disability is a personal misfortune, and that exclusion is an appropriate way to 'deal with' disabled people, the social model assumes that the 'disability' is located in the structures – which may be physical, or attitudinal and social – that disable people who have particular needs due to an impairment. Although the disability movement coined the phrase 'Nothing about us without us', the voices of people with disabilities are also often relatively silent, especially if they are also elderly (Cattan *et al.*, 2009a, b, 2012).

'Learning disability' is the term used in the UK to describe those with a significantly reduced ability to understand new or complex information or to learn new skills, and a reduced ability to cope independently. Learning disabled people thus have impaired intelligence and impaired social functioning, which has affected their development since childhood (DOH, 2001a). Statistical data of those with learning disabilities are difficult to come by, but in England an estimated 2% of the population has learning disabilities (Emerson *et al.*, 2011). They experience poorer health than the general population due to poorer access to health services, reduced health literacy, issues associated with causes of the learning disability itself, and exposure to risky behaviours. These inequalities were investigated in the UK by an independent inquiry (Michael, 2008). As a group, they are often left out of health promotion initiatives.

These categories – age, 'race', gender, dis/ability – are useful but they render invisible other forms of discrimination. 'Travellers', a term used to describe gypsies, those of Romany origin and travelling families, occupy one of the most discriminated against positions in Europe, with appalling health statistics. They are subjected to unfair laws, are excluded from the services provided to the rest of society and their mistreatment is condoned in ways that would be unacceptable even in conservative societies if they were simply black or women. Huge gains have been made by gay and lesbian people in much of the industrialized world, but these gains are fragile and easily rescinded. Homophobia is still a feature of all societies, and the deaths of gay activists in Africa, such as that of David Kato in Uganda in 2011 shows that people still lose their lives simply for being who they are and for standing up for their rights.

Whilst many writers tend to focus on single areas of discrimination, what is useful for us, in the messiness and complexity of the real world, is to see how these areas intersect and overlap, and how marginalization can be compounded. Thus the black, working class, disabled woman living in a deprived area of London or the black, rich, upper class man living in a 'nice' neighbourhood in Kampala occupy social niches that defy easy analysis. To help with this analysis, feminist theory has described 'intersectionality' as the interaction between gender, race and other categories of difference. The concept of intersectionality allows a thorough examination of 'difference'. As Morris and Bunjun (2007) argue, multiple social categories create a unique social location, and not only does this influence a person's ability to navigate the social world, but it is *only* from this location that people can negotiate that world. Hankivsky *et al.* (2009) further suggest that intersectionality can provide a progressive research and policy paradigm, and thus a theoretical foundation for pursuing social justice, given that history, social and economic structures work in tandem to reinforce the status quo and thus prevent progress for marginalized groups such as women (Morris and Bunjun, 2007). Corbin and Bonde (2012) writing about HIV suggest that,

> In a complex arena, intersectionality gives us more than the social determinants of health approach: it advances the examination of the 'causes of the causes' by providing a systematic way of inquiring about which social determinants are of concern for a particular group of people based on their experience of privilege or oppression on several interlocking fronts.

Marginality can lead to social exclusion, defined by Levitas *et al.* (2007, p. 9) as,

> … a complex and multi-dimensional process. It involves the lack or denial of resources, rights, goods and services, and the inability to participate in the normal relationships and activities available to the majority of people in a society, whether in economic, social, cultural or political arenas. It affects both the quality of life of individuals and the equity and cohesion of society as a whole.

The Bristol Social Exclusion Matrix captures this diagrammatically (Fig. 6.1).

Combating oppression and social exclusion are clearly major challenges of the 21st century. We now turn to other challenges of the new century. We cannot present an exhaustive list, but we present here a few of the main problems as we see them.

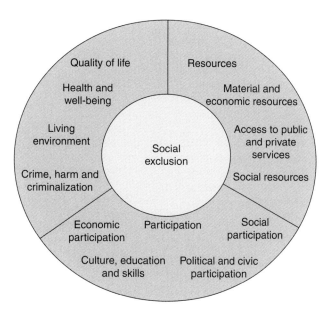

Fig. 6.1. The Bristol Social Exclusion Matrix (from Levitas *et al.*, 2007; © University of Bristol).

Understanding the Challenges of the 21st Century

The fourth role of the academic community is to throw light on the 'big questions' facing the global community. Arguably, globalization, the environment and new public health issues are among these.

Globalization

Debate about the positive and negative impacts of globalization centres on its impact on health (McClean, 2003), and whether it is an important mechanism for addressing inequality. Wolf (2004) argues that globalization is *the* solution to poverty and inequality; it increases growth and wealth and as a result decreases poverty (Labonte, 2010). Similarly, the World Bank argues that current poverty is residual, in that the benefits associated with globalization have yet to reach those in the poorest parts of the world excluded thus far from economic development. Bhagwati (2004) cites an impressive, lessened inequality and increased positive global governance. He argues that it is domestic policy rather than globalization that is particularly damaging. Stiglitz (2006) offers an optimistic perspective on globalization, suggesting that it *can* 'work'.

However, one of the 'particularly disturbing' aspects of globalization according to Khor (2001, p. 18) is increased inequality. He suggests that rapid liberalization has caused greater inequality by favouring certain income groups over others. He notes the increasing disparities between skilled and unskilled workers (in both the global North and South); the disparities between those with capital and those with just their labour; the rise of the new *rentier* class (i.e. those with unearned income) partly due to the rapid rise of debt servicing, which redistributes income from the poor to the rich; and the agricultural pricing system favouring traders rather than farmers, resulting in farmers becoming poorer.

He also argues that most developing countries are ill-equipped to cope with the forces of globalization and furthermore have seen a decline in their independent policy-making capacity, whilst having to accept the policies made by outside agencies. Given that the key economic players and most influential agencies driving globalization reside in the global North (such as the IMF, World Bank and WTO), power and control are vested here. In contrast, the global South lacks bargaining and negotiating strength. The anti-globalization theorists do appear to have more evidence for their case, and appear to be more vocal in marshalling their arguments. Bhagwati (2004) suggests that anti-globalization is much more prevalent in the richer countries, whereas people in the global South are more likely to see its benefits.

Moghadam (2005) suggests that globalization has expanded gender equality, and that the globalization of politics and international NGOs has allowed women's movements to grow globally. According to Martell (2010), globalization exposes women to more education and information, leading to empowerment and greater equality. Others see positive aspects of globalization. Scholte (2000) for example, discusses the continued growth of global consciousness as a positive outcome resulting from globalization, leading to ideas about the importance of global neighbourhoods and the common global social problems faced by the entire world.

The relationship between the processes of globalization and health are complex and go beyond what we are able to discuss here. Not only is there a large amount of literature arguing that globalization has exacerbated inequality, therefore worsening health for some but there has also been a globalization of health trends, due to the globalization of unhealthy lifestyles (McClean, 2003). Globalized marketing has meant that products such as soft drinks like Coca-Cola can be found in the remotest villages, tobacco is promoted throughout the world, and marketing of formula feeding of babies is prevalent (Labbock and Nazro, 1995; MacDonald, 2006). Consumption of processed food and cigarettes has increased consistently in poorer countries (Graham, 2008). In Bangladesh, although 80% of the population live on less than US$2 per day, smoking rates amongst 35–49-year-old men are over 70% (World Bank, 2002).

HIV, whilst seemingly a globalized disease, is experienced very differently by people in different parts of the world. It is particularly disproportionately experienced by those in southern Africa, with some reports suggesting a thousand deaths per day. Average life expectancy fell (declining to less than 40 years) in Angola, Botswana, Rwanda and Zambia, as a result of the HIV/AIDS epidemic (MacDonald, 2006). The latest epidemiological data indicating that *globally* the spread of the disease peaked in 1996 and that the epidemic has significantly stabilized since then (UNAIDS, 2009) detracts from the ongoing crisis presented by HIV in a country such as Zambia. Whereas in the UK HIV has become almost a manageable, albeit long-term, condition, it remains a matter of life and death in Africa, particularly if funding for ARVs is reduced in the future.

Globalization clearly raises key issues for the global governance of health, making it both necessary and possible. Gostin (2007) began the discussions about the importance of a Framework Convention on Global Health (FCGH) and more recently has made practical suggestions for such a framework together with a Global Plan for Justice. He makes a persuasive argument that,

> The global community has widely accepted the normative value of health. Despite this recognition, unsettling disparities persist between the world's rich and poor. Donors' geostrategic goals and philanthropists' idiosyncratic interests perpetuate these disparities because they do not align with populations' dominant health needs. A new approach, therefore, is necessary.
>
> (Gostin, 2010, p. 3)

He then outlines the Framework:

> The FCGH contains five primary objectives: (1) prioritizing basic survival needs, (2) building country capacity for enduring, effective health systems, (3) engaging all relevant stake-holders to leverage their resources and expertise, (4) coordinating and harmonizing activities among global health actors, and (5) establishing minimal funding levels for international development assistance for health and requiring accountability for those commitments.

His work outlines in some detail how such a framework can be operationalized (Gostin, 2010, p. 3).

Sustainable development, the environment and climate change

Globally agreed frameworks for health governance are perhaps overshadowed by the need for such agreements on how to tackle climate change and environmental issues. From the discussion of the development of health promotion in Chapter 1, it is clear that a concern with the environment, ecosystems and sustainability has been present from the outset. The Ottawa Charter stated, 'The protection of the natural and built environment and the conservation of natural resources must be addressed in any health promotion strategy' (WHO 2009a, p. 3). Baum (2009, p. 73), commenting that 'Lifestyles in rich countries carry a huge ecological footprint', argues that the environment represents the key health issue of the 21st century. Ron Labonte argued over a decade ago that 'Health professionals should not wait to be invited into sustainable development discussions. They must invite themselves' (Labonte, 1997, p. 267). Conventionally, the definition of sustainability is taken from the World

Commission on Environment and Development (1987), to mean 'development that meets the needs of the present without compromising the ability of future generations to meet their needs'. Jenny Griffiths has become a central voice in trying to persuade health professionals to take seriously the idea that climate change is *the* key health problem facing the planet, and Griffiths *et al.* (2009) set out the arguments regarding the threats of climate change. More importantly, their book also provides a practical guide to how health professionals can be part of tackling climate change by planning sustainable communities and facilitating behaviour change towards the environment. With case studies and clear sets of guidance, this book in its *Part Two: Action* provides nine chapters of practical steps to organizing and creating communities, which not only contribute to tackling environmental challenges, but are even healthier because they have adopted sustainable lifestyles.

New public health challenges

Globalization has led to the perception of 'global' health issues. For example, the increase in the prevalence of obesity during the last two or three decades has arisen so rapidly that the World Health Organization has described it as a 'global epidemic' (WHO, 1997a). There has been a major shift from it primarily being a public health concern of the most affluent societies to now being seen in less industrialized countries and in particular, those undergoing economic transition, such as the Gulf states (Seidell, 2000; Prentice, 2006; Candib, 2007). Current figures suggest that 250 million people worldwide are obese and by 2025 this is estimated to rise to 300 million (WHO, 1997a). The rise among children has been equally dramatic in developed countries, with a scramble to see what interventions might work (Campbell *et al.*, 2002), and childhood obesity was documented as emerging in 'developing' countries over a decade ago (De Onis and Blossner, 2000). The preschool age has shown particular rises in obesity over the past 20 years (Reilly *et al.*, 2001; Ogden *et al.*, 2002). An Australian study indicates that one in six children aged 2–4 is overweight or obese (Zuo *et al.*, 2006). Sproston and Primatesta (2003) suggest that one in four children aged 2–5 in the UK might be obese, but data on this age group are lacking. The Child Growth Foundation (Fry, 2007) has called for this data to be collected

routinely, and if this is started in a range of countries, more information about the scale of the 'global epidemic' will be available in the future. Ironically, it has been tackling other health concerns facing children that has had unhealthy consequences. For example, Dixey (1998b) has discussed how tackling concerns about child pedestrian safety in England has led to increases in obesity and reductions in physical exercise. It has also led to increased mental distress for parents and a moral panic about 'stranger danger' (Dixey, 1999a).

This increasing prevalence in children raises concern about the creation of a growing health and economic burden for the next generation particularly as there is evidence that obesity in childhood persists into adulthood (Serdula *et al.*, 1993; Guo *et al.*, 1994; Parsons *et al.*, 1999; Freedman *et al.*, 2001). Data from 'developing' or transition countries indicate that the association between a child's socio-economic status and the patterns of obesity are complex. In China, Wang *et al.* (2000) reported that children from urbanized, affluent families had higher prevalence of obesity than those from more disadvantaged backgrounds. However, in Brazil, women in the lowest socio-economic group show the highest prevalence of both obesity and underweight (Caballero, 2005). Other countries are showing similar patterns. For instance in Madagascar, childhood obesity has risen from 1.6% in 1992 to 6.2% in 2004, yet there are still around 36% underweight and roughly half were stunted (IRINnews, 2009). In countries undergoing epidemiological transition, there will be the 'old' problems of infectious diseases alongside the newer diseases created by changing lifestyles. The literature on the discourse of obesity has become an interesting area in its own right but suffice it to say that it seems to be a potent symbol of the malaise of the 21st century world that one half of the world is obese whilst the other half still faces food insecurity. Moreover, apart from news-worthy 'famines', the day-to-day hunger, which is debilitating but not life threatening and affects so many of the world's poor, appears to have slipped off the global health community's radar.

Epidemiological Transition and the 'Double Burden'

Attention has turned recently to the effects on health of development, and as countries become more 'developed', they go through demographic as well as epidemiologic transitions. The data on these transitions is patchy. Surveillance data on non-communicable disease in West Africa, according to Abubakari *et al.* (2009, p. 610), 'are rare'. They found high rates of inactivity and obesity among women in West Africa, and suggest that 'in the near future', West Africa will have rates of diabetes comparable with wealthier industrialized countries (Abubakari *et al.*, 2009, p. 611).

Cancer screening, cancer prevention measures and better quality care for cancer have received growing attention due to the rising rates in developing nations (Kanavos, 2006; Igene, 2008; Galukande and Kiguli-Malwadde, 2010; Hanna and Kangolle, 2010), with a 'call to action' on cancer care and control (Farmer *et al.*, 2010). Farmer *et al.* (2010) note the exceedingly small spend on cancer care in African countries.

Whilst these 'newer' diseases are undoubtedly important – and under-resourced (Ozgediz and Riviello, 2008) – there is a need to reflect on whether this concern shifts too much attention away from the key health issues of less developed countries. Whilst globally a move from a concern with communicable disease (which accounts for 32% of global deaths), to non-communicable disease (which accounts for 59%) would seem sensible, this split is not what is found in developing countries, where the respective figures are nearer to 77% and 15%. Gwatkin (1997) thought that this shift in WHO emphasis would disadvantage poorer countries. It is important not to forget that the more common causes of death are the same – diarrhoea, malaria, acute respiratory infections and so on. Certainly, the emerging non-communicable diseases require urgent attention but so do these other main killers. Too many children in Africa do not survive long enough to go on to become the adults at risk of non-communicable diseases, and many millions do not have safe water or enjoy the dignity of having adequate toilets (Bartram and Cairncross, 2010). Significant causes of ill health are neglected in the global agenda, such as exposure to pesticides (Kuye *et al.*, 2007) or work-related injuries (Culp *et al.*, 2007) in countries such as The Gambia. Additionally, there is often not the data available in poorer countries to describe the emerging inequalities in health between social groups (Chopra, 2005).

Neglected Diseases

Many issues do not appear to be high on the health promotion agenda. Arguably, the 'global crisis' of HIV/AIDS has skewed the international agenda, leaving certain issues such as access to family planning further down that agenda. Several issues are not prioritized but are essential to well-being and the ability to function as a normal member of society. Our late colleague John Hubley was passionate about eye health. One of the last papers John wrote was on prevention of blindness in developing countries, where the majority of blindness occurs. It was published in the prestigious *British Journal of Ophthalmology* (Hubley and Gilbert, 2006) and provided practical steps to reaching the target of 'Vision 2020: the right to sight', which aims to prevent 100 million cases of blindness by the year 2020. John called for more qualitative research to explain people's behaviour such as not going for treatment for curable eye diseases even when health services are available, a common feature in West Africa. More research is needed on effective communication methods to promote basic eye care, and on why this highly important issue does not appear higher up the list of global health priorities. There are 45 million blind people in the world (58% of them in Asia), and 135 million with serious visual impairment. The number of blind people increases by 1 million every year, and obviously has devastating effects on people's ability to earn an income and live an independent life.

Sleeping sickness is a further example of 'neglected' disease that still affects many people. According to WHO, sleeping sickness is second only to diseases like malaria in the global ranking of the parasitic infections, ranking seventh in sub-Saharan Africa in terms of disability-adjusted years. In the 1970s, the disease resurged into the continent's most remote countries, yet is hardly addressed by national and international health authorities, resulting in a WHO estimate that 60 million people in 36 African countries are at risk of developing the disease. Between 300,000 and 500,000 people are estimated to be affected by the disease in Africa, but only 5–10% of them currently have access to relevant treatments (WHO, 2002). This reflects the global unjust distribution of access to medicines, with approximately 80% of the World's population living without access to essential medication (Leach *et al.*, 2005). Shuklenk (2003) writes that only 5% of the funding for medical research and drugs goes to health issues faced by the poorer countries, and of the 1400 drugs launched in the last few years, only four have been for malaria and just 13 for 'tropical' diseases (Kaufmann, 2009).

This focus on disease here makes the point that diseases are an essential aspect of health promotion endeavour, as they can devastate people's lives. We take up the theme later of newer approaches to positive health in the final section of this chapter. We now turn to discuss what particular role universities can play in taking forward the development of health promotion.

The Role of Universities

Universities play vital roles in knowledge exchange and innovation, and in thinking about the environment, sustainability and health (Orme and Dooris, 2010). Universities (and the higher education sector generally) can play a vital role in developing health promotion. At least four roles for universities can be outlined:

1. Carrying out health promotion research, which makes a difference.
2. Capacity building for health promotion.
3. Engaging with communities.
4. Developing as health-promoting universities and thereby modelling a settings approach.

Health Promotion Research

Watson (2000) provides an overview of the state of health promotion research, albeit now over a decade ago. Lahtinen *et al.* (2005) have written a useful paper contributing to an understanding of the distinctive nature of health promotion research, and of how to assess its quality. Although presented as a 'Finnish approach', it has far wider relevance. They suggest that there are three factors that mark health promotion research out from research in other disciplines. First, health promotion research is 'research on action'; in other words, health promotion research aims at making changes for better health, either at individual, organizational or environmental levels. It is concerned with processes of change, rather than merely providing detailed 'state of the art' or descriptive accounts of phenomena. Health promotion research implicitly therefore, is concerned with making a difference for the better. Secondly, health promotion research is multidisciplinary, moving beyond

the 'guild-like' (Lahtinen *et al.*, 2005, p. 3) research of separate disciplines with their clear boundaries. Whilst not rejecting intra-disciplinary research, health promotion research does maintain openness and 'makes simultaneous use of several different scientific disciplines, such as theology, biomedicine, behavioural sciences, pedagogy, nursing science, social sciences and economics' (Lahtinen *et al.*, 2005, p. 4). The third feature is the way in which health promotion research incorporates the value base of health promotion, and as such, the health promotion practitioner's values are also those of the researcher's. Health promotion research must 'practice what it preaches' and therefore explicitly incorporate participation, inclusion, empowerment, transparency, sustainable development and emphasize 'the importance of working with people in respectful partnership, in contrast to a style in which "experts" know best' (Lahtinen *et al.*, 2005, p. 4).

A piece of research we are currently engaged in at Leeds Met illustrates these three distinctive features. Our systematic review on peer-led interventions in prison settings aims at understanding the evidence for the success of these approaches and thus improving access to health promotion in prisons; it is multidisciplinary, including economists, sociologists, health promotion specialists, policy analysts, as well as methodology experts. Finally, it is inclusive and participative, as the methodology includes expert hearings or symposia, and interviews with prisoners, prison officers, and those familiar with the workings of the criminal justice system, plus a range of other key stakeholders. As a systematic review, this is a relatively straightforward piece of research, and if conventionally undertaken would merely involve a desk review. Instead, it takes up Lahtinen *et al.*'s exhortation that health promotion research must show 'appreciation of people's wisdom and experience, listening to people's expressions about needs and solutions, and respect for the significance of the community in people's lives' (2005, p. 7). Lay involvement in health promotion research, and the training of lay people as researchers is an established aspect of research at the Centre for Health Promotion Research at Leeds Met (Newell and South, 2009).

The 'Finnish approach' has seven health promotion research criteria, followed by seven criteria for general research quality. The first seven relate to health promotion relevance, values, innovation, discourse, practice, action and context. Taken together, these seven areas ensure that health promotion

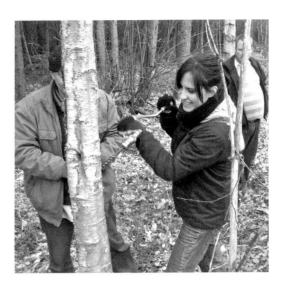

Leeds Met Researcher Karina Kinsella working with users in the Wye Wood Mental Health Project.

Capacity Development

As well as research, universities and other HEIs have teaching as a core function, and a major role in educating health workers in their initial training as well as in continuing professional development and 'life-long learning'. Three universities in England were asked in 1972 to develop courses for specialist health educators, later described as health promotion specialists. (As mentioned earlier, Leeds Met was one of these three.) There are now up to 30 such courses in the UK, although not all currently have health promotion in their title. Specialist courses abound in other parts of the world, though principally in countries of the global North. Health promotion is normally also found as an aspect of courses in nursing, environmental health, physiotherapy, occupational therapy, teaching and so on.

Professional development is one of the eight 'tracking indicators' proposed by the Bangkok conference for national capacity building in health promotion. Professional development would require national level education and training programmes, and a professional association. Another of the eight is performance monitoring, which would comprise national level research and evaluation, plus information systems to monitor and report on relevant indicators to health promotion policies and priorities. Both these 'tracking indicators' have implications for the role of higher education. (The tracking indicators are in Box 6.1; Catford, 2005.)

The need to invest in the training and education of health promotion practitioners and other workers

research is related to the body of ideas, values and priority areas outlined by the epistemic community, is appropriate to the context and ensures action. The general quality criteria relate to scientific quality, defined scope, anticipated outcomes, operationalization, feasibility, process evaluation, and documentation and dissemination. These latter seven ensure that health promotion research is well designed and scientifically sound, is workable, with a feasible plan of evaluation, and the results are properly fed back into the arena to inform future practice.

Box 6.1. Tracking indicators.

1. National policies and plans: national government policies and plans for health promotion priorities, which embrace the underlying concepts of the five Ottawa Charter strategies.
2. National leadership: core of expertise and leadership within the national Ministry of Health for health promotion development, coordination and partnerships.
3. Joined up government: coordinating mechanisms within the Ministry of Health and across national government for policy development and plan implementation for health promotion priorities.
4. Programme delivery: delivery structures and mechanisms for health promotion priorities at national and/or sub-national levels, including support for intersectoral partnerships.

5. National partnerships: national partnerships among NGOs, civil society, private sector and government for health promotion priorities.
6. Professional development: national-level advanced education and training programmes, and a professional association for health promotion practitioners, policy makers and researchers.
7. Performance monitoring: national-level research and evaluation, and information systems to track and report on health indicators relevant to health promotion policy, priorities and programmes.
8. Sustainable financing: transparent and sustainable source of public financing for health promotion priorities at national or sub-national levels.

(Catford, 2005, p. 4)

---

so that they have the required competencies and skills to address complex health issues within rapidly changing social and political contexts seems obvious. Strengthening the capacity of academic health promotion at international level is vital in this respect, as it will provide a solid scientific base for the development of knowledge-based practice and the facility to critically determine current and future health promotion needs (Barry, 2008).

In Chapter 5, we argued that current and future health challenges demand new and changing competencies and skills, and these need to be identified in order to inform the basis of education and training development. Barry (2008) has argued that there is a need to consider critically what skills and competencies are required by health promoters in addressing current health challenges, such as tackling health inequities and SDH, promoting healthy ageing and positive mental health. The MDGs and the WHO Commission on Social Determinants of health call for actions that require a complex mix of technical skills, expertise and leadership.

Hawe *et al.* (1998) described capacity building as the 'invisible work' of health promotion. Capacity building is defined as an approach to the development of sustainable skills, structures, resources and commitment to health improvement in health and other sectors to prolong and multiply health gains many times over (Hawe *et al.*, 2000). Working collaboratively with other sectors is required, but is often missed when organizations do not have the capacity to initiate and sustain involvement – building capacity requires action from within organizations as well as between them. Workforce development strategies represent an important component of building the capacity for public health work and for health promotion in particular, but strategic thinking is often lacking given the crisis management nature of many health systems in poorer countries, and the continual change in structures in some counties of the North, such as the UK's NHS. As Barry (2008) points out, investment in the human resources to support implementation of structures for health promotion is very variable, with significant gaps.

Carrington and Detragiache (1999) asked the question back in the 1990s as to whether the universities and training institutions of Africa were servicing the demands of *developed* countries, due to the outpouring of health professionals trained in Africa leaving to work in developed nations. However, in health promotion, with a lack of

capacity to educate health promotion workers in many countries of the global South, health promotion courses are accessed in those countries of the global North where courses are run. Mittelmark (2003) describes such an approach, where the Norwegian national development agency, NORAD, provides funding for students to access public health education in Norway. Several of the Nordic and western European countries, such as the Netherlands, have such schemes, and this forms an important aspect of development assistance.

Studying overseas is an expensive way of gaining qualifications. Distance learning is an alternative, but there can be a loss of a sense of an academic community (Postman, 1995), leading to the isolated learner being vulnerable (Bennett, 1998). More recently, online communities have overcome some of these issues, with e-learning and m-learning. An evaluation of e-learning in South Africa suggests that while there are advantages, such as ease of access to materials, there were also substantial disadvantages, including unequal access to computers and disjointed communication. The study concluded that more face-to-face interaction was required (Rohleder *et al.*, 2008). Many countries do not yet enjoy a level of Internet connectivity that makes online learning possible.

Although students learn enormously by studying overseas (Dixey, 2001), they usually return to their post in an unchanged organization, and can then face bureaucratic inertia, and/or a lack of opportunity to act on their learning. If new learning is not translated into practice, demoralization can ensue. The same is true where a student studies in their country, is enthused with new ideas but returns to find colleagues who are 'stuck in their ways'. Edwards and Collinson (2002) suggest that for employees to feel empowered at work, they need to have clear broad objectives, they need the right of access to the means of achieving the objectives; they need to be enabled to use their own initiative, and they need 'participatory power' – the right to challenge and debate goals and methods. These conditions are not present in many of the contexts in which health workers (as potential health promoters) work, such as in Ministries of Health, especially in countries where it is not the norm to challenge those above in the organizational hierarchy. It is noticeable that many graduates (from our UK course) move from government posts to find work with international agencies and NGOs in their home country, partly because of better remuneration

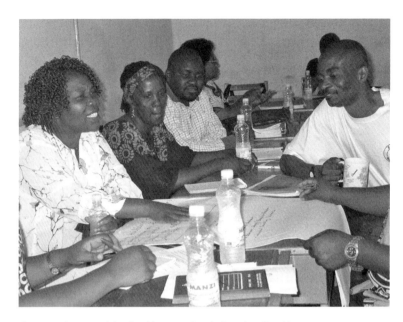

Leeds Met postgraduate students studying health promotion in Lusaka, Zambia.

packages, but also because of the certainty that their ideas will find support and that these non-governmental agencies are more dynamic. Rather than educating one or two workers per year (by sending them overseas on expensive courses), the aim needs to be to create a critical mass of health promotion practitioners capable of driving change from the 'middle ground'. The middle ground is that which can close the implementation gap by facilitating dialogue between strategic direction and local action – between the policy makers at 'the top' and local communities on the ground (Attwood *et al.*, 2003). Health promotion rests on the idea of putting communities at the centre of change, in the belief that top-down, programmatic approaches to change do not work. The same is true when attempting to change the approach to health promotion within any country wishing to change the way it tackles health issues – it is not likely that change imposed from above will be successful.

An approach to capacity building is thus needed which attempts to address the implementation gap by addressing the 'grassroots delivery mechanisms'. There is a lack of a *community* of practice capable of effecting change. Lave and Wenger (1998), who developed the concept of communities of practice, felt that such communities are built through

'apprenticeship' – learning how to be a member, participating and gradually taking on the professional identity, language and practices of that community, and thus enabling a new identity of public health/health promotion worker. According to Attwood *et al.* (2003), communities of practice are useful to individuals but, more importantly, 'are collectively valuable as repositories of knowledge and learning' (p. 147). One aim therefore, must be to create communities of practice, with learning shared in multidisciplinary groups, helping to break down the professional competitiveness highlighted above by Nyamwaya (2003). Development of health promotion is likely to be inhibited where organizations are structured into 'silos', with little shared understanding or communication across disciplines (Attwood *et al.*, 2003).

Given the lack of capacity in some parts of the world, the challenges facing universities in the global South (Bourne, 2000) and the expense of students accessing courses in the global North, universities have responded by delivering work in partnership in those parts of the world in need of infrastructure and capacity building. Jackson *et al.* (2007) describe the impressive amount of capacity development work undertaken by Canadian universities and other bodies, in Latin America, Africa and emerging European countries. Canada is acknowledged as a leader in terms of its impact on the development of health promotion (Dupere, 2007). The experience of running our Leeds Met Masters' course in Zambia, as a means of strengthening capacity for health promotion, to widen access, and to provide more cost-effective education can be found in Dixey and Green (2009).

Engaging with Communities

Universities, even in the current cash-strapped climate, are important resources for the communities that surround them. Universities in developed countries are wealthy institutions with all kinds of physical, social and knowledge capital. Knowledge transfer partnerships are usually developed in the hope of financial gain for the university and, cynically, partnerships with communities are fostered in the hope that this will lead to student recruitment. However, we would hope that there are other reasons, some based on altruism and some on a wish to tackle inequalities, that universities espouse.

Two examples of our engagement with communities are, first, a long-term relationship with the Hamara Centre in Leeds and, secondly, our partnership with two HEIs in Tanzania and Zambia, which enables them to strengthen partnership working with communities on solid waste management. This demonstrates working both locally and globally. Hamara is an example of a thriving and energetic NGO making a valuable contribution to the lives of ethnic minorities in Leeds, including asylum seekers and refugees, plus providing a service to the traditional, local white neighbourhoods. The Health Promotion Group at Leeds Met has provided technical support, on activities such as bid writing, project planning and evaluation, facilitated student volunteers and also carried out evaluations of projects. Over time, the role has evolved into that of a critical friend, and the partnership has enriched the working life of Leeds Met too.

Hamara, a name that means 'ours' in Urdu, is a voluntary sector organization based in Leeds, UK, which is working to improve the health and well-being of minority ethnic communities across the city, but particularly the South Asian community in the locality where the centre is based. Hamara is involved in range of activities around women's empowerment, older people's health, youth activities and inter-faith work as well as providing a community gym and café in the Centre itself. University staff in the Centre for Health Promotion

Research have forged strong links with Hamara, with collaborative activities spanning over a decade. In the first instance, assistance was provided in designing and analysing a community health needs assessment that helped secure funding to develop the centre. In 2007, the university undertook a collaborative evaluation of Hamara, looking at the health impact with service users and in the wider community. The evaluation involved both academic researchers and the centre staff working together to design a survey, and jointly carry out data collection. The developing partnership work was supported through a university public engagement funding and led to a large stakeholder event – 'One Community' – celebrating Hamara's achievements and the importance of community cohesion. Both organizations have continued to identify opportunities for dialogue and joint working. For example, through the partnership, connections were made with a service providing antenatal and postnatal support for women from minority ethnic communities, including asylum seekers and refugees. The university facilitated a consultation event bringing together professional stakeholders with women using the service. This event demonstrated the added value of partnership working as the university team brought skills around facilitation and report writing, while Hamara offered the facilities of the centre, a culturally appropriate setting that many of the service users were familiar with, and provided organizational support to the event.

A long-term partnership between the Centre for Health Promotion Research and Hamara has been of benefit to both organizations. Access to academic skills in research, critical thinking and programme planning and evaluation, have enhanced the capacity of Hamara to secure funding and to develop as an organization committed to addressing health inequalities. From a university perspective, the partnership has brought better understanding of the health issues facing minority ethnic communities, it has given staff experience of working with a grassroots community organization, new research opportunities have been identified and the university is seen to demonstrate respect for the diversity of languages, faiths and cultures in the city. Overall, the work with Hamara provides an example of how community–campus partnerships need to be built over time, and are ultimately based on good communication, mutual learning and relationships founded on trust.

Our second example involves negotiating the tricky waters of North/South relationships, with two former British colonies. Despite the focus on sustainable 'partnerships' in the discourse of development, and its emphasis in funding calls suggesting that donor agencies value partnerships, there is little literature on the processes and operationalization of such types of collaboration (Jentsch, 2004). Brehm (2001) suggests that whilst the financial power is held by the 'Northern' partner, there is little hope that a partnership can mean true equality and the sharing of responsibilities. Manji (2006) likewise is sceptical about there being sufficient trust between North and South partners for true partnerships to develop. Some of the ingredients of successful partnerships are discussed in our paper on working with a college in Zambia (Dixey and Green, 2009).

Our role as an HEI formed a valuable addition to a partnership between Dar-es-Salaam Institute of Technology in Tanzania and Chainama College in Lusaka, Zambia, which had both been tasked with providing training support to community-based organizations and small and medium enterprises who had been awarded contracts for collecting waste from households in their respective communities. Our role was to develop participative methodologies for the training and participative methods for researching the effect on gender, empowerment and income generation. As outsiders, we were able to suggest research questions that were 'taken for granted' by our African colleagues, and also to bring in novel ways of asking those questions and writing up the research.

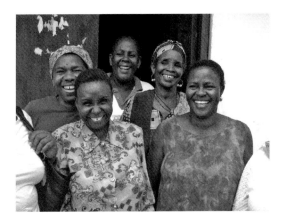

Women in a solid waste management cooperative in Dar-es-Salaam, Tanzania.

The fourth role of universities, to model a settings approach by working towards becoming a health-promoting university, will not be explored fully here. Dooris has written much about settings, including university settings (Dooris, 2001; Dooris and Martin, 2002; Doherty and Dooris, 2006). Earlier, Tsouros *et al.* (1998) provided a comprehensive guide to developing healthy universities, and the idea has been taken up in Germany (Stock *et al.*, 2010) and China (Tian *et al.*, 2003). Latterly, Dooris and Doherty (2010a, b) have provided an overview of progress towards developing universities as settings for health.

Towards the Future of Health Promotion

Understanding 'healthworlds'

As has been discussed elsewhere in this book, and in keeping with the social model of health, health promotion efforts should aim to privilege lay 'voices' and perspectives. In order for this to happen, voices must be 'heard'. Often lay opinion is not in tandem with public health and health promotion opinion. Robertson (1998) has commented that 'Health promotion makes room for the stories which individuals and communities tell about their everyday experience of health, which legitimizes them as being important to our understanding of health as statistics on morbidity and mortality rates.' Some of this 'room' was made in Chapter 1; in moving towards greater room for lay involvement in creating health, and lay epidemiologies, we show the importance of a 'constructionist epistemology' – in other words, knowledge (in this case, understandings of 'health') are constructed by interactions between people in the real world. These meaning are not 'given', but alter and develop over time. These meanings are what health promoters need to start with, not try to change or suggest that they are 'wrong'. Fox and Ward (2006, p. 476) point out that 'health must be acknowledged to be a highly contextualized outcome of the lived body/self and its relation with the material and psychosocial environment'. Radley and Billig (1996) make a similar point when they stress that ideas about health and illness 'articulate a person's situation in the world and, indeed, articulate that world in which the individual will be held accountable to others' (p. 221). A recent contribution to this perspective is that of Germond and

Cochrane (2010) in their use of the concept of 'healthworlds'. They write:

> The healthworld relates to people's conceptions of health, to their health-seeking behaviour, and to their conditions of health. Individuals' healthworlds are shaped by, and simultaneously affect, their social shared healthworld constituted by the collective search for health & well-being. (p. 309)

They also point out that while health worlds may be patterned in a coherent way at a community level, often people utilize differing healing systems and explanations for health. This suggests that a real danger is to overemphasize such beliefs and practices as 'determined'. Biographical factors and changing circumstances mean that people may change their ideas, and this element of agency is important to bear in mind.

Calnan and Williams (1991) commented on the salience of health, and pointed out that health concerns were often not primary factors in people's behaviour, indeed health tends to be taken for granted unless it fails. And even if people see the advice they receive as important and apt, they may not be able to act on it, given their circumstances; the impact of resources on health has been the focus of a number of studies (for example, in much recent work on food poverty, such as Dowler (1998) and Dowler *et al.* (2007). It is also a theme in Backett (1992) and in accounts of lay perceptions of factors in health:

> Smoking and drinking and drug taking. I put it down to one thing … until money is spent on these areas … there doesn't seem to be much point in trying to stop people smoking and what else. As long as the environment is going down the pan the people will go down with it.
>
> (Williams *et al.*, 1995, pp. 123, 125; as cited in Williams, 2003, p. 147)

Thus people have a clear idea of social determinants, and of these not merely being bound up with individual lifestyle choices. However, in their study of post-soviet citizens, Abbott *et al.* (2006) highlight the focus on the environment and poverty in people's accounts of the causes of illness: 'Informants' talk about their lives suggested a complex understanding of health that recognizes the influence of factors over which they have little control' (p. 234). Yet interestingly they found these factors were not stressed when respondents discussed responsibility for health, where they emphasized the role of the individual in terms of coping, strength of will and behaviour. Similarly, Blaxter

(1997) found that whilst people identified many factors important in health and illness, what they stressed as most important was behaviour. What links these two studies is the suggestion in both that people in deprived and difficult circumstances are those most likely to stress behaviour as important in preventing illness; indeed Blaxter (1997) found that the middle class respondents in the Health & Lifestyles Surveys were the most likely to see structural factors such as poverty as important in health and illness. Her explanation for this is that accounts of health and illness are strongly linked to identity and thus those whose lives are indeed most affected by lack of income and other structural factors do not want to talk about their risk status, and instead stress not giving in to illness and the moral responsibility to cope:

> I think if they eat the right foods and do have a proper balanced diet, I mean, even the poorest people can be just as healthy as the other … I wouldn't say that a poor person suffers more with their health just because they are poor.
>
> (Blaxter, 1997, p. 752)

Similar findings are reported by Popay *et al.* (2003), where those in deprived circumstances were reluctant to attribute ill health to those circumstances, even when their accounts of their own lives and health suggested how important they were. These ideas are not incompatible with other studies, which stress working class people as feeling that the causes of illness are not under their control (e.g. Pill and Stott, 1982). Very often health is seen as something one can influence, to build what Herzlich calls 'health as reserve', the better to cope with illness when it occurs.

The work on people's perceptions and understandings of health tell us that people see health and its social determinants in complex ways. They are thus likely to react to health communication, messages about risk and healthy lifestyles, in complex ways too. Health promotion has begun to embrace the idea of complexity theory (Pisek and Greenhalgh, 2001; Walby, 2007) and insert it into its theory and practice (McQueen, 2000; Campbell, 2011), but there remains to be a proper marrying of the sociology of lay health beliefs and health promotion theory. What we have to be clear about in health promotion is that the relativist and critical standpoint adopted logically leads to seeing health as based on historical, contextual and subjective exigencies, and thus leads to better understanding of the complexities of 'health'. The health beliefs literature, however, does resonate with some of the new agendas for health, particularly in the emerging ideas of well-being and happiness, and this is explored in the next section.

Well-being and Happiness – New Paradigms for the 21st Century?

Recent times have seen a move towards a new paradigm of health, with the concepts well-being, happiness and wellness emerging in the health discourse. The New Economics Foundation has launched its Happy Planet Index and the government of Bhutan has launched a measure of Gross National Happiness (GNH) to replace GNP (Gross National Product). These moves key into the zeitgeist where hypercapitalism is being scrutinized, and the claims that economic growth necessarily lead to 'development' and 'progress' are questioned. These developments in the 21st century are logical extensions of, and accelerate, changes that began to emerge in the last century. The 20th century saw major breaks with how things used to be seen in the past – a series of 'paradigm shifts' occurred, which transformed science and ways of thinking. In a nutshell, these changes could be seen as a reaction against the Enlightenment notions of rationality and positivism, where 'science' was split off from 'emotions', where 'objectivity' was prized over the 'merely' subjective. As Outram (2006, p. 6) suggests, the Enlightenment was where 'Man gained control over nature, and then over other human beings, by controlling them "rationally" through the use of technology … Enlightenment in this view is ultimately totalitarian in the sense that it abandons the quest for meaning and simply attempts to exert power over nature and the world. The Enlightenment relies on "rationality", reasoning that is free from superstition, mythology, fear and revelation, which is often based on mathematical "truth", which calibrates ends to means, which is often therefore technological, and expects solutions to problems which are objectively correct.' For some, the logical end of this process (of Enlightenment) was the Nazi extermination camps, where people were 'treated as mere objects to be administered' (Outram, 2006, p. 7).

The new ways of looking at the world challenged the idea that there was one universal truth waiting to be discovered; quantum theory suggested that matter was not solid or static and Einstein presented his ideas about relativity, turning upside down ideas about space and time. Rather than reality being 'objective', and available to all, it began to be seen that 'reality' depends on where you happen to be standing. The newer, more interactive understanding of reality placed the observer centrally – developing the notion that we bring about our own reality. This systemic or interactive (or ecological) view replaced a linear view of how things work, with a circular view – that systems maintain stability by feedback, and that every system is connected to other systems in a process of reciprocal determinism. As Gerhardt (2004, p. 9), puts it: 'How one person behaves affects how another behaves and his or her behaviour then influences the original person in a circular process. Cause and effect depend on your vantage point, on where you start in the loop, and how much information you include or exclude. There is not one truth, but several possible truths.'

The ideas of many possible truths resonates with postmodern ideas of the importance of listening to multiple voices, of the reintegration of the emotional, the subjective, the lived experience, not only into social science but also into the popular imagination, and the valuing of the plurality of cultures, faiths and ways of life that make up our globalizing world. In certain disciplines such as psychology, it has led to the development of critical psychology, which challenges the dominant stress on cognitions and the ability to measure quantitatively people's attitudes, feelings and emotional states. In geography, the paradigm shift can be exemplified by the move into understanding how people perceive the world, with their own 'mental maps' based on gender, ethnicity, age and ability – these are more 'real' than the actual physical manifestation of the geography on the ground as drawn by 'objective' map makers. It has brought about a major new field of qualitative research based on phenomenology, social interactionism and other methods, which attempt to understand the world from the point of view of the people who inhabit that world. In terms of understanding health, it led to the seminal work of the late Mildred Blaxter, whose work on lay beliefs of health has challenged the dominant medical ways of understanding 'health'. Thus whereas the Enlightenment scientists saw emotion as getting in the way of seeing the world 'properly', the 20th century began to see a real reintegration of the importance of the emotional and subjective, such that in the 21st century, this has become a more dominant paradigm. It is not surprising, perhaps, that it was in the immediate post-war period that the WHO's radical definition of health emerged, questioning as it does, the purely medical, scientific concept of health, and establishing the importance not only of holistic health, but of the inter-subjective state of emotional, social and mental health. This was precisely when the role of technology as a means to bring about human health and happiness was beginning to be questioned.

This worldview challenges the notion of 'experts' – now the people who are the experts on their health are those living with their own bodies, with their own homes and neighbourhoods, and not the outside professionals who do not share the same lived experiences. Thus 'experts by experience' has become a common catchphrase. The challenge for health promotion 'experts' was discussed in Chapter 5.

The stage appears to be set for the emergence of a politics of well-being, although there is still a great deal of focus on the importance of economic growth, higher standards of living, consumerism and materialism in bringing about greater health and happiness. Well-being is in the UN Declaration on the Right of Development: '... development is a comprehensive economic, social, cultural and political process, which aims at the constant improvement of the well-being of the entire population on the basis of their active, free and meaningful participation in development and the fair distribution of benefits' (UN, 1986).

The Organisation for Economic Co-Operation and Development (OECD), hardly a radical organization, has recently decided to look again at how to measure 'progress'. The London School of Economics, an old-established institute of higher education in London, has launched its Wellbeing Programme, headed by Richard Layard, whose book *Happiness: Lessons from a New Science* (Layard, 2011) and previous work (Layard, 2006) have brought about some of this changed thinking in policy circles. The prime minister of the UK has developed a project to create a set of National Wellbeing Indicators. The Centre for Well-being at the new economics foundation hopes that the emerging interest in what makes people genuinely happy and able to live flourishing lives will counter the ecologically unsound growth paradigm, and academics working there have begun to suggest policy changes to make the vision come to fruition. Marks (2011), for example, writes of the urgency

to reform our financial and banking systems, develop an education system that moves away from the obsession with measuring performance and more towards developing children's full potential and well-being and, finally, take a radically different approach to the built environment, so that neighbourhoods properly work for people. The latter has been taken up by CABE, a UK NGO, in its concern with the relationship between spaces and health. (Unfortunately CABE was closed down by the current government.) Marks (2011) further comments on work that the new economics foundation carried out to produce evidence-based actions, which illustrate the causal pathways to greater happiness and well-being. If people are well connected, with strong personal relationships, are physically active, aware and taking notice of what is happening, feel they are learning, are able to give and be generous, then they have higher levels of well-being. It does appear that what makes most people happy is the quality of their relationships with friends, family and work colleagues, and the most important factor is belonging to the local community (Anielski, 2007). Research into altruism ('other-regarding') indicates that this is positively linked to better health and well-being (Post, 2005, p. 66). This makes the focus on social capital within health promotion, and the importance to health of 'connectedness', seem well placed. Anielski though, suggests that social capital is only one aspect of capital. If social capital represents relationships, there are four other important types of capital – human capital (people), natural capital (natural resource and the environment), built capital (the built environment) and financial capital (money). That 'natural capital' has a bearing on health has been well documented, and features largely in people's own accounts of what makes them feel alive; contact with nature can recharge batteries, reduce stress and produce greater mental well-being (Bird, 2007).

Research by Abdel-Khalek (2006) demonstrated that good mental health was predictive for happiness whilst good physical health did not have the same effect. In this study, the strongest predictor for happiness was religion, but as the sample was all Kuwaiti Muslim undergraduate students, there are limits as to the conclusions drawn! Genetic and environmental factors also appear to play a part in subjective well-being and perceptions of health (Roysamb *et al.*, 2006). Diener and Chan (2011) carried out a review of more than 160 studies and

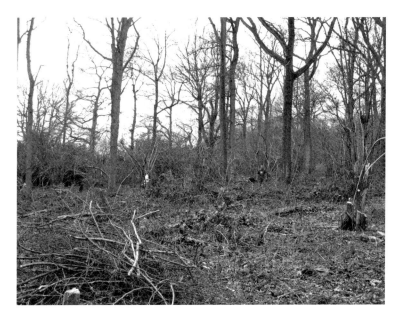

Tackling mental health problems by working outdoors, Wye Wood Project, UK.

concluded that happy people live longer, and have better health, than unhappy people. In an interview about the study Diener stated that 'it may be time to add "be happy and avoid chronic anger and depression" to the list of health recommendations currently comprising avoidance of obesity, eating well, not smoking and taking exercise'.

A wealth of activity in this area is trying to develop scales to measure happiness and feelings of well-being, for example, the 'Happiness Measures' index (Fordyce, 2005). Clearly, there are some theoretical and methodological issues with exploring these dimensions of human existence in a positivist and reductionist way, and using more exploratory, qualitative methods is arguably more appropriate. However, happiness surveys do consistently demonstrate a clear statistical relationship between happiness and health – and significantly, this is stronger than the relationship between happiness and wealth (Graham, 2008). Whilst much of this literature has been generated from the positive psychology and community psychology disciplines, there has not been as much activity attempting to establish the social conditions required to produce such optimal functioning and happiness (Gable and Haidt, 2005) and neither is there understanding of how these vary across cultures (Kovess-Masfety *et al.*, 2005).

This new discourse is in danger of being a Eurocentric/North Atlantic phenomenon, though 'Southern' voices have been calling for a changed conception of 'development' from that espoused by the global North for some time, and the fact that Bhutan is leading the way in switching from measures of economic growth towards measures of happiness suggest that these ideas are not luxuries promulgated by richer countries. It has been known for decades that western ideas of development do not necessarily bring about improved conditions for the urban and rural poor of 'developing' countries. Kwame Nkrumah, the first President of independent Ghana said, 'We shall measure our progress by the improvement in the health of our people. The welfare of our people is our chief pride, and it is by this that (we) ask to be judged' (Nkrumah, 1957). Sen's notion of development as freedom is a major strand of the development discourse, based on the idea that development can be measured by the removal of 'unfreedoms', which are those things that leave people with little choice and no ability to exercise their 'reasoned agency' (Sen, 1999, p. xii). Similarly, ul Haq points out that development indices do not always capture what is important for people:

The basic purpose of development is to enlarge people's choices. In principle, these choices can be infinite and can change over time. People often value achievements that do not show up at all, or not immediately, in income or growth figures: greater access to knowledge, better nutrition and health services, more secure livelihoods, security against crime and physical violence, satisfying leisure hours, political and cultural freedoms and sense of participation in community activities. The objective of development is to create an enabling environment for people to enjoy long, healthy and creative lives.

(Human Development Report, 2011, p. 1)

Furthermore, Sen's idea of the 'capability framework' (Sen, 1980) can be used to measure quality of life; it 'suggests that quality of life should be measured by focussing on people's capabilities, namely their real opportunities to lead the life that they have reason to value'. Implicitly, it

> ... criticizes approaches to the measurement of quality of life exclusively based on resources, such as income, or, in the case of health-related quality of life, health status, and mental states, such as satisfaction, happiness, and desire fulfilment.
>
> (Giuntoli, 2010)

None of these approaches provides comprehensive accounts of quality of life. Both Sen (1993) and Nussbaum (2000) stress the importance of freedom to quality of life, to capability and thus to health. The opportunities and liberties available to individuals allow them to function as full human beings, rather than merely subsisting. These opportunities, which enable greater control and choice, have clear implications for empowerment.

A number of academics have argued that the world adults have created has affected children's quality of life, and that it is not a healthy one in which children flourish. Guldberg's (2009) book critiquing our safety-obsessed society has the title 'Reclaiming childhood: freedom and play in an age of fear', reflecting the debates about the impacts on childhood and healthy development of those trends which have curtailed children's independence, reduced their exposure to the outdoors and placed more stress on them to perform well so that they can compete later in an increasingly complex labour market. Guldberg attempts to demolish some of the myths about the fragility of children and points out how children and young people's lives *have* improved in many ways. Possibly the most outspoken critic is Frank Furedi (1997, 2001) who argues that a culture of fear has been promulgated to the extent that parents are now 'paranoid'.

Parents now perceive themselves as subjected to surveillance, and have lost confidence in their abilities to parent in a situation where the state has intervened to say what standards of good parenting are (for example, several developed nation-states have laws about whether parents can smack their children).

New Models of Health?

This discussion raises the issue of whether models of health conventionally adopted by the epistemic health promotion community adequately fulfil the needs of the new century, given that definitions of health are subjective, culture-bound and change over time. One of the key dimensions which is mentioned in students' discussions of Labonte's model (presented in Chapter 1) is the lack of a spiritual circle. Vader (2006) notes that spiritual health is almost totally absent from discussions in European public health, despite an attempt nearly 30 years ago by the WHO to include spiritual health in its definition. He calls on the public health community to take spiritual health seriously if health improvements are to occur (see Box 6.2). In contrast, Aboriginal Australians place spiritual health at the forefront: '... Health does not just mean the physical well-being of the individual but refers to the social, emotional, spiritual and cultural well-being of the whole community. This is a whole of life view and includes the cyclical concept of life-death-life' (National Health and Medical Research Council, 1996).

The post-Enlightenment reintegration of the emotional into everyday life affects the way we build our models of health. For example, O'Donnell's (2009) definition of health, which has been adopted by the *American Journal of Health Promotion* (http://www.healthpromotionjournal.com/), includes spiritual, emotional, intellectual and social health in an outer wheel, with physical health at the centre.

There have been attempts to define spiritual health and also to develop health promotion interventions to improve spiritual health (Hawks *et al.*, 1995), and perhaps this is one of the ways in which the concepts developed in the last century no longer fully and adequately serve the needs of the 21st – the most quoted definition of health is still that proposed by the WHO in 1946. Saracci (1997) has called on the WHO to reconsider it; apart from the lack of mention of spiritual health, many see the WHO's idea as utopian and unachievable, given the stress on a 'complete' state of physical, mental and social health. However, it is still important to assert that health is *not* merely about *not* being ill or diseased. It is much more than that. The WHO's definition also implicitly suggests that health is a dynamic process of development, where we can become all that we want to be.

Spiritual health includes the dimensions of fulfilment, meaning and well-being, and despite the decline of organized religion in many 'developed' countries in particular, Inglehart's research on changes in 43 countries shown that 'Spiritual concerns are not vanishing: on the contrary, we find a consistent cross-national tendency to spend more time thinking about the meaning and purpose of life' (Ingelhart, 1997, p. 328). Perhaps this is one area where lay perspectives need to be incorporated rather more into definitions of what it means to be a healthy, well-integrated and happy person in the 21st century!

Some would view spiritual health as one aspect of mental health. Margaret Barry (2001, 2009) has made an important contribution to developing ideas about positive mental health and its social determinants. She calls for the mobilization of public demand for greater policy focus on well-being and mental health, which resonates well with current trends outlined above.

Thinking Afresh and Developing New Paradigms

The discussion above, about the disciplinary base of health promotion and in the previous chapters, shows how in a number of areas of study, there has been a rejection of simple, linear models of human behaviour. This is very evident in communication theory and in the psychology of behaviour change. New ways of conceptualizing behaviour change suggest that what is more important than concentrating on the 'choices' individuals make, is rather to focus on how shared social practices are initiated, sustained and become normalized. This would shift the area of focus from health behaviours to health practices, and from behaviour change to practice change, and implicitly from individualized 'choices' to the social construction of daily life. Behavioural economics is currently in vogue, perhaps as it rejects some of the mechanistic ways of seeing people as rational beings and implicitly critiques such simple notions as 'nudge'.

One of the initiatives to think afresh about public health in the 21st century comes from the website www.afternow.org.uk. The group at Glasgow University who set up the website think tank include Phil Hanlon, Gerry McCartney, Sandra Carlisle, and they call for a new mindset in public health, which takes up the key issues facing the globe, such as climate change, the peaking of oil, growing inequalities, addictions and well-being. They call for a 'fifth wave', and for radically different ways of thinking about the world we want to create, a world which challenges consumerism and which would create true health. We cannot do justice here to the many ideas presented but we recommend exploration of the publications on the website.

Meanwhile others have set out to turn other concepts such as justice, on their head. For example, Danny Dorling (2011) has set out to redefine 'injustice'. He argues that 'The five tenets of

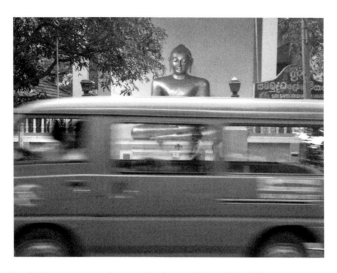

Religion is part of everyday life for many people, contributing to their spiritual life.

injustice are that: elitism is efficient, exclusion is necessary, prejudice is natural, greed is good and despair is inevitable.' Also in terms of the social justice agenda, Wrigley *et al.* (2011) show how social justice is integral to educational reforms and raising standards of schooling to bring about greater democracy and informed citizenship.

Finally, Gregg and O'Hara (2007a) have attempted to outline the value base of health promotion in the 21st century and to suggest a model that fits the zeitgeist, in their Red Lotus model. First, they produced a useful overview of the values and principles found in current health promotion practice, showing the continuum of values spanning conventional health promotion and the newer, holistic, ecological and salutogenic health promotion (Table 6.1).

After presenting the challenges of working with those values in practice, they go on, in a second paper, to present a new model of health promotion for 'holistic, ecological and salutogenic health promotion practice', which they call the 'red lotus model' (Gregg and O'Hara, 2007b). Having argued that existing health promotion planning models do not explicitly use values and principles systematically, they show how their model enables incorporation of the central values in each stage of the planning cycle for health promotion activities. They suggest that there are three domains: the philosophical, ethical and technical, and these are presented here (Tables 6.2, 6.3 and 6.4).

These three tables contain a huge number of ideas and as such embrace some of the complexity we have mentioned previously, providing links between principles and practice. We cannot do justice here to the full use of the symbolism of the red lotus flower, and we suggest that you read the paper to appreciate this. We also do not present Gregg and O'Hara's work as the only or 'best' way of conceptualizing the values of health promotion, but as one device to enable readers to think about the important issue of the values and principles base of health promotion.

Final Thoughts

Health promoters see in the world around them systemic inequalities in the capabilities (Sen, 1993) of entire continents, nations and the communities and individuals, to lead lives with value and meaning to themselves. If health is about living a meaningful life, then this is surely our primary concern and starting point. In a world of global plenty, where resources are not an issue (but the distribution of them is), then our engagement must be with an attempt to re-shape the lived-experience of those struggling in the margins between mere existence and a meaningful life. Socio-economic and political inequalities restrict people's freedoms and capabilities, capacity for self-determination and independence and ability to develop their personhood. They cannot be, in Maslow's terms, self-actualized beings.

Table 6.1. The continuum of values and principles evident in current health promotion practice (Gregg and O'Hara, 2007a, pp. 8–9).

Focus of value or principle	Holistic, ecological, salutogenic health promotion value or principle	Description of each end of the values and principles continuum	Conventional health promotion value or principle
Worldview	Organic	Seeing the world as a living, breathing, dynamic whole as opposed to seeing the world as an unchanging, static machine	Mechanistic
Epistemology	Constructionist, Subjectivist	Acknowledging that all people are connected and that collectively they construct knowledge and understanding about their world, as distinct from believing that there is only one truth that is ascertained by an objective observer	Objectivist
Science	Ecological	Using the science of ecology, which recognizes that people exist in multiple ecosystems, from the individual level, to the family group, community and population level. All parts within the whole system affect each other, and the whole is greater than the sum of the parts. Ecological science incorporates the tenets of connectedness, complementarity, uncertainty and non-locality. This principle is distinct from reductionism or positivism, in which understanding about the whole comes from simply understanding each part	Reductionist, positivist
Health paradigm	Holistic	Understanding that health is a complex concept that includes aspects of well-being that relate to the whole person, rather than seeing heath as an absence of disease or 'unhealthy' behaviours, as reflected in the biomedical and behavioural health paradigms	Biomedical, behaviourist
Emphasis	Health and well-being	Emphasizing factors that create and support health, well-being, happiness and meaning in life, as distinct from emphasis on risk factors for disease	Rates of disease and risk behaviours
Motivation for health	Health as a resource for living, sense of purpose and enjoyment of life	Recognizing that health provides a sense of purpose and enables greater enjoyment of life and is not an end in itself. This is distinct from believing that fear about the consequences of unhealthy behaviours are the primary motivators for people to develop long-term sustainable changes	Fear about consequences of unhealthy behaviours
Assumptions about people	People are naturally healthy	Assuming that when left to their own devices, people will do the best they can for themselves, their families and their communities, given their circumstances and available resources. This is distinct from assuming that left to their own devices, people will naturally adopt 'unhealthy' lifestyles	People are naturally unhealthy
Health promotion strategies	Participatory processes that enable and empower people	Using participatory processes that enable and empower people to connect with their inner wisdom and gain control over their lives and the determinants of their health. This is distinct from using disempowering interventions that target 'at risk' people and educations and their 'unhealthy' behaviours	Target 'at risk' people with behaviour change strategies
Population focus	Determined by equality	Prioritizing work with communities that are most marginalized, vulnerable, disadvantaged and often regarded as 'hard to reach' based on considerations of equity. This is distinct from working with more visible groups or whole populations, or the less vulnerable and more accessible populations	Whole groups or populations

Continued

Table 6.1. Continued.

Focus of value or principle	Holistic, ecological, salutogenic health promotion value or principle	Description of each end of the values and principles continuum	Conventional health promotion value or principle
Power	Participatory, egalitarian	Facilitating participatory and egalitarian processes that assist with the redistribution of power, rather than processes that have their foundations in patriarchy and domination	Patriarchal, dominator
Change processes	Active participation of people affected by the issue	Ensuring that people most affected by an issue are an integral part of all components of a health promotion change process that addresses the issue, as distinct from being targeted as recipients of decisions made external to them	Passive recipients of external decisions
	Processes do not impinge on personal autonomy	Ensuring that all relevant parties consent to health promotion change processes and acknowledging and respecting that not all people will choose the same actions, rather than processes that expect all people to adopt the same actions, irrespective of their own processes	Universal processes that restrict personal autonomy
	Maximum beneficence	Actively considering what the benefits of any health promotion change process may be to the full range of beneficiaries, as distinct from processes that only consider a limited range of beneficiaries	Limited beneficence
	Non-maleficence is a priority consideration	Actively considering what the potential harms of any health promotion change process may be; who may be harmed by the change processes and in what way; taking steps to minimize or avoid this harm; communicating risks involved in a truthful and open manner. This is distinct from change processes that do not assess the full range of potential harms due to a belief that health promotion processes will result in positive health outcomes	Scope of malefi-cence not fully considered
Basis for practice	Practice based on evidence of need and effectiveness, and sound theoretical foundations	Ensuring that needs assessment process incorporate the perspectives of all stakeholders, and that health promotion practice is based on sound evidence of need, evidence of effectiveness, and appropriate theoretical foundations. This is distinct from practice that is based on a selective use of evidence and/or political motives	Practice based on selec-tive use of evidence, or on political imperatives
Strategy approach	Multiple strategies	Using multiple strategies incorporating all action areas of the Ottawa Charter, as opposed to reliance on one or two strategies, particularly legislation and regulation, and developing personal skills for behaviour change	One or two strategies
Governance and decision making	Collaborative models of governance and decision making	Using models of governance and decision making that facilitate active and meaningful participation by all stakeholders, as distinct from non-democratic governance and decision making	Health worker led and/or imposed from outside
Professional role	Ally	Working with a person as an ally and a resource, who is on tap for the community, as distinct from working on top of people as an outside expert who assumes they know what's best for the community	Expert
Evaluation objects of interest	Sustainable changes to determinants of health	Ensuring that evaluation focuses on assessing the sustainable changes in the range of factors that enable people to increase control over the determinants of their health, as distinct from evaluating changes in rates of 'unhealthy' behaviours and diseases	Behaviour changes and disease rates

Table 6.2. Values and principles in the philosophical domain (Gregg and O'Hara, 2007b, p. 14).

Value	Principle	Explanation
Organic worldview	The existence of an organic universe	Seeing the world as a living, breathing, dynamic whole
Constructionist epistemology	The construction of knowledge through interactions within and between health promotion practitioners and communities	Acknowledging that all people are connected and that collectively they construct knowledge and understanding about their worlds
Ecological science	The science underpinning health promotion is ecological	Using the science of ecology, which recognizes that people exist in multiple ecosystems, from the individual level, to the family group, community and population level. Health is determined by complex interactions between people (including their biological status, such as age, gender and genetics, state of health and well-being, socio-economic status, attitudes, values, beliefs and behaviours) and their social, economic, political, built and natural environments. All parts within the whole system affect each other, and the whole is greater than the sum of the parts. Ecological science incorporates the tenets of connectedness, complementarity, uncertainty and non-locality
Holistic health paradigm	The concept of health includes interrelated dimensions of spiritual, mental, social and physical health and well-being	Understanding that health is a complex concept that includes aspects of well-being that relate to the whole person or communities of people
Salutogenic focus	Focusing on the creation of health	Emphasizing factors that create and support health, well-being, happiness and meaning in life
Health is purposeful	The motivation for health is as a resource for living	Recognizing that health provides a sense of purpose and enables greater enjoyment of life and is not an end in itself
Assumption of positive intentions	Assume that people have a natural desire to do the best for themselves, their families and their communities	Assuming that when left to their own devices, people will do the best they can, given their circumstances and available resources
Empowering health promotion strategies	Participatory processes that enable and empower people	Using participatory processes that enable and empower people to connect with their inner wisdom, and gain control over their lives and the determinants of their health

The modest aims of the MDGs are being threatened by a global recession, which impacts the excessive lifestyles of the global rich, leading the Secretary General of the United Nations to proclaim that it could prevent the promises of the rich nations being kept, 'plunging millions more into poverty and posing a risk of social and political unrest' (Ban Ki-Moon, in UN, 2009, p. 3).

Globalization has meant that 'the sense of spatial distance which separated and insulated people from the need to take into account all the other people which make up what has become known as humanity has become eroded' (Featherstone, 1993, p. 169).

In summing up Ricoeur's ideas of the ethical life, Rutherford asserts that the aim of living encompasses a sense of justice (Rutherford, 2007). Ricouer felt that the essence of an ethical life is the necessity of interdependence (in Rutherford, 2007). Kubow *et al.* (2000, p. 134) simply say that if we are to be effective citizens, global challenges 'are part of our individual and social responsibility to address'. A global ethic is at the heart of health promotion, where universal norms and values are shared. These are outlined in the many declarations and statements produced over the years by the health promotion community. Dower has elaborated on the idea of a global ethic suggesting it includes '… a norm of global responsibility according to which agents have responsibilities to promote what is good anywhere in the world (or, as often as not, to oppose what is bad)' (Dower, 2003, p. 18). Promoting what is good and living well together as

Table 6.3. Values and principles in the ethical domain (Gregg and O'Hara, 2007b, p. 15).

Value	Principle	Explanation
Equity-based priority communities	Prioritize action with the most vulnerable or disadvantaged communities	Prioritizing work with communities that are the most marginalized, vulnerable, disadvantaged and often regarded as 'hard to reach' based on considerations of equity
Equitable distribution of power	Power is distributed equitably between stakeholders	Facilitating participatory and egalitarian processes that assist with the redistribution of power
Ethical change processes	Change processes enable active participation of people affected by the issue	Ensuring that people most affected by an issue are an integral part of all components of a health promotion change process that addresses the issue, as distinct from being targeted as recipients of decisions made external to them
	Processes do not impinge on people's personal autonomy	Ensuring that all relevant parties consent to health promotion change processes and acknowledging and respecting that not all people will choose the same actions
	Beneficence is a priority consideration	Actively considering what the benefits of any health promotion change process may be and who may be the beneficiaries
	Non-maleficence is a priority consideration	Actively considering what the potential harms of any health promotion change process may be, who may be harmed by the change processes and in what way. Taking steps to minimize or avoid this harm. Communicating risks involved in a truthful and open manner
Evidence-based practice	Practice is based on evidence of need and effectiveness, and sound theoretical foundations	Ensuring that needs assessment processes incorporate the perspectives of all stakeholders, and that health promotion practice is based on sound evidence of need, evidence of effectiveness, and appropriate theoretical foundations

a global community sits well not only with our moral intuitions but also with Rawls' famous phrase, 'the justice of fairness' (Rawls, 1971). Health promoters thus embody a personal ethic with global scope and a will to act to make the world a 'better place', invoking Karl Marx's famous maxim that the point is not only to understand the world, but to change it. Health promoters clearly go further than say, traditional epidemiologists, whose role is to describe the world (of disease and illness), as a fundamental part of the role of the health promoter is to change the world.

Following McGregor (2004, pp. 98–99), it is essential that health promoters have 'an engagement in how we are involved in reproducing power imbalances, oppression, and difference between ourselves and others'. This *political* awareness necessarily moves us away from the language of 'helping' and towards 'working alongside', 'joining together' in an empathic identification with others (Peterson, 2007).

Health promoters with their personal ethic of social justice and equity may appear to be relentlessly optimistic about the role of health promotion as a means to save the world from health injustices. Health promotion is a profession of hope and it does place at its centre a hopeful view of people and the enduring qualities of what it means to be human. The fact that the Commission on the Social Determinants of Health was set up *and* that it has achieved a great deal of attention at the highest levels fuels this optimism. The SDH are well known and tackling the major ones is relatively straightforward; other areas are less tangible and thus more difficult, but Barry (2009) has argued for example in the case of mental health, that we have robust evidence from systematic reviews about the effectiveness of interventions tackling social determinants. The use of policy to tackle the social determinants is also becoming a refined science (Exworthy, 2008). We thus have no excuse for not taking action – we know what to do.

Table 6.4. Values and principles in the technical domain (Gregg and O'Hara, 2007b, p. 16).

Value	Principle	Explanation
Comprehensive actions	Portfolio of multiple strategies is used to address complex issues	Using multiple strategies incorporating all action areas of the Ottawa Charter
Democratic governance	Collaborative models of governance and decision making	Using models of governance and decision making that facilitate active and meaningful participation by all stakeholders
Practitioner is a resource	Work with communities as an ally	Working with communities as an ally and a resource on tap for communities
System-level evaluation	Evaluate sustainable changes to systems that support people to increase control over their health	Ensuring that evaluation focuses on assessing the changes in the range of factors that enable people to increase control over the determinants of their health

Similarly, the application of settings approaches has become much more sophisticated in terms of design, implementation and evaluation (Poland *et al.*, 2009).

However, optimism needs to be tempered with realism, and we have to be realistic about what *can* be achieved. We can perhaps pause here to reflect on what are the most important things for health promoters to do, in the absence of being able to do everything. What then are the most important things on the health promoter's 'to do list'?

To Do List

- Recognize that networks are stronger than hierarchies, and work to build coalitions, networks and means of enabling the marginalized to access these too.
- Remind the major global players that whilst the discourse on health has moved into newer ways of conceptualizing health and development to include less easily measured factors such as happiness, satisfaction and well-being, there are many whose basic needs are not being met. There is therefore still a need for focus on the basic social indicators of development such as life expectancy at birth, maternal mortality, literacy rates, access to safe water and so on.
- Given that social capital is crucial to communities taking charge of their own affairs, work to maintain and build social capital in innovative and creative ways.
- Develop the evidence base on the success of attempts to tackle social determinants and how these affect health.

- Develop settings as a practical means of 'doing' health promotion, thus creating enabling environments for true transformation, whilst also recognizing that there are interstitial spaces where often the most marginalized live their lives.
- Continue to develop methods for authentic participation.

Summary

This book summarizes our thinking on health promotion and is presented as *one* contribution to the field. It's important the readers find other views and also follow up ideas that we have only been able to skim over here. Fields of endeavour apart from health promotion also struggle with the goals of empowerment, equality, justice, and are also contemplating how to deal with challenges of the 21st century, such as complexity, globalization and social capital. These fields might include education, criminal justice, social work, sport, development, and so provide rich and relevant avenues for further reading. Much of our work is fuelled by the sense of injustice exemplified by the obscene levels of wealth in the global North and the continuing, pernicious and crippling levels of poverty in parts of the global South, in tandem with the inequalities seen *within* countries. The result is that people cannot become all they are capable of becoming, they live in conditions which are not dignified, and their human rights are not respected. If health promotion is essentially about enabling people to take control of the determinants of their health, we can only too plainly see that many people, perhaps the majority in global terms, are not in charge of their own destinies. Those destinies are determined, rather, by those in charge of global markets. There is a groundswell movement towards challenging those powers and creating a global world where health and human happiness are prioritized. We need to put a halt to unsustainable development, and learn lessons from those middle-income countries that have developed decent living standards and good levels of health for their populations. Nothing short of a transformation is needed in the way that global priorities are set and in the way that power and wealth are distributed. There do appear to be openings for such transformations at the start of the 21st century, with more room to hear the voices of civil society in calling for different ways of measuring well-being, happiness and development, and in challenging the power of the corporations, governments and other powerful interests who wish to subjugate and silence those voices. It remains to be seen whether these opportunities for creating a more just world will materialize, but health promotion, as a movement for health justice, needs to keep creating a place for itself at the global debating table, whilst continuing to practice at grassroots level to bring small but significant changes to people's lives.

Further Reading

Fisher, W.F. and Ponniah, T. (eds) (2003) *Another World Is Possible: Popular Alternatives to Globalization at the World Social Forum.* Zed Books, London.

Gaventa, J. and McGee, R. (2010) *Citizen Action and National Policy Reform: Making Change Happen.* Zed Books, London.

Haworth, J. and Hart, G. (2012) *Well-Being: Individual, Community and Social Perspectives.* Palgrave Macmillan, London.

Smith, S. (2011) *Equality and Diversity – Value Incommensurability and the Politics of Recognition.* The Policy Press, London.

Wilkinson, R. and Pickett, K. (2010) *The Spirit Level.* Penguin, London.

References

Abbott, P.A., Turmov, S. and Wallace, C. (2006) Health world views of post-soviet citizens. *Social Science & Medicine* 62, 228–238.

Abdel-Khalek, A.M. (2006) Measuring happiness with a single-item scale. *Social Behaviour and Personality* 34, 139–149.

Abercrombie, N., Hill, S. and Turner, B.S. (2006) *Penguin Dictionary of Sociology*. Penguin Books Ltd, London.

Abraham, C. and Sheeran, P. (2005) The health belief model. In: Conner, M. and Norman, P. (eds) *Predicting Health Behaviours*, 2nd edition. Open University Press, Buckingham, UK, pp. 28–80.

Abroms, L. and Maibach, E. (2008) The effectiveness of mass communication to change public behaviour. *Annual Review of Public Health* 29, 219–234.

Abubakari, A.R., Lauder, W., Jones, M.C., Kirk, A., Agyemang, C. and Bhopal, R.S. (2009) Prevalence and time trends in diabetes and physical inactivity among adult West African populations: the epidemic has arrived. *Public Health* 123, 602–614.

Acheson, D. (1998) *Independent Inquiry into Inequalities in Health Report*. Stationery Office, London.

Aday, R.H. and Kehoe, G. (2008) Working in old age: benefits of participation in the Senior Community Service Employment Program. *Journal of Workplace Behavioral Health* 23, 1–2.

Adeleye, O.A. and Ofili, A.N. (2010) Strengthening intersectoral collaboration for primary health care in developing countries: can the health sector play broader roles? *Journal of Environmental and Public Health*, article ID 272896, doi: 10.115/2010/272896.

Aidoo, M. and Harpham, T. (2001) The explanatory models of mental health amongst low income women and health care practitioners in Lusaka, Zambia. *Health Policy and Planning* 16, 206–213.

Airhihenbuwa, C. and Obregon, R. (2000) A critical assessment of theories/models used in health communication for HIV/AIDS. *Journal of Health Communication* 5 (Supplement), 5–15.

Airhihenbuwa, C.O. (2007) 2007 SOPHE Presidential Address: On being comfortable with being uncomfortable: centering an Africanist vision in our gateway to global health. *Health Education Behavivour* 34, 31.

Ajayi, J.E.A., Lameck, K.H., Goma, G. and Ampah, J. (1996) *The African Experience with Higher Education*. Association of African Universities, Accra, Ghana.

Ajzen, I. (1988) *Attitudes, Personality and Behaviour*. Open University Press, Milton Keynes, UK.

Ajzen, I. (1991) The theory of planned behaviour. *Organizational Behavior and Human Decision Processes* 50, 179–211.

Albery, I.P. and Munafò, M. (2008) *Key Concepts in Health Psychology*. Sage, London.

Albrecht, G., Freeman, S. and Higginbotham, N. (1998) Complexity and human health: the case for a transdisciplinary paradigm. *Culture, Medicine and Psychiatry* 22, 55–92.

Alcock, P. (2003) *Social Policy in Britain*. Palgrave, Basingstoke, UK.

Alderson, P. (2000) School students' views on school councils and daily life at school. *Children and Society* 14, 121–134.

Allah Nikkhah, H. and Redzuan, M. (2009) Participation as a medium of empowerment in community development. *European Journal of Social Sciences* 11, 170–176.

Allegrante, J.P., Barry, M., Airhihenbuwa, C.O., Auld, E., Collins, J.L., Lamarre, M-C., Magnusson, G., McQueen, D.V., Maurice, B. and Mittelmark, M. on behalf of the Galway Consensus Conference (2009) Domains of core competency, standards, and quality assurance for building global capacity in health promotion: the Galway Consensus Conference Statement. *Health Education & Behavior* 36, 476–482.

Allmark, P. and Tod, A. (2006) How should public health professionals engage with lay epidemiology? *Journal of Medical Ethics* 32, 460–463.

Amunyunzu-Nyamongo, M. and Nyamwaya, D. (eds) (2009) *Evidence of Health Promotion Effectiveness in Africa*. African Institute for Health, Nairobi.

Amunyunzu-Nyamongo, M., Jones, C. and McQueen, D. (2009) Repositioning health promotion in Africa. In: Amunyunzu-Nyamongo, M. and Nyamwaya, D. (eds) (2009) *Evidence of Health Promotion Effectiveness in Africa*. African Institute for Health, Nairobi.

Angell, M. (2004) *The Truth About the Drug Companies: How They Deceive Us and What to Do About It*. Random House, New York.

Anielski, M. (2007) *The Economics of Happiness: Building Genuine Wealth*. New Society Publishers, Grabiola Island, Canada.

Anme, T. and McCall, M.E. (2011) Empowerment in health and community settings. In: Muto, T., Nakahara, T. and Woo Nam, E. (eds) *Asian Perspectives and Evidence on Health Promotion and Education*. Springer, London.

Antoniades, A. (2003) Epistemic communities, epistemes and the construction of world politics. *Global Society* 17, 21–38.

Antonovksy, A. (1996) The salutogenic model as a theory to guide health promotion. *Health Promotion International* 11, 11–18.

Appiah, K.A. (2006) *Cosmopolitanism: Ethics in a World of Strangers*. Norton, New York.

Araujo, N. (2011) Health Promotion Awards 2011: recognising today's health promotion. *Perspectives on Public Health* 132, 14–15.

Archer, M. (2007) *Making our Way Through the World. Human Reflexivity and Social Mobility*. Cambridge University Press, Cambridge.

Armstrong, J.R.M., Abdulla, S., Nathan, R., Mulasa, O., Marchant, T.J., Kikumbuh, N., Mushi, A.K., Mponda, H., Minja, H., Mshinda, H., Tanner, M. and Lengeler, C. (2001) Effect of large-scale social marketing of insecticide-treated nets on child survival in rural Tanzania. *The Lancet* 357, 1241–1247.

Armstrong, R., Waters, E., Crockett, B. and Keleher, H. (2007) The nature of evidence resources and knowledge translation for health promotion practitioners. *Health Promotion International* 21, 76–83.

Arneson, H. and Ekberg, K. (2005) Evaluation of empowerment processes in a workplace health

promotion intervention based on learning in Sweden. *Health Promotion International* 20, 351–359.

Arnott, D., Dockrell, M., Sandford, A. and Willmore, I. (2007) Comprehensive smoke free legislation in England: how advocacy won the day. *Tobacco Control* 16, 423–428.

Arnstein, S. (1969) A ladder of citizen participation. *Journal of the American Institute of Planners* 35, 216–24.

Arroyo, H. (2005) Health promotion in Latin America. In: Scriven, A. and Garmen, S. (eds) *Promoting Health: Global Perspectives*. Palgrave Macmillan, Basingstoke, UK, pp. 179–186.

Asbridge, M. (2004) Public place restrictions on smoking in Canada: assessing the role of the state, media, science and public health advocacy. *Social Science & Medicine* 58, 13–24.

Asthana, S. and Halliday, J. (2006) *What Works in Tackling Health Inequalities? Pathways, Policies and Practice through the Lifecourse*. The Policy Press, Bristol, UK.

Atkinson, R. and Kintrea, K. (2004) Opportunities and despair, it's all there; practitioner experiences and explanations of area effects and life chances. *Sociology* 38, 437–455.

Attree, P., Clayton, S., Karunanithi, S., Nayak, S., Popay, J. and Read, D. (2011) NHS health trainers: a review of emerging evaluation evidence, *Critical Public Health*. DOI: 10.1080/ 09581596.2010.549207. Available at: http:// dx.doi.org/10.1080/09581596.2010.549207

Attwood, M., Pedler, M., Pritchard, S. and Wilkinson, D. (2003) *Leading Change. A Guide to Whole Systems Working*. The Policy Press, Bristol, UK.

Aubel, J., Touré, I. and Diagne, M. (2004) Senegalese grandmothers promote improved maternal and child nutrition practices: the guardians of tradition are not averse to change. *Social Science & Medicine* 59, 945–959.

Bach, S., Haynes, P. and Smith, J.L. (2007) *Online Learning and Teaching in Higher Education*. Open University Press, London.

Backett, K. (1992) Taboos and excesses: lay health moralities in middle class families. *Sociology of Health and Illness* 7, 110–117.

Baistow, K. (1994) Liberation and regulation? Some paradoxes of empowerment. *Critical Social Policy* 14, 34–46.

Ballantyne, D. (2000) Internal relationship marketing: a strategy for knowledge renewal. *International Journal of Bank Marketing* 18, 274–286.

Bambra, C., Fox, D. and Scott-Samuel, A. (2005) Towards a politics of health. *Health Promotion International* 20, 187–193.

Bambra, C., Gibson, M., Sowden, A., Wright, K., Whitehead, M. and Petticrew, M. (2010) Tackling the wider social determinants of health and health inequalities: evidence from systematic reviews. *Journal of Epidemiology & Community Health* 64, 284–291.

Bandura, A. (1986) *Social Foundations of Thought and Action: a Social Cognitive Theory*. Prentice Hall, Englewood Cliffs, New Jersey.

Barić, L. (1992) Health promoting hospitals. *Journal of the Institute of Health Education* 30, 141–148.

Barić, L. (1993) The settings approach – implications for policy and strategy. *Journal of the Institute of Health Education* 31, 17–24.

Barić, L. (1994) *Health Promotion and Health Education in Practice: Module 2 – the Organisational Model*. Barns Publications, Altrincham, UK.

Barić, L. (1995) Implications for policy and strategy. In: Theaker, T. and Thompson, J. (eds) *The Settings Based Approach to Health Promotion: Conference Report*. Hertfordshire Health Promotion, Welwyn Garden City, UK.

Barić, L. (1998) *People in Settings*. Barns Publications, Altrincham, UK.

Barić, L. and Barić, L. (1995) *Health Promotion and Health Education: Module 3 – Evaluation, Quality, Audit*. Barns Publications, Altrincham, UK.

Baric´, L. and Blinkhorn, A. (2007) Consumer-driven embedded health promotion and health education. *International Journal of Health Promotion and Education* 45, 87–92.

Barker, K. Lowe, C.M. and Reid, M. (2006) *The Use of Mass Media Interventions for Health Care Messages about Back Pain: What do Members of the Public Think?* Nuffield Orthopaedic Centre NHS Trust, Oxford, UK.

Barnekow, V., Buijs, G., Clift, S., Bruun Jensen, B., Paulus, P., Rivett, D. and Young, I. (2006) *Health-promoting Schools: a Resource for Developing Indicators*. European Network of Health Promoting Schools, Copenhagen.

Barnes, B. (2000) *Understanding Agency*. Sage, London.

Barnes, M. and Walker, A. (1996) Consumerism versus empowerment: a principled approach to the involvement of older service users. *Policy and Politics* 24, 375–393.

Barrett, E., Heycock, M., Hick, D. and Judge, E. (2003) Issues in access for disabled people: the case of the Leeds transport strategy. *Policy Studies* 4, 227–242.

Barry, J. and Doherty, B. (2001) The Greens and social policy. *Social Policy and Administration* 35, 387–609.

Barry, M. (2001) Promoting positive mental health: theoretical frameworks for practice. *International Journal of Mental Health Promotion* 3, 25–34.

Barry, M. (2008) Capacity building for the future of health promotion. *Global Health Promotion* 15, 56–58.

Barry, M. (2009) Addressing the determinants of positive mental health: concepts, evidence and practice. *International Journal of Mental Health Promotion* 11, 4–17.

Barry, M., Allegrante, J., Lamarre, M-C., Auld, E. and Taub, A. (2009) The Galway Consensus Conference: international collaboration on the development of core competencies for health promotion and health education. *Global Health Promotion* 16, 5–11.

Bartram, J. and Cairncross, S. (2010) Hygiene, sanitation and water: forgotten foundations of health. *PLoS Medicine* 7(11), e1000367.

Baum, F. (1999) The role of social capital in health promotion: Australian perspectives. *Health Promotion Journal of Australia* 9, 171–178.

Baum, F. (2001) Health, equity, justice and globalisation: some lessons from the People's Health Assembly. *Journal of Epidemiology and Community Health* 55, 613–616.

Baum, F. (2002) Health and greening the city. Setting for health promotion: the importance for an evidence base. *Journal of Epidemiology and Community Health* 56, 897–898.

Baum, F. (2003) *The New Public Health*, 2nd edition. OUP, South Australia.

Baum, F. (2007) Cracking the nut of health equity: top down and bottom up pressure for action on the social determinants of health. *Promotion & Education* 14, 90–95.

Baum, F. (2009) Envisioning a healthy and sustainable future: essential to closing the gap in a generation. *Global Health Promotion Supplement* 1, 72–80.

Baum, F. and Sanders, D. (1995) Can health promotion and primary health care achieve Health for All without a return to their more radical agenda? *Health Promotion International* 10, 149–160.

Baum, F. and Simpson, S. (2006) Building healthy and equitable societies – what Australia can contribute to and learn from the Commission on the Social Determinants of Health. *Health Promotion Journal of Australia* 17, 173–1797.

Baxter Magolda, M. (2001) *Making their Own Way: Narratives for Transforming Higher Education to Promote Self-development.* Stylus, Sterling, Virginia.

BBC News (2011) David Cameron's NHS 'support' claim disputed by staff. BBC News Online, 7 September: Available at: http://www.bbc.co.uk/news/uk-politics- 14829485

Beattie, A. (1991) Knowledge and control in health promotion: a test case for social policy and social theory. In: Gabe, J., Calnan, M. and Bury, M. (eds) *The Sociology of the Health Service.* Routledge and Kegan Paul, London.

Begum, H. (2003) *Social Capital in Action: Adding Up Local Connections and Networks. A Pilot Study in London.* Centre for Civil Society and NCVO, London.

Bellis, M.A., Hughes, K. and Lowey, H. (2002) Healthy nightclubs and recreational substance use. From a harm minimisation to a healthy settings approach. *Addictive Behaviors* 27, 1025–1035.

Bengel, J., Strittmatter, R. and Willmann, H. (1999) What keeps people healthy? The current state of discussion and the relevance of Antonovsky's salutogenic model of health. *Research and Practice of Health Promotion*, 4, Federal Centre for Health Education, Cologne, Germany.

Bennett, P. (1998) The heart of distance learning: a student's perspective. *International Journal of Lifelong Education* 17, 51–60.

Bennett, P. and Murphy, S. (1997) *Psychology and Health Promotion.* Open University Press, Buckingham, UK.

Bensberg, M. and Kennedy, M. (2002) A framework for health promoting emergency departments. *Health Promotion International* 17, 179–188.

Berkman, L.F., Leo-Summers, L. and Horwitz, R.I. (1992) Emotional support and survival after myocardial infarction: a prospective, population-based study of the elderly. *Annals of Internal Medicine* 117, 1003–1009.

Berman, Y. and Phillips, D. (2003) Indicators for social cohesion. Paper submitted to the European Network on Indicators of Social Quality of the European Foundation on Social Quality, Amsterdam.

Berne, E. (1964) *Games People Play.* Penguin Books, New York.

Berry, D. (2007) *Health Communication: Theory and Practice.* Open University Press, Maidenhead, UK.

Best, S. and Kellner, D. (1997) *The Postmodern Turn.* Guilford Press, New York.

Bhagwati, J. (2004) *In Defence of Globalisation.* Oxford University Press, Oxford.

Billings, J. and Hashem, F. (2009) *Literature Review: Salutogenesis and the Promotion of Positive Mental Health in Older People.* EU Thematic conference 'Mental Health and Wellbeing in Older People – Making it Happen' 19–20 April 2010, European Commission Directorate-General for Health and Consumers and the Spanish Ministry of Health and Social Affairs with support of the Spanish Presidency of the European Union, Madrid.

Bird, L., Hayton, P., Caraher, M., McGough, H. and Tobutt, C. (1999) Mental health promotion and prison health-care staff in young offenders' institutions in England. *The International Journal of Mental Health Promotion* 1, 16–24.

Bird, W. (2007) *Natural Thinking: Investigating the Links between the Natural Environment, Biodiversity and Mental Health.* A report for the Royal Society for the Protection of Birds, Sandy, UK.

Bissell, P., May, C.R. and Noyce, P.R. (2004) From compliance to concordance: barriers to accomplishing a re-framed model of health care interactions. *Social Science & Medicine* 40, 851–862.

Blake, G., Robinson, D. and Smerdon, M. (2006) *Living Values: A Report Encouraging Boldness in Third Sector Organisations.* Common Links, London.

Blakemore, K. and Griggs, E. (2007) *Social Policy. An Introduction.* Open University Press, Maidenhead, UK.

Blaxter, M. (1990) *Health and Lifestyles.* Routledge, London.

Blaxter, M. (1997) Whose fault is it? People's own conceptions of the reasons for health inequalities. *Social Science & Medicine* 44, 747–56.

Blaxter, M. (2004) *Health.* Polity Press, Cambridge, UK.

Blumler, J.G. and Katz, E. (eds) (1974) *The Use of Mass Communications: Current Perspectives on Uses and Gratifications Research.* Sage, Newbury Park, California.

Bodenheimer, T.S. (1985) The transanational pharmaceutical industry and the health of the world's people. In: McKinley, J.B. (ed.) *Issues in the Political Economy of Health Care*. Tavistock, London.

Boseley, S. (2003) Sugar industry threatens to scupper WHO. *The Guardian*, 21 April 2003.

Boster, F.J. and Mongeau, P.A. (1984) Fear arousing persuasive messages. In: Bostrom, R. (ed.) *Communication Year Book*, Volume 8. Sage, Newbury Park, California, pp. 330–375.

Bourdieu, P. (1986) The forms of capital. In: Richardson, J. (ed.) *Handbook of Theory and Research for the Sociology of Education*. Greenwood Press, New York, pp. 241–258.

Bourdieu, P. (1999) *The Weight of the World: Social Suffering in Contemporary Society*. Cambridge University Press, Cambridge.

Bourne, R. (ed.) (2000) *Universities and Development*. Association of Commonwealth Universities, London.

Boyle, D., Coote, A., Sherwood, C. and Slay, J. (2010) Right Here, Right Now Taking co-production into the Mainstream, NESTA. Available at: http://www.neweconomics.org/publications/right-here-right-now (accessed 23 July 2010).

Bracht, N. and Tsouros, A. (1990) Principles and strategies of effective participation. *Health Promotion International* 5, 199–208.

Bradley, S. (1994) *How People Use Pictures*. IIED/British Council, London.

Brannen, J. and Storey, P. (1996) *Child Health in Social Context: Parental Employment and the Start of Secondary School*. Health Education Authority, London.

Branscum, P. and Sharma, M. (2010) A review of motivational interviewing-based interventions targeting problematic drinking among college students. *Alcoholism Treatment Quarterly* 28, 63–77.

Brautigam, D. (2000) *Interest Groups, Economic Policy, and Growth in Sub-Saharan Africa*, African Economic Policy Discussion Paper No. 40, Washington, DC, United States Agency for International Development Bureau for Africa.

Brehm, M.V. (2001) *Promoting Effective North–South NGO Partnerships*. Occasional paper series Number 35. INTRAC, Oxford, UK.

British Institute of Learning Disability (2005) No need to scream: good practice made easy. *Advocacy News*, Issue 20.

Britten, N. (2003) Does a prescribed treatment match a patient's priorities? *British Medical Journal* 327, 840.

Brodie, D.A. and Inoue, A. (2005) Motivational interviewing to promote physical activity for people with chronic heart failure. *Journal of Advanced Nursing* 50, 518–527.

Brooks, W. and Heath, R. (1985) *Speech Communication*. W.C. Brown, Dubuque, Iowa; cited in Hargie, O., Saunders, C. and Dickson, D. (1994) *Social Skills in Interpersonal Communication*, 3rd edition. Routledge, London and New York.

Brooks-Gunn, J., Duncan, G., Klebanov, P. and Sealane, N. (1993) Do neighbourhoods influence child and adolescent development? *American Journal of Sociology* 99, 353–393.

Brown, P., Zavestoski, S., McCormick, S., Mayer, B., Morello-Frosch, R. and Altman, R.G. (2004) Embodied health movements: new approaches to social movements in health. *Sociology of Health & Illness* 26, 50–80.

Brown, P.A. and Piper, S.M. (1993) Perpetuating the status quo: a response to Jeff French and Sue Milner. *Health Education Journal* 52, 256–258.

Brownson, R.C., Baker, E.A., Leet, T.L. and Gillespie, K.N. (2003) *Evidence Based Public Health*. Oxford University Press, Oxford.

Brownson, R.C., Fielding, J.E. and Maylahn, C.M. (2009) Evidence-based public health: a fundamental concept for public health practice. *Annual Review of Public Health* 30, 175–201.

Bruhn, J.G. and Wolf, S. (1979) *The Roseto Story: An Anatomy of Health*. University of Oklahoma Press, Norman, Oklahoma.

Buckley, J. and O Tuama, S. (2010) 'I send the wife to the doctor' – men's behaviour as health consumers. *International Journal of Consumer Studies* 34, 587–595.

Bull, F.C., Adams, E.J., Hooper, P.L. and Jones, C.A. (2008) *Well@Work: A Summary Report and Calls to Action*. British Heart Foundation, London.

Bunton, R. (2002) Health promotion as social policy. In: Bunton, R. and Macdonald, G. (eds) *Health Promotion. Disciplines, Diversity and Developments*, 2nd edition. Routledge, London, pp. 129–157.

Bunton, R. and MacDonald, G. (1992) *Health Promotion: Disciplines and Diversity*. Routledge, London.

Bunton, R., Nettleton, S. and Burrows, R. (1996) *The Sociology of Health Promotion: Critical Analyses of Consumption, Lifestyle and Risk*. Routledge, London.

Bunton, R., Baldwin, S., Flynn, D. and Whitelaw, S. (2000) The 'stages of change' model in health promotion: science and ideology. *Critical Public Health* 10, 55–70.

Burgoyne, J. (1992) *Creating a Learning Organization*. Royal Society of the Arts Paper, London.

Burke, B., Arkowitz, H. and Menchola, M. (2003) The efficacy of motivational interviewing: a meta analysis of controlled clinical trials. *Journal of Consulting and Clinical Psychology* 74, 943–954.

Burns, M. and Gavey, N. (2004) 'Healthy weight' at what cost? 'Bulimia' and a discourse of weight control. *Journal of Health Psychology* 9, 549–565.

Bury, M. (1994) Health promotion and lay epidemiology: a sociological view, *Health Care Analysis* 2, 23–30.

Caballero, B. (2005) A nutrition paradox: underweight and obesity in developing countries. *New England Journal of Medicine* 352, 1514–1516.

Cacioppo, J. and Patrick, W. (2008) *Loneliness: Human Nature and the Need for Social Connection*. WW Norton and Co., London.

Cairney, P. (2009) The role of ideas in policy transfer: the case of UK smoking bans since devolution. *Journal of European Public Policy* 11, 57–77.

Calman, K. (2009) Beyond the 'nanny state': stewardship and public health. *Public Health* 123, 6–10.

Calnan, M. (1987) *Health and Illness: the Lay Perspective*. Tavistock Publications, London.

Calnan, M. and Williams, S. (1991) Style of life and the salience of health. *Sociology of Health and Illness* 13, 506–516.

Campbell, C. (1999) *Social Capital and Health*. Health Education Authority, London.

Campbell, C. (2001) Social capital and health: contextualizing health promotion within local community networks. In: Baron, S., Field, J. and Schuller, T. (eds) *Social Capital: Critical Perspectives*. Oxford University Press, Oxford, pp. 182–196.

Campbell, C. (2011) Embracing complexity: towards more nuanced understandings of social capital and health. *Global Health Action* 4, 1–3.

Campbell, C. and Scott, K. (2011) Retreat from Alma Ata?: the WHO's report on task shifting to community health workers for AIDS care in poor countries. *Global Public Health* 6, 125–138.

Campbell, K., Waters, E., O'Meara, S., Kelly, S. and Summerbell, C. (2002) Interventions for preventing obesity in children. *Cochrane Database of Systematic Reviews*, 2, D001871.

Canadian Health Services Research Foundation (2007) Incorporate lay health workers to promote health and prevent disease, Evidence Boost for Quality September 2007, Ontario, Canadian Health Services Research Foundation. Available at: http://www.chsrf.ca/publicationsandresources/pastseries/evidenceboost/07-09-01/b672cd4e-564a-4f10-8f96-679c1109eb41.aspx

Candib, L.M. (2007) Obesity and diabetes in vulnerable populations: reflections on proximal and distal causes. *Annals of Family Medicine* 5, 547–556.

Capstick, S., Norris, P., Sopoaga, F. and Tobata, W. (2009) Relationship between health and culture in Polynesia: a review. *Social Science & Medicine* 68, 1341–1348.

Caraher, M., Dixon, P., Hayton, P., Carr-Hill, R., McGough, H. and Bird, L. (2002) Are health-promoting prisons an impossibility? Lessons from England and Wales. *Health Education* 102, 219–229.

Carlisle, S. (2000) Health promotion, advocacy and health inequalities. *Health Promotion International* 15, 369–376.

Carr, D. (2004) *Improving the Health of the World's Poorest People*. Health Bulletin, 1. Population Reference Bureau, Washington, DC.

Carrington, W. and Detragiache, E. (1999) How extensive is the brain drain? *Finance and Development, A quarterly magazine of the IMF*, 36(2).

Carter, M., Karwalajtys, T., Chambers, L., Kaczorowski, J., Dolovich, L., Gierman, T., Cross, D. and Laryea, S. (2009) Implementing a standardised community-based cardiovascular risk assessment program in 20 Ontario communities. *Health Promotion International* 24, 325–333.

Carvalho, A.I. Westphal, M.F. and Pereira Lima, V.L.G. (2005) Health promotion in Brazil. *Promotion and Education* (Special Edition) 1, 7–12.

Casiday, R. Kinsman, E. and Bambra, C. (2008) Volunteering and health: what impact does it really have? Report to Volunteering England. Available at: http://www.volunteering.org.uk/WhatWeDo/Projects+and+initiatives/volunteeringinhealth/hsc.ht (accessed 19 November 2011).

Catford, J. (1998) Social entrepreneurs are vital for health promotion – but they need supportive environments too. *Health Promotion International* 13, 95–97.

Catford, J. (2005) The Bangkok conference: steering countries to build national capacity for health promotion. *Health Promotion International* 20, 1–6.

Catford, J. (2010) Editorial: Implementing the Nairobi Call to Action: Africa's opportunity to light the way. *Health Promotion International* 25, 1–4.

Cattan, M. (2009a) Loneliness, interventions. In: Reis, H. and Sprecher, S. (eds) *The Encyclopedia of Human Relationships*. Sage, London.

Cattan, M. (ed.) (2009b) *Mental Health and Wellbeing in Later Life*. McGraw-Hill/Open University Press, Maidenhead, UK.

Cattan, M. (2010) *Preventing Social Isolation and Loneliness among Older People*, VDM Publishing, Saarbrücken, Germany.

Cattan, M. (2012) Mental health issues for older people. In: Reed, J., Clarke, C. and MacFarlane, A. (eds) *Nursing Older Adults*. Open University Press/McGraw-Hill, Maidenhead, UK.

Cattan, M. and Tilford, S. (2006) *Mental Health Promotion: A Lifespan Approach*. McGraw-Hill, Maidenhead, UK.

Cattan, M., White, M., Bond, J. and Learmouth, A. (2005) Preventing social isolation and loneliness among older people: a systematic review of health promotion intervention. *Ageing and Society* 25, 41–67.

Cattan, M., Woodward, J., Marsden, G. and Jopson, A. (2009) Will anyone listen to me? The older traveller and transport planning. *Access by Design* 118, 31–36.

Cattaneo, L.B. and Chapman, A.R. (2010) The process of empowerment: a model for use in research and practice. *American Psychologist* 65, 646–659.

Cattell, V. (2001) Poor people, poor places and poor health: the mediating role of social networks and social capital. *Social Science & Medicine* 52, 1501–1516.

Chapman, J., Edwards, C. and Hampson, S. (2009) *Connecting the dots*. Demos, London. Available at: http://www.demos.co.uk/publications/connecting-the-dots (accessed 6 November 2012).

Chapman, N., Emerson, S., Gough, J., Mepani, B. and Road, N. (2000) *Views of Health 2000*. Save the Children, London Development Team.

Chen, H., Tu, S.P., The, C.Z., Yip, M.P., Choe, J.H., Hislop, T.G., Taylor, V.M. and Thompson, B. (2006) Lay beliefs about hepatitis among North American Chinese: implications for hepatitis prevention. *Journal of Community Health* 31, 94–112.

Chen, M., Jhabvala, R., Kanbur, R. and Richards, C. (eds) (2007) *Membership-based Organisations of the Poor*. Routledge, New York.

Chen, M.C. (2007) Rethinking the informal economy: linkages with the formal economy and the formal regulatory environment. DESA Working Paper No 46, UN Department of Economic & Social Affairs. Available at: http://www.un.org/esa/desa/papers (accessed 6 November 2012).

Chopra, M. (2005) Inequalities in health in developing countries: challenges for public health research. *Critical Public Health* 15, 19–26.

Christakis, N.A. and Fowler, J.H. (2007) The spread of obesity in a large social network over 32 years. *New England Journal of Medicine* 357, 370–379.

Christakis, N.A. and Fowler, J.H. (2008) The collective dynamics of smoking in a large social network. *New England Journal of Medicine* 358, 2249–2258.

Chronin de Chavez, A., Backett-Milburn, K., Parry, O. and Platt, S. (2005) Understanding and researching well-being: its usage in different disciplines and potential for health research and health promotion. *Health Education Journal* 64, 70–87.

Chu, C. (2003) *Assessment of Health Promotion in Indonesia*. Report for WHO, Geneva.

CIESIN – Center for International Earth Science Information Network (2005) *Poverty Mapping project: Global Subnational Infant Mortality Rates*. Columbia University, New York. Available at: http://sedac.ciesin.columbia.edu

Clay, E.J. and Schaffer, B.B. (1986) *Room for Manoeuvre. An Explanation of Public Policy in Agriculture and Rural Development*. Heinemann, London.

Colby, S.M., Monti, P.M., Barnett, N.P., Rohsenow, D.J., Weissman, K., Spririto, A., Woolard, R.H. and Lewander, W.J. (1999) Brief motivational interviewing in a hospital setting for adolescent smoking: a preliminary study. *Journal of Consulting and Clinical Psychology* 66, 574–578.

Cole, M. (2000) Learning through reflective practice: a professional approach to effective continuing professional development among healthcare professionals. *Research in Post-Compulsory Education* 5, 23–38.

Colebatch, H.K. (2002) *Policy*, 2nd edition. Open University Press, Philadelphia, Pennsylvania.

Coleman, J.S. (1990) *Foundations of Social Theory*. The Belknap Press of Harvard University Press, Cambridge, Massachusetts.

Coleman, J.S. (1998) Social capital in the creation of human capital. *American Journal of Sociology* 94, 95–120.

Collier, P. (2007) *The Bottom Billion: Why the Poorest Countries are Failing and what can be done about it*. Oxford University Press, Oxford.

Colvin, C.J. (2011) Think locally, act globally: developing a critical public health in the global South. *Critical Public Health* 21, 253–256.

Colvin, N. and Wargalla, K. (2011) What we're doing here. *The Guardian*, 24 October, p. 28.

Commission on Social Determinants of Health (2008) *Closing the Gap in a Generation: Health Equity through Action on the Social Determinants of Health. Final Report of the Commission on Social Determinants of Health*. WHO, Geneva.

Conner, M. and Norman, P. (eds) (2005) *Predicting Health Behaviours*, 2nd edition. Open University Press, Buckingham, UK.

Conrad, D. and White, A. (eds) (2007) *Men's Health: How to Do It*. Radcliffe Publishing, Oxford, UK.

Conrad, D. and White, A. (2010) *Promoting Men's Mental Health*. Radcliffe Publishing, Oxford, UK.

Cooper, R.J., Bissell, P., Warde, P., Murphy, E., Anderson, C., Avery, T., James, V., Lymn, J., Guillaume, L., Hutchinson, A. and Ratcliffe, J. (2011) Further challenges to medical dominance? The case of nurse and pharmacist supplementary prescribing. *Health* 20, 1–19.

Corbin, J. and Bonde, L.T. (2012) Intersections of context and HIV/AIDS in sub-Saharan Africa: what can we learn from feminist theory? *Perspectives in Public Health* 132(8), DOI: 10.1177/1757913911430909.

Corcoran, N. (2007) *Communicating Health: Strategies for Health Promotion*. Sage, London.

Corcoran, N. (2011) *Working on Health Communication*. Sage, London.

Corcoran, N. and Bone, A. (2007) Using settings to communicate health promotion. In: Corcoran, N. (ed.) *Communicating Health Strategies for Health Promotion*. Sage, London.

Cornish, F. and Campbell, C. (2010) *How can Community Health Programmes build Enabling Environments for Transformative Communication?: Experiences from India and South Africa*. HCD Working Papers 1, London School of Economics and Political Science, London.

Crabb, J. and Ratinckx, L. (2005) *The Healthy Stadia Initiative*. UCLan/DOH, Preston, UK.

Craig, J.V. and Smyth, R.L. (2002) *The Evidence Based Practice Manual for Nurses*. Churchill Livingstone, London.

Craig, R.L., Felix, H.C., Walker, J.F. and Phillips, M.M. (2010) Public health professionals as policy entrepreneurs: Arkansas's childhood obesity policy experience. *American Journal of Public Health* 100, 2047–2052.

Crawford, R. (1984) A cultural account of health: control, release and the social body. In: McKinlay, J.B. (ed.) *Issues in the political economy of health*. Tavistock, London, pp. 60–103.

Cribb, A. and Duncan, P. (2002) *Health Promotion and Professional Ethics*. Blackwell, Oxford, UK.

Crinson, I. (2009) *Health Policy: A Critical Perspective*. Sage, London.

Critical Appraisal Skills Programme (no date) *Resources and Tools*. CASP, Oxford, UK.

Cross, R., Milnes, K., Rickett, B. and Fylan, F. (2011) Risking a stigmatised identity: a discourse analysis of young women's talk about health and risk. *Qualitative Methods in Psychology* 12, 22–29.

Crossley, M.L. (2001) The 'Armistead' project: an exploration of gay men, sexual practices, community health promotion and issues of empowerment. *Journal of Community & Applied Social Psychology* 11, 111–123.

Crossley, M.L. (2002) The perils of health promotion and the 'barebacking' backlash. *Health* 6, 47–68.

Crossley, N. (2001) Citizenship, intersubjectivity and the lifeworld. In: Stevenson, N. (ed.) *Culture and Citizenship*. Sage, London, pp. 33–46.

Crundall, I. and Deacon, K. (1997) A prison-based alcohol use education program: evaluation of a pilot study. *Substance Use & Misuse* 32, 767–777.

Culp, K., Kuye, R., Donham, K., Rautiainen, R., Umbarger-Mackey, M. and Marquez, S. (2007) Agricultural-related injury and illness in The Gambia. *Clinical Nursing Research* 16, 170–188.

Curtis, V., de Barra, M. and Aunger, R. (2011) Disgust as an adaptive system for disease avoidance behaviour. *Philosophical Transactions of the Royal Society B: Biological Sciences* 366, 389–401.

D'Houtaud, A. and Field, M.G. (1984) The image of health: variations in perception by social class in a French population. *Sociology of Health and Illness* 6, 30–60.

Dahlgren, G. and Whitehead, M. (1991) *Policies and Strategies to Promote Social Equity in Health*. Institute of Futures Studies, Stockholm.

Dahlgren, G. and Whitehead, M. (2006) *European Strategies for Tackling Social Inequities in Health: Levelling up Part 1*. WHO, Copenhagen.

Dahlgren, G. and Whitehead, M. (2007) *Policies and Strategies to Promote Social Equity in Health*. Background document to WHO – Strategy paper for Europe, Institute for Futures Studies, Stockholm.

Daley, B.J. (2001) Learning and professional practice: a study of four professions. *Adult Education Quarterly* 52, 39–54.

Dalyrymple, J. and Burke, B. (2001) *Anti-oppressive Practice: Social Care and the Law*. Open University Press, Buckingham, UK.

Darzi, A. (2008) *High Quality Care for All: NHS Next Stage Review Final Report*. DOH, London, Cmd 7432.

Davies, R. (2002) Monitoring and evaluation NGO achievements. In: Desai, V. and Potter, R.B. (eds) *The Companion to Development Studies*. Arnold, London.

Davies, S.E. (2010) *Global Politics of Health*. Polity, Cambridge, UK.

Davison, C., Davey-Smith, G. and Frankel, S. (1991) Lay epidemiology and the prevention paradox. *Sociology of Health and Illness* 13, 1–19.

Davison, C., Frankel, S. and Davey Smith, G. (1992) The limits of lifestyle: re-assessing fatalism in the popular culture of illness prevention. *Social Science and Medicine* 34, 675–685.

Daykin, J. and Naidoo, N. (1995) Feminist critiques of health promotion. In: Bunton, R., Nettleton, S. and Burrows, R. (eds) *The Sociology of Health Promotion: Critical Analysis of Consumption, Lifestyle and Risk*. Routledge, London and New York, pp. 59–69.

De Leeuw, E. (2000) Commentary – beyond community action: communication arrangements and policy networks. In: Poland, B., Green, L.W. and Rootman, I. (eds) *Settings for Health Promotion*. Sage, Thousand Oaks, California.

De Leeuw, E. (2010) Online tool for network participants, stakeholders, social and policy entrepreneurs to map policy networks. Available at: http://evelynedeleeuw.net

De Leeuw, E. and Skovgaard, T. (2005) Utility-driven evidence for healthy cities: problems with evidence generation and application. *Social Science & Medicine* 61, 1331–1341.

De Onis, M. and Blossner, M. (2000) Prevalence and trends of overweight among preschool children in developing countries. *American Journal of Clinical Nutrition* 72, 1032–1039.

de Viggiani, N. (2006) Surviving prison: exploring prison social life as a determinant of health. *International Journal of Prisoner Health* 2, 71–89.

de Viggiani, N. (2009) *A Healthy Prison Strategy for HMP Bristol. Project report*. University of the West of England, Bristol, UK.

De Villiers, W.A. (2008) The learning organisation: validating a measuring instrument. *The Journal of Applied Business Research* 24, 11–20.

De Vos, P., Malaise, G., De Ceukelaire, W., Perez, D., Lefevre, P. and Van der Stuyft, P. (2009) Participation and empowerment in Primary Health Care: from Alma Ata to the era of globalization. *Social Medicine* 4, 121–127.

Dean, M. (2011) *Democracy under attack – How the Media Distort Policy and Politics*. The Policy Press, Bristol, UK.

De-Graft Aikins, A., Boynton, P. and Atanga, L.L. (2010) Developing chronic disease interventions in Africa: insights from Ghana and Cameroon. Globalization and Health 6, 6. Available at: http://www.globalizationandhealth.com/content/6/1/6

Deiner, E. and Chan, M.Y. (2011) Happy people live longer: subjective well-being contributes to health and longevity. *Applied Psychology: Health and Well-Being* 3, 1–43.

Delaney, F. (1994) Muddling through the middle ground: theoretical concerns in intersectoral collaboration and health promotion. *Health Promotion International* 9, 217–225.

Denman, S., Moon, A., Parsons, C. and Stears, D. (2002) *The Health Promoting School: Policy, Research and Practice*. Routledge, London.

DOH (Department of Health) (1992) *The Health of the Nation: a Strategy for Health in England*. HMSO, London.

DOH (2001a) *The Expert Patient: a New Approach to Chronic Disease Management for the 21st Century*. DOH, London.

DOH (2001b) *Valuing People: a New Strategy for Learning Disability for the 21st Century*. DOH, London.

DOH (2002) *Health Promoting Prisons: a Shared Approach*. Crown, London.

DOH (2004) *Choosing Health: Making Healthier Choices Easier*. The Stationery Office, London.

DOH (2005) *Shaping the Future of Public health: Promoting health in the NHS*. Department of Health and Welsh Assembly, Crown, London.

DOH (2009) *Improving health, supporting justice: the national delivery plan of the health and criminal justice programme board*. DOH, London.

DOH (2010) *Healthy Lives, Healthy People. White Paper: Our strategy for public health in England*. DOH, London.

Dewey, J. (1916) *Democracy and Education*. Macmillan, Old Tappan, NJ. In: Brookfield, S.D. and Preskill, S. (1999) *Discussion as a way of Teaching – Tools and Techniques for University Teachers*. The Society for Research into Higher Education and Open University Press, London.

Diener, E. and Chan, M.Y. (2011) Happy people live longer: subjective well-being contributes to health and longevity. *Applied Psychology: Health and Well-Being*, DOI: 10.1111/j.1758-0854.2010.01045.x.

Dixey, R. (1999b) 'Fatalism', accident causation and prevention: issues for health promotion from an exploratory study in a Yoruba town, Nigeria. *Health Education Research* 14, 197–208.

Dixey, R. (2001) The experience of postgraduate study in the UK. *Africa Health* 2001, 6–7.

Dixey, R. (2010) Health promotion and occupational therapy. In: Curtin, M., Molineux, M. and Supyk-Mellson, J. (eds) *Occupational Therapy and Physical Dysfunction: Enabling Occupation*, 6th edition. Churchill-Livingstone/Elsevier, London.

Dixey, R. and Green, M. (2009) Sustainability of the health care workforce in Africa: a way forward in Zambia. *The International Journal of Environmental, Cultural, Economic and Social Sustainability* 5, 301–310.

Dixey, R. and Woodall, J. (2012) The significance of 'the visit' in an English category-B prison: views from prisoners, prisoners' families and prison staff. *Community, Work and Family* 15, 29–48.

Dixey, R., Sahota, P., Atwal, S. and Turner, A. (2001a) Children talking about healthy eating: data from focus groups with 300 nine to eleven year olds. *British Nutrition Foundation Bulletin* 26, 71–79.

Dixey, R., Sahota, P., Atwal, S. and Turner, A. (2001b) 'Ha ha, you're fat, we're strong'; a qualitative study of boys' and girls' perceptions of fatness, thinness, social pressures and health using focus groups. *Health Education* 101, 206–216.

Dixey, R., Rudolf, M.C.J. and Murtagh, J. (2006) WATCH IT obesity management for children: a qualitative exploration of the views of parents. *International Journal of Health Promotion and Education* 44, 131–137.

Dixey, R.A. (1998a) Healthy eating in schools, overweight and 'eating disorders': are they connected? *Educational Review* 50, 29–35.

Dixey, R.A. (1998b) Improvements in child pedestrian safety: have they been gained at the expense of other health goals? *Health Education Journal* 57, 60–69.

Dixey, R.A. (1999a) Keeping children safe: the effect on parents' daily lives and psychological well-being. *Journal of Health Psychology* 4, 45–57.

Dixon-Woods, M., Agarwal, S., Young, B., Jones, D. and Sutton, A. (2004) *Integrative Approaches to Qualitative and Quantitative Evidence*. Health Development Agency, London.

Doherty, S. and Dooris, M. (2006) The healthy settings approach: the growing interest within colleges and universities. *Education and Health* 24, 42–43.

Dooris, M. (2001) The 'health promoting university': a critical exploration of theory and practice. *Health Education* 101, 51–60.

Dooris, M. (2004) Joining up settings for health: a valuable investment for strategic partnerships? *Critical Public Health* 14, 37–49.

Dooris, M. (2005) Healthy settings: challenges to generating evidence of effectiveness. *Health Promotion International* 21, 55–65.

Dooris, M. (2006) Health promoting settings: future directions. *Promotion & Education* 13, 4–6.

Dooris, M. and Doherty, S. (2010a) Healthy universities – time for action: a qualitative research study exploring the potential for a national programme. *Health Promotion International* 25, 94–106.

Dooris, M. and Doherty, S. (2010b) Healthy universities: current activity and future directions – findings and reflections from a national-level qualitative research study. *Global Health Promotion* 17, 6–16.

Dooris, M. and Hunter, D.J. (2007) Organisations and settings for promoting public health. In: Lloyd, C.E., Handsley, S., Douglas, J., Earle, S. and Spurr, S. (eds) *Policy and Practice in Promoting Public Health*. Sage, London.

Dooris, M. and Martin, E. (2002) Developing a health promoting university initiative within the context of inter-sectoral action for sustainable public health: reflections from the University of Central Lancashire. *Promotion & Education* Supplement 1 – Special Edition, 16–24.

Dooris, M. and Thompson, J. (2001) Health-promoting universities: an overview. In: Scriven, A. and Orme, J. (eds) *Health Promotion: Professional Perspectives*, 2nd edition. Palgrave, London.

Dooris, M., Dowding, G., Thompson, J. and Wynne, C. (1998) The settings-based approach to health promotion. In: Tsouros, A., Dowding, G., Thompson, J. and Dooris, M. (eds) *Health Promoting Universities: Concept, Experience and Framework for Action*. WHO, Copenhagen.

Dooris, M., Poland, B., Kolbe, L., Leeuw, E.D., McCall, D. and Wharf-Higgins, J. (2007) Healthy settings. Building evidence for the effectiveness of whole system health promotion – challenges and future directions. In: McQueen, D.V. and Jones, C.M. (eds) *Global Perspectives on Health Promotion Effectiveness*. Springer, New York.

Dorling, D. (2011) *Injustice: Why Social Inequality Persists*. The Policy Press, Bristol, UK.

Douglas, J. (1995) Developing anti-racist health promotion strategies. In: Bunton, R., Nettleton, S. and Burrows, R. (eds) *The Sociology of Health Promotion*. Routledge, London.

Douglas, J. (1997) Developing health promotion strategies with black and minority ethnic communities which address social inequalities. In: Sidell, M., Jones, L., Katz, J. and Peberdy, A. (eds) *Debates and Dilemmas in promoting health*. Macmillan Press, Basingstoke, UK.

Douglas, R. (1998) A framework for healthy alliances. In: Scriven, A. (eds) *Alliances in Health Promotion. Theory and Practice*. Macmillan, Basingstoke, UK, pp. 3–17.

Dovlo, D. (2003) The brain drain and retention of health professionals in Africa. A case study prepared for a regional training conference on *Improving Tertiary Education in Sub-Saharan Africa: Things that Work!* 23–25 September 2003, Accra, Ghana.

Dovlo, D. (2005) Wastage in the health force: some perspectives from African countries. *Human Resources for Health*, 3(6).

Dower, N. (2003) *An Introduction to Global Citizenship*. Edinburgh University Press, Edinburgh, UK.

Dowler, E. (1998) Food poverty and food policy. *IDS Bulletin* 29, 58–65.

Dowler, E., Caraher, M. and Lincoln, P. (2007) Inequalities in food and nutrition: challenging 'lifestyles'. In: Dowler, E. and Spencer, N. (eds) *Challenging Health Inequalities: from Acheson to Choosing Health*. The Policy Press, Bristol, UK, pp. 127–155.

Dowling, B., Powell, M. and Glendinning, C. (2004) Conceptualising successful partnerships. *Health and Social Care in the Community* 12, 309–317.

Downie, R.S., Fyfe, C. and Tannahill, A. (1990) *Health Promotion: Models and Values*, 1st edition. Oxford University Press, Oxford.

Downie, R.S., Tannahill, C. and Tannahill, A. (1996) *Health Promotion. Models and values*. Oxford University Press, Oxford.

Doyal, L. (1995) *What Makes Women Sick: Gender and the Political Economy of Health*. Rutgers University Press, New Brunswick, New Jersey.

Doyal, L. with Pennell, I. (1979) *The Political Economy of Health*. Pluto, London.

Draper, A., Hewitt, G. and Rifkin, S. (2010) Chasing the dragon: developing indicators for the assessment of community participation in health programmes. *Social Science & Medicine* 71, 1102–1109.

Draper, R. (1998) Healthy public policy: a new political challenge. *Health Promotion* 2, 217–218.

Duncan, P. (2007) *Critical Perspectives on Health*. Palgrave Macmillan, Basingstoke, UK.

Duncan, P. and Cribb, A. (1996) Helping people change – an ethical approach? *Health Education Research* 11, 339–348.

Dupere, S. (2007) Views on the international influence of Canadian health promotion. In: O'Neil, M., Pederson, A., Dupere, S. and Rootman, I. (eds) *Health Promotion in Canada: Critical Perspectives*. Canadian Scholars Press Inc., Toronto.

Durie, M. (2004) An indigenous model of health promotion. *Health Promotion Journal of Australia* 15, 181–185.

Eade, D. (ed.) (2006) *Development, NGOs and Civil Society*. Oxfam, Oxford, UK.

Eakin, J.M. (2000) Commentary. In: Poland, B.D., Green, L.W. and Rootman, I. (eds) *Settings for Health Promotion. Linking Theory and Practice*. Sage, Thousand Oaks, California.

Earle, S. (2007) Promoting public health: exploring the issues. In: Earle, S., Lloyd, C.E., Sidell, M. and Spurr, S. (eds) *Theory and Research in Promoting Public Health*. Sage, London, pp. 1–36.

Easton, P., Monkman, K. and Miles, R. (2003) Social policy from the bottom up: abandoning FGC in sub-Saharan Africa. *Development in Practice* 13, 445–458.

EC (2011) *The State of Men's Health in Europe: Extended Report*. The European Commission, DG Sanco, Luxembourg. Available at: http://ec.europa.eu/health/population_groups/docs/men_health_extended_en.pdf

Economic Commission for Africa (2005) *Economic Report on Africa 2005: Meeting the Challenges of Unemployment and Poverty in Africa*. Economic Commission for Africa, Addis Ababa.

Edwards, P. and Collinson, M. (2002) Empowerment and managerial labor strategies: pragmatism regained. *Work and Occupations* 29, 272, DOI: 10.1177/ 0730888402029003002.

Egan, M., Bambra, C. and Thomas, S. (2007) The psychosocial and health effects of workplace reorganisation: a systematic review of interventions that aim to increase employee participation or control. *Journal of Epidemiology & Community Health* 61, 945–954.

Egolf, B., Lasker, J., Wolf, S. and Potvin, L. (1992) The Roseto effect: a 50-year comparison of mortality rates. *American Journal of Public Health* 82, 1089–1092.

El Ansari, W., Phillips, C.J. and Zwi, A.B. (2002) Narrowing the gap between academic professional wisdom and community lay knowledge: partnerships in South Africa. *Public Health* 116, 151–159.

Ellen, I. and Turner, M. (1997) Does neighbourhood matter? Assessing review evidence. *Housing Policy Debate* 8, 833–866.

Emerson, E., Baines, S., Allerton, L. and Welch, V. (2011) *Health Inequalities and People with Learning Disabilities in the UK 2011*. Improving Health and Lives Learning Disabilities Observatory, Durham, UK.

Emslie, C. and Hunt, K. (2008) The weaker sex? Exploring lay understandings of gender differences in life expectancy: a qualitative study. *Social Science & Medicine* 67, 808–816.

Emslie, C., Hunt, K. and Watt, G. (2001) Invisible women? The importance of gender in lay beliefs about heart problems. *Sociology of Health and Illness* 23, 203–233.

Epstein, S. (1996) *Impure Science: AIDS, Activism and the Politics of Knowledge*. University of California Press, Berkeley, California.

Eraut, M. (2001) Do continuing professional development models promote one-dimensional learning? *Medical Education* 35, 8–11.

Eraut, M. (2004) Informal learning in the workplace. *Studies in Continuing Education* 26, 247–273.

Eriksson, M. and Lindström, B. (2008) A salutogenic interpretation of the Ottawa Charter. *Health Promotion International* 23, 190–199.

Esping-Anderson, G. (1990) *The Three Worlds of Welfare Capitalism*. Polity Press, Cambridge, UK.

European Environment Agency (2002) *Late Lessons from Early Warnings: the Precautionary Principle 1896–2000*. Environmental issue report No. 22, European Environment Agency.

European Network for Health Promotion Agencies (2001) *The Role of Health Promotion in Tackling Inequalities in Health*. European Commission.

Evans, L. (2008) Professionalism, professionality and the development of education professionals. *British Journal of Educational Studies* 56, 20–38.

Everingham, C. (2003) *Social Justice and the Politics of the Community*. Ashgate, Aldershot, UK.

Ewles, I. and Simnett. (2003) *Health Promotion, Practical Approaches*. Elsevier Health Sciences, London.

Ewles, L. and Simnett, I. (1985) *Promoting Health: A Practical Guide to Health Education*. John Wiley & Sons, Chichester, UK.

Exworthy, M. (2008) Policy to tackle the social determinants of health: using conceptual models to understand the policy process. *Health Policy and Planning* 23, 318–327.

Eyer, J. (1985) Capitalism, health, and illness. In: McKinley, J.B. (ed.) *Issues in the Political Economy of Health Care*. Tavistock, London, pp. 23–59.

Farmer, P., Frenk, J. and Knaulet, F.M. (2010) Expansion of cancer care and control in countries of low and middle income: a call to action. *Lancet*, epub 16 Aug, 2.

Farquhar, S.A., Wiggins, N., Michael, Y.L., Luhr, G., Jordan, J. and Lopez, A. (2008) 'Sitting in different chairs': roles of the community health workers in the Poder es Salud/Power for Health Project. *Education for Health* 21, 39.

Farrant, W. (1997) Addressing the contradictions: health promotion and community health action in the United Kingdom. In: Sidell, M., Jones, L.,

Katz, J. and Peberdy, A. (eds) *Debates and Dilemmas in Promoting Health*. Macmillan Press, Basingstoke, UK.

Featherstone, M. (1993) Global and local cultures. In: Bird, J., Curtis, B., Putnam, T., Robertson, G. and Tickner, L. (eds) *Mapping the Future: Local Cultures, Global Change*. Routledge, London and New York.

Federation of Community Development Learning (undated) A summary of good practice standards for CD work. Available for download from: http://www.fcdl.org.uk

Feste, C. and Anderson, R.M. (1995) Empowerment: from philosophy to practice. *Patient Education and Counseling* 26, 139–144.

Fidler, D.P. (2007) Architecture amidst anarchy: global health's quest for governance. *Global Health Governance* 1, 1–17.

Finn, P. (1981) Teaching students to be lifelong peer educators. *Health Education* 12, 13–16.

Fisher, B.J. and Gosselink, C.A. (2008) Enhancing the efficacy and empowerment of older adults through group formation. *Journal of Gerontological Social Work* 51, 1–2.

Fisher, W.F. (1997) DOING GOOD? The politics and antipolitics of NGO practices. *Annual Review of Anthropology* 26, 439–464.

Fitzpatrick, R., Newman, S., Archer, R. and Shipley, M. (1991) Social support, disability and depression a longitudinal study. *Social Science & Medicine* 33, 605–611.

Fletcher, C.M. (1973) *Communication in Medicine*. Nuffield Provincial Hospital Trust, London.

Flora, J.L. (1998) Social capital and communities of place. *Rural Sociology* 63, 481–506.

Fordyce, M.W. (2005) A review of research on the happiness measures: a sixty second index of happiness and mental health. *Social Indicators Research Series* 26, 373–399.

Foster, S., Dixey, R., Oberlin, A. and Nkhama, E. (2012) 'Sweeping is women's work': employment and empowerment opportunities for women through engagement in solid waste management in Tanzania and Zambia. *International Journal of Health Promotion and Education* 50, 203–217.

Fowler, A. (1998) *NGOs in Africa: achieving comparative advantage in relief and micro development*, IDS Discussion Paper 249. Institute of Development Studies, Brighton, UK.

Fowler, J.H. and Christakis, N.A. (2008) Dynamic spread of happiness in a large social network: longitudinal analysis over 20 years in the Framingham heart study. *British Medical Journal* 337, 1–9.

Fox, N. and Ward, K. (2006) Health identities: from expert patient to resisting consumer. *Health: An Interdisciplinary Journal for the Social Study of Health, Illness and Medicine* 10, 461–479.

Fraser, C. and Restrepo-Estrada, S. (1998) *Communicating for Development: Human Change for Survival*. I.B. Tauris, London.

Fraser, H. (2005) Four different approaches to community participation. *Community Development Journal* 40, 286–300.

Freedman, D.S., Khan, L.K., Dietz, W.H., Srinivasan, S.R. and Berenson, G.S. (2001) Relationship of childhood obesity to coronary heart disease risk factors in adulthood: the Bogalusa Heart Study. *Pediatrics* 108, 712–718.

Freire P (1972) *Pedagogy of the Oppressed*. Penguin, London.

Freire, P. (2000) *Pedagogy of the Oppressed*, 30th anniversary edition, translated by Myra Bergman Ramos, with introduction by Macedo. Continuum, London and New York.

French, J. (2007) The market-dominated future of public health? In: Douglas, J., Earle, S., Handsley, S., Lloyd, C.E. and Spurr, S. (eds) *A Reader in Promoting Public Health: Challenge and Controversy*. Sage, London, pp. 19–25.

French, J. and Milner, S. (1993) Should we accept the status quo? *Health Education Journal* 52, 98–101.

French, J., Blair-Stevens, C., McVey, D. and Merritt, R. (2010) *Social Marketing and Public Health: Theory and Practice*. Oxford University Press, Oxford.

Freudenberg, N. (2005) Public health advocacy to change corporate practices: implications for health education, practice and research. *Health Education and Behaviour* 32, 298–319.

Freudenberg, N. (2007) Health research behind bars: a brief guide to research in jails and prisons. In: Greifinger, R.B., Bick, J. and Goldenson, J. (eds) *Public health behind bars. From prisons to communities*. Springer, New York.

Friedman, A. and Philips, M. (2004) Continuing professional development: developing a vision. *Journal of Education Work* 17, 361–376.

Friel, S., Bell, R., Houweling, A.J. and Marmot, M. (2009) Calling all Don Quixotes and Sancho Panzas: achieving the dream of global health equity through practical action on the social determinants of health. *Global Health Promotion Supplement* 1, 9–13.

Frosh, S. (2001) Psychoanalysis, identity and citizenship. In: Stevenson, N. (ed.) *Culture and Citizenship*. Sage, London, pp. 62–73.

Fry, T. (2007) A growing concern: soon the UK will adopt new World Health Organization growth charts based on measurements of breastfed babies. Available at: http://findarticles.com/p/articles/mi_m1SFS/is_5_80/ai_n25006311/ (accessed 10 February 2012).

Fukuyama, F. (1999) Social Capital and Civil Society. Conference paper prepared for the IMF Conference on Second Generation Reforms.

Fukuyama, F. (2001) Social capital, civil society and development. *Third World Quarterly* 22, 7–20.

Furudi, F. (1997) *The Culture of Fear: Risk Taking and the Morality of Low Expectations*. Cassell, London.

Furudi, F. (2001) *Paranoid Parenting: Abandon your Anxieties and be a Good Parent*. Allen Lane, London.

Gable, S.L. and Haidt, J. (2005) What and why is positive psychology? *Review of General Psychology* 9, 103–110.

Gage, A.J. (2007) Barriers to the utilisation of maternal health care in rural Mali. *Social Science & Medicine* 65, 1666–1682.

Galea, G., Powis, B. and Tamplin, S.A. (2000) Healthy islands in the Western Pacific-international settings development. *Health Promotion International* 15, 169–178.

Galer-Unti, R.A., Tappe, M.J.K. and Lachenmayr, S. (2004) Advocacy 101: getting started in health education advocacy. *Health Promotion Practice* 5, 280–288.

Galukande, M. and Kiguli-Malwadde, E. (2010) Rethinking breast cancer screening strategies in resource-limited settings. *African Health Sciences* 10, 89–92.

Gamarnikow, E. and Green, A. (1999) Developing social capital: dilemmas, possibilities and limitations in education. In: Hayton, A. (ed.) *Tackling Disaffection and Social Exclusion*. Kogan Page, London, pp. 44–64.

Gambling, T.S. (2003) A qualitative study into the informational needs of coronary heart disease patients. *International Journal of Health Promotion and Education* 41, 68–76.

Gerdtham, U. and Johannesson, M. (2001) The relationship between happiness, health, and socio-economic factors: results based on Swedish microdata. *Journal of Socio-Economics* 30, 553–557.

Gerhardt, S. (2004) *Why Love Matters; How Affection Shapes a Baby's Brain*. Routledge, London and New York.

Germond, P. and Cochrane, J. (2010) Healthworlds: conceptualising landscapes of health & healing. *Sociology* 44, 307–324.

Gibbon, M. (2000) The health analysis and action cycle: an empowering approach to women's health. *Sociological Research Online*, 4.

Gibson, A. (2006) Health and community: is the concept of social capital helpful? PhD thesis, Faculty of Health and Social Care, Open University, Milton Keynes, UK.

Gibson, A. (2010) Does social capital have a role to play in the health of communities? In: Douglas, J., Earle, S., Handsley, S., Jones, L., Lloyd, C.E. and Spurr, S. (eds) *A Reader in Promoting Public Health. Challenge and Controversy*, 2nd edition. Sage, London.

Giuntoli, G. (2010) Understanding quality of life through Sen's capability framework: an application to people living with HIV/AIDS. PhD thesis, The Australian National University, Canberra.

Godhino, J. (2005) Public health in the former Soviet Union. In: Scriven, A. and Garman, S. (2005) *Promoting Health: Global Perspectives*. Palgrave Macmillan, Basingstoke, UK.

Goldstein, M. (1999) *Alternative Health Care: Medicine, Miracle or Mirage?* Temple University Press, Philadelphia, Pennsylvania.

Gostin, L. (2007) A proposal for a framework convention on global health. *Journal of International Economic Law* 10, 989–1008.

Gostin, L. (2010) Transforming global governance through broadly imagined global health governance. *McGill Journal of Law and Health* 4, 3–16.

Grace, V. (1991) The marketing of empowerment and the construction of the health consumer: a critique of health promotion. *International Journal of Health Services* 21, 329–343.

Graham, C. (2008) Happiness and health: lessons – and questions – for public policy. *Health Affairs* 27, 72–87.

Grant, A.M., Christianson, M.K. and Price, R.H. (2007) Happiness, health, or relationships? Managerial practices and employee well-being tradeoffs. *Academy of Management Perspectives* August, 51–63.

Grant, M. (1994) *Propaganda and the role of the state in inter-war Britain*. Clarendon Press, Oxford, UK.

Green, G., Grimsley, M., Syolcas, A., Prescott, M., Jowitt, T. and Linacre, R. (2000) *Social Capital, Health and Economy in South Yorkshire Coalfield Communities*. Centre for Regional Economic and Social Research, Sheffield Hallam University, Sheffield, UK.

Green, J. and South, J. (2006) *Evaluation*. Open University Press, Maidenhead, UK.

Green, J. and Tones, K. (1999) Towards a secure evidence base for health promotion. *Journal of Public Health Medicine* 21, 133–139.

Green, J. and Tones, K. (2010) *Health Promotion: Planning and Strategies*, 2nd edition. Sage, London.

Green, L.W., Poland, B.D. and Rootman, I. (2000) The settings approach to health promotion. In: Poland, B.D., Green, L.W. and Rootman, I. (eds) *Settings for Health Promotion. Linking Theory and Practice*. Sage, Thousand Oaks, California.

Gregg, J. and O'Hara. (2007a) Values and principles evident in current health promotion practice. *Health Promotion Journal of Australia* 18, 7–11.

Gregg, J. and O'Hara. (2007b) The Red Lotus Health Promotion Model: a new model for holistic, ecological and salutogenic health promotion practice. *Health Promotion Journal of Australia* 18, 12–19.

Griffiths, J. and Reynolds, A. (2009) How to help organisations to take action. In: Griffiths, J., Rao, M., Adshead, F. and Thorpe, A. (2009) *The Health Practitioner's Guide to Climate Change, Diagnosis and Cure*. Earthscan, London.

Griffiths, J., Blair-Stevens, C. and Thorpe, A. (2008) Social marketing for health and specialised health promotion: stronger together – weaker apart. A paper for debate. Shaping the Future of Health Promotion, Royal Society of Public Health, National Social Marketing Centre, London.

Griffiths, J., Rao, M., Adshead, F. and Thorpe, A. (2009) *The Health Practitioner's Guide to Climate Change, Diagnosis and Cure*. Earthscan, London.

Grinstead, O., Zack, B. and Faigeles, B. (2001) Reducing postrelease risk behavior among HIV seropositive prison inmates: the health promotion program. *AIDS Education and Prevention* 13, 109–119.

Groot, E. (2011) Use of evidence in WHO health promotion declarations: overview, critical analysis, and personal reflection. *Reflective Practice* 12, 507–513.

Groves, R., Middleton, A., Murie, A. and Broughton, K. (2003) *Neighbourhoods That Work. A Study of the Bournville Estate, Birmingham*. The Policy Press, Bristol, UK.

Grunau, G.L., Ratner, P. and Hossain, S. (2008) Ethnic and gender differences in perceptions of mortality risk in a Canadian urban centre. *International Journal of General Medicine* 1, 41–50.

Guareschi, P. and Jovchelovitch, S. (2004) Participation, health and the development of community resources in southern Brazil. *Journal of Health Psychology* 9, 311–322.

Guldberg, H. (2009) *Reclaiming Childhood: Freedom and Play in an Age of Fear*. Routledge, London.

Guldbrandsson, K. and Fossum, B. (2009) An exploration of the theoretical concepts policy windows and policy entrepreneurs at the Swedish public health arena. *Health Promotion International* 24, 434–444.

Gunn, L.A. (1978) Why is implementation so difficult? *Management Services in Government* 33, 169–176.

Guo, S.S., Roche, A.F., Chumlea, W.C., Gardner, J.D. and Siervogel, R.M. (1994) The predictive value of childhood body mass index values for overweight at age 35 years. *American Journal of Clinical Nutrition* 59, 810–819.

Gureje, O. and Alem, A. (2000) Mental health policy development in Africa. *Bulletin of the World Health Organization* 78, 475–482.

Gustafson, P. (2001) Meanings of place: everyday experience and theoretical conceptualisations. *Journal of Environmental Psychology* 21, 5–16.

Gutiérrez, L. (1991) Empowering women of color: a feminist model. In: Bricker-Jenkins, M., Hooyman, N.R. and Gottlieb, N. (eds) *Feminist Social Work Practice in Clinical Settings*. Sage, London.

Gwatkin, D.R. (1997) Global burden of disease. *The Lancet* 350, 141.

Haas, P. (1989) Do regimes matter? Epistemic communities and Mediterranean pollution control. *International Organization* 43, 377–403.

Hale, J. and Dillard, J.P. (1995) Fear appeals in health promotion campaigns: too much, too little or just right? In: Maibach, E. and Parrott, R. (eds) *Designing Health Messages*. Sage, Thousand Oaks, California.

Hall, J. and Taylor, R. (2003) Health for all beyond 2000: the demise of the Alma-Ata Declaration and primary care in developing countries. *The Medical Journal of Australia* 178, 17–20.

Halpern, D. (2005) *Social Capital.* Polity Press, Cambridge, UK.

Hancock, R.E.E., Bonner, G. and Madden, A.M. (2011) A qualitative examination of patient experiences of dietetic consultations. *Journal of Human Nutrition and Dietetics* 24, 284–285.

Hancock, T. (1999) Creating health and health promoting hospitals: a worthy challenge for the twenty-first century. *International Journal of Health Care Quality Assurance* 12, 8–19.

Hankivsky, O., Cormier, R. and Merich, D.D. (2009) *Intersectionality: Moving Women's Health Research and Policy Forward.* Women's Health Research Network, Vancouver.

Hanna, T. and Kangolle, C. (2010) Cancer control in developing countries: using health data and health services research to measure and improve access, quality and efficiency. *BMC International Health and Human Rights* 10: 24. Available at: http://www.biomedcentral.com/1472-698X/10/24 (accessed 3 November 2012).

Harden, A., Weston, R. and Oakley, A. (1999) *A Review of the Effectiveness and Appropriateness of Peer-delivered Health Promotion Interventions for Young People.* EPPI Centre, London.

Hargie, O., Saunders, C. and Dickson, D. (1994) *Social Skills in Interpersonal Communication,* 3rd edition. Routledge, London and New York.

Harkins, C. (2010) The Portman Group – Lobby Watch column. *British Medical Journal* 340, b5659.

Harper, R. (2001) *The Measurement of Social Capital in the United Kingdom.* Office for National Statistics, London.

Harper, R. and Kelly, M. (2003) *Measuring Social Capital in the United Kingdom.* Office for National Statistics, London.

Harris, T.A. (2004) *I'm ok – You're ok.* Quill, New York.

Harvey, D. (1973) *Social Justice and the City.* Arnold, London.

Hastings, G. and Stead, M. (2006) Social marketing. In: MacDowall, W., Bonell, C. and Davies, M. (eds) *Health Promotion Practice.* Open University Press, Maidenhead, UK, pp. 139–151.

Hawe, P., King, L., Noort, M., Gifford, S. and Lloyd, B. (1998) Working invisibly: health workers talk about capacity building in health promotion. *Health Promotion International* 13, 285–295.

Hawe, P., King, L., Noort, M., Jordens, C. and Lloyd, B. (2000) *Indicators to help with capacity building in health promotion.* NSW Health Department, Sydney.

Hawks, S.R., Hull, M.L., Thalman, R.L. and Richins, P.M. (1995) Review of spiritual health: definition, role, and intervention strategies in health promotion. *American Journal of Health Promotion* 9, 371–378.

Hazelwood, A. (2008) Using text messaging in the treatment of eating disorders. *Nursing Times* 104, 28–29.

Health Empowerment Leverage Project (no date) Available at: http://www.healthempowerment group.org.uk/

Health Scotland (2005) *Competencies for Health Promotion Practitioners.* NHS Health Scotland, Edinburgh, UK.

Henderson, J. (2010) Expert and lay knowledge: a sociological perspective. *Nutrition and Dietetics* 67, 4–5.

Heritage, Z. and Dooris, M. (2009) Community participation and empowerment in healthy cities. *Health Promotion International* 24, 45–55.

Herzlich, C. (1973) *Health and Illness.* Academic Press, New York.

Hibbitt, K., Jones, P. and Meegan, R. (2001) Tackling social exclusion: the role of social capital in urban regeneration on Merseyside – from mistrust to trust. *European Planning Studies* 9, 141–161.

Hilhorst, D. (2003) *The Real World of NGOs: Discourses, Diversity and Development.* Zed Books, London.

Hill, K., Thomas, K., Abouzahr, C., Walker, N., Say, L., Inoue, M. and Suzuki, E., on behalf of the Maternal Mortality Working Group. (2007) Estimates of maternal mortality worldwide between 1900 and 2005: an assessment of available data. *Lancet* 370, 1311–1319.

Hill, M. (1997) *The Policy Process in the Modern Society,* 3rd edition. Prentice Hall, London.

Hillsden, M. (2006) Motivational interviewing in health promotion. In: MacDowall, W., Bonell, C. and Davies, M. (eds) *Health Promotion Practice.* Open University Press, Maidenhead, UK, pp. 74–85.

Hoeijmakers, M., De Leeuw, E., Kenis, P. and de Vries, N.K. (2007) Local health policy development processes in the Netherlands: an expanded toolbox for health promotion. *Health Promotion International* 22, 112–121.

Hogwood, B. (1987) *From Crisis to Complacency? Shaping Public Policy in Britain*. Clarendon, Oxford.

Hogwood, B. and Gunn, L. (1984) *Policy Analysis for the Real World*. Oxford University Press, Oxford.

Holroyd, C. (2000) Are assessors professional? *Active Learning in Higher Education* 1, 28–44.

Hooge, M. and Stolle, D. (eds) (2003) *Generating Social Capital. Civil Society and Institutions in Comparative Perspective*. Palgrave Macmillan, Basingstoke, UK.

Horsely, K. (2007) Storytelling, conflict and diversity. *Community Development Journal* 10, 109.

Horsman, D. (2004) An investigation of the extent to which the University of Bradford compares to other higher education institutions (HEIs) in the UK in developing a learning and knowledge management climate. MEd Thesis, University of Bradford, UK.

Hubley, J. (1993) *Communicating Health: An Action Guide to Health Education and Health Promotion*. Macmillan Press, London.

Hubley, J. (2002) Health empowerment, health literacy and health promotion–putting it all together. Available at: http://www.hubley.co.uk/ (accessed 23 August 2010).

Hubley, J. (2006) Patient education in the developing world – a discipline comes of age. *Patient Education and Counselling* 61, 161–164.

Hubley, J. and Copeman, J. (2008) *Practical Health Promotion*. Polity Press, Cambridge, UK.

Hubley, J. and Gilbert, C. (2006) Eye health promotion and the prevention of blindness in developing countries: critical issues. *British Journal of Ophthalmology* 90, 279–284.

Huddart, J. and Picazo, O. (2003) *The Health Sector Human Resources Crisis in Africa: an Issues Paper*. USAID Bureau for Africa, Office of Sustainable Development, Washington, DC.

Hudson, B. (2002) Interprofessionality in health and social care: the Achilles' heel of partnership? *Journal of Interprofessional Care* 16, 7–17.

Hudson, J. and Lowe, S. (2004) *Understanding the Policy Process. Analysing Welfare Policy and Practice*. The Policy Press, Bristol, UK.

Hudson, J., Kuhner, S. and Lowe, S. (2008) *The Short Guide to Social Policy*. The Policy Press, Bristol, UK.

Hughner, R.S. and Kleine, S.S. (2004) Views of health in the lay sector: a compilation and review of how individuals think about health. *Health: An Interdisciplinary Journal for the Social Study of Health, Illness and Medicine* 8, 395–422.

Human Development Report (2011) Sustainability and Equity: A Better Future for All. Available at: http://hdr.undp.org/en/humandev (accessed 30 January 2012).

Hylton, K. (2010) How a turn to critical race theory can contribute to our understanding of 'race', racism and anti-racism in sport. *Sociology of Sport* 45, 335–354.

Hyung Hur, M. (2006) Empowerment in terms of theoretical perspectives: exploring a typology of the process and components across disciplines. *Journal of Community Psychology* 34, 523–540.

IDeA (2010) *A glass half-full: how an asset approach can improve community health and well-being*.

Ife, J. (2000) *Community Development: Community Based Alternatives in an Age of Globalisation*. Longman, Melbourne, Australia.

Igene, H. (2008) Global health inequalities and breast cancer: an impending public health problem for developing countries. *The Breast Journal* 14, 428–434.

Illich, I. (1976) *Limits to Medicine*. Marion Boyars, London.

ILO (2006) *Employment Creation in Municipal Service Delivery in Eastern Africa – Improving Living Conditions and Providing Jobs for the Poor* (Project Terminal Evaluation Report). ILO, Rome.

ILO (2010) Brief Profile on Informal Economy: Employment for Social Justice and a Fair Globalization. Available at: http://www.ilo.org/employment/Whatwedo/Publications/WCMS_140951/lang—en/index.htm (accessed 12 July 2011).

Ingelhart, R. (1997) *Modernisation and Postmodernisation: Cultural, Economic and Political Change in 43 Societies*. Princeton University Press, Princeton, New Jersey.

IRINnews (2009) Africa: Fighting the 'double whammy' of obesity and hunger. Available at: http://www.IRINnews.org (accessed 8 October 2009).

Ishikawa, H., Nomura, K., Sato, M. and Yano, E. (2008) Developing a measure of communicative and critical health literacy: a pilot study of

Japanese office workers. *Health Promotion International* 23, 269–274.

Jackson, S.F., Ridde, V., Valenti, H. and Gierman, N. (2007) Canada's role in international health promotion. In: O'Neil, M., Pederson, A., Dupere, S. and Rootman, I. (eds) *Health Promotion in Canada: Critical Perspectives.* Canadian Scholars Press Inc., Toronto.

Jacobs, G. (2006) Imagining the flowers, but working the rich and heavy clay: participation and empowerment in action research for health. *Educational Action Research* 14, 569–581.

Jaggar, A. (ed.) (2010) *Thomas Pogge and his Critics.* Polity Press, Cambridge, UK.

Janis, I.L. and Fresbach, S. (1953) Effects of fear arousing communications. *Journal of Abnormal and Social Psychology* 48, 78–92.

Jencks, C. (2007) *Critical Modernism: Where is Postmodernism Going?* John Wiley & Sons, London.

Jencks, C. and Mayer, S. (1990) The social consequences of growing up in a poor neighbourhood. In: Lynn, L. and McGeary, M. (eds) *Inner City Poverty in the United States.* National Academic Press, Washington, DC, pp. 111–186.

Jentsch, B. (2004) Making Southern realities count: research agendas and design in North-South collaborations. *International Journal of Social Research Methodology* 7, 259–269.

Jewkes, R. and Murcott, A. (1998) Community representatives: representing the 'community'? *Social Science & Medicine* 46, 843–858.

Jochum, V. (2003) *Social Capital: Beyond the Theory.* NCVO Publications, London.

Joffe, M. and Mindell, J. (2004) A tentative step towards health public policy. *Journal of Epidemiology and Community Health* 58, 966–968.

Johnson, A. and Baum, F. (2001) Health promoting hospitals: a typology of different organizational approaches to health promotion. *Health Promotion International* 16, 281–287.

Jolanki, O. (2004) Moral argumentation in talk about health and old age. *Health: An Interdisciplinary Journal for the Social Study of Health, Illness and Medicine* 8, 483–503.

Juma, C. and Clark, N. (1995) Policy research in sub-Saharan Africa: an exploration. *Public Administration and Development* 15, 121–137.

Kalnins, I., Hart, C., Ballantyne, P., Quartaro, G., Love, R., Sturis, G. and Pollack, P. (2002) Children's perceptions of strategies for resolving community health problems. *Health Promotion International* 17, 223–232.

Kanavos, P. (2006) The rising burden of cancer in the developing world. *Annals of Oncology* 17, viii15–viii23, doi: 10.1093/annonc/mdl983.

Karsten, S., Kubow, P., Matrai, Z. and Pitiyanuwat, S. (2000) Challenges facing the twenty-first century citizen: views of policy makers. In: Cogan, J.J. and Derricott, R. (eds) *Citizenship for the 21st Century: An International Perspective in Education.* Kogan Page, London, pp. 109–130.

Katz, E. and Lazarfeld, P.F. (1955) Personal influence. In: McQuail, D. and Windahl, S. (eds) (1993) *Communication Models: for the Study of Mass Communications,* 2nd edition. Longman, London.

Kaufmann, S. (2009) *The New Plagues. Pandemics and Poverty in a Globalised World.* Haus Publishing, London.

Kawachi, I. and Berkman, L. (2001) Social ties and mental health. *Journal of Urban Health –Bulletin of the New York Academy of Medicine* 78, 458–467.

Kawachi, I. and Kennedy, B.P. (1999) Income inequality and health: pathways and mechanisms. *Health Services Research* 34, 215–227.

Kawachi, I., Kennedy, B.P., Lochener, K. and Prothrow-Stith, D. (1997) Social capital, income inequality and mortality. *American Journal of Public Health* 87, 1491–1498.

Keating, D. (2000) Social capital and developmental health: making the connection. *Journal of Developmental and Behavioural Pediatrics* 21, 50–52.

Kebaabetswe, P.M. (2007) Barriers to participation in the prevention of mother to child HIV transmission programme in Gaborone, Botswana, a qualitative approach. *AIDS Care* 19, 355–360.

Keleher, H. (2004) Why build a health promotion evidence base about gender? *Health Promotion International* 19(3), doi: 10.1093/heapro/dah313.

Kelly, M., Swann, C., Killoran, A., Naidoo, B., Barnett-Paige, E. and Morgan, A. (2002) *Methodological Problems in Constructing the Evidence Base in Public Health.* Health Development Agency, London.

Kemm, J. (2001) Health impact assessment: a tool for healthy public policy. *Health Promotion International* 16, 79–85.

Keneally, T. (2011) *Three Famines: Starvation and politics.* Perseus, Reading, Massachusetts.

Kennedy, B.P., Kawachi, I. and Brainerd, E. (1998) The role of social capital in the Russian mortality crisis. *World Development* 26, 2029–2043.

Kettunen, T., Poskiparta, M. and Liimatainen, L. (2001) Empowering counselling, a case study: nurse patient encounter in a hospital. *Health Education Research* 16, 227–238.

Kettunen, T., Poskiparta, M. and Karhila, P. (2003) Speech practices that facilitate patient participation in health counselling – a way to empowerment? *Health Education Journal* 62, 326–340.

Khor, M. (2001) *Rethinking Globalisation: Critical Issues and Policy Choices*. Zed Books, London and New York.

Kickbusch, I. (1995) An overview to the settings based approach to health promotion. In: Theaker, T. and Thompson, J. (eds) *The Settings Based Approach to Health Promotion: Conference Report*. Hertfordshire Health Promotion, Welwyn Garden City, UK.

Kickbusch, I. (2005) Foreword. In: Scriven, A. and Garman, S. (eds) *Promoting Health: Global Perspectives*. Palgrave Macmillan, Basingstoke, UK, pp. xiii–xv.

Kickbusch, I., Draper, R. and O'Neill, M. (1990) Healthy public policy: a strategy to implement the Health for All philosophy at various governmental levels. In: Evers, A., Farrant, W. and Trojon, A. (eds) *Healthy Public Policy at the Local Level*. European Centre for Social Welfare Policy and Research, Vienna, pp. 1–6.

Kiger, A. (2004) *Teaching for Health*, 3rd edition. Churchill Livingstone, London.

Kime, N., South, J. and Lowcock, D. (2008) *An Evaluation of the Bradford District Health Trainers Programme – Phase 2*. Centre for Health Promotion Research, Leeds Metropolitan University, Leeds, UK.

Kinder, G., Cashman, S.B., Siefer, S.D., Inouye, A. and Hagopian, A. (2000) Integrating healthy communities concepts into health professions training. *Public Health Reports* 115, 266–270.

Kindhauser, M.K. (2003) *Communicable Diseases 2002: Global Defence Against the Infectious Disease Threat*. WHO/CDS/2003.15. WHO, Geneva.

King, L. (1998) The settings approach to achieving better health for children. *New South Wales Public Health Bulletin* 9, 128–129.

Kingdon, J.W. (1995) *Agendas, Alternatives and Public Policy*. Harper, New York.

Kinsella, K., White, J. and South, J. (2011) *East Riding Health Trainer Service: an Evaluation Report*. Bridlington, UK.

Kirschenbaum, H. and Henderson, V.L. (1989) *The Carl Rogers Reader*. Houghton Mifflin, Boston, Massachusetts.

Kleinman, A. (1980) *Patients and Healers in the Context of Culture*. University of California Press, London.

Knowles, M. (1980) *The Modern Practice of Adult Education*. Association Press, Chicago, Illinois.

Kobasa, S., Hiker, R. and Maddi, S. (1979) Who stays healthy under stress? *Journal Occupational Medicine* 21, 595–598.

Koenig, M., Hossain, M.B. and Whittaker, M. (1997) The influence of quality of care upon contraceptive use in rural Bangladesh. *Studies in Family Planning* 28, 278–289.

Kokko, S., Kannas, L. and Villberg, J. (2006) The health promoting sports club in Finland – a challenge for the settings-based approach. *Health Promotion International* 21, 219–229.

Kotter, J.P. (1996) *Leading Change*. Harvard Business School Press, Boston, Massachusetts.

Kovess-Masfety, M., Murray, M. and Gureje, O. (2005) Positive mental health. In: Herrman, H., Saxena, S. and Moodie, R. (eds) *Promoting Mental Health: Concepts, Emerging Evidence, Practice*. A report of the WHO, Department of Mental Health and Substance Abuse and the Victorian Health Promotion Foundation and University of Melbourne. WHO, Geneva.

Kreuter, M.T. and McClure, S.M. (2004) The role of culture in health communication. *Annual Review of Public Health* 25, 439–455.

Kreuter, M.W., Lukwago, S.N., Bucholtz, D.C., Clark, E.M. and Sanders-Thompson, V. (2003) Achieving Cultural appropriateness in health promotion programs: targeted and tailored approaches. *Health Education and Behavior* 30, 133.

Krumeich, A., Weitjts, W., Reddy, P. and Meijer-Weitz, A. (2001) The benefits of anthropological approaches for health promotion research and practice. *Health Education Research* 16, 121–130.

Kubow, P., Grossman, D. and Ninomiya, S. (2000) Multidimensional citizenship: educational policy for the 21st century. In: Cogan, J. and Derricot, R. (eds) *Citizenship for the 21st Century: An International Perspective on Education*. Kogan Page, London, pp. 131–150.

Kuye, R., Donham, K., Marquez, S., Sanderson, W., Fuortes, L., Rautiainen, R., Jones, M. and Culp, K. (2007) Pesticide handling and exposures among cotton farmers in The Gambia. *Journal of Agromedicine* 12, 57–69.

Kwok, C. and Sullivan, G. (2007) Health seeking behaviours among Chinese-Australian women: implications for health promotion programmes. *Health: An Interdisciplinary Journal for the Social Study of Health, Illness and Medicine* 11, 401–415.

Kymlicka, W. (1995a) *Multicultural Citizenship.* Clarendon Press, Oxford, UK.

Kymlicka, W. (ed.) (1995b) *The Rights of Minority Cultures.* Open University Press, Oxford, UK.

Kymlicka, W. and Norman, W. (1995) Return of the citizen: a survey of recent work on citizenship theory. In: Beiner, R. (ed.) *Theorizing Citizenship.* State University of New York Press, Albany, New York, pp. 283–322.

Labbock, M. and Nazro, J. (1995) *Breastfeeding: Protecting a Natural Resource,* Institute for Reproductive Health, Washington, DC; cited in Macdonald, T. (2005) *Third World Hostage to First World Health.* Radcliffe Publishing, Oxford, UK.

Labonte, R. (1997) Econology: integrating health and sustainable development. Guiding Principles for decision making. In: Sidell, M., Jones, L., Katz, J. and Peberdy, A. (eds) *Debates and Dilemmas in Promoting Health: A Reader.* Open University Press, Basingstoke, pp. 260–270.

Labonte, R. (2010) Health promotion, globalisation and health. In: Douglas, J., Earle, S., Handsley, S., Jones, L., Lloyd, C.E. and Spurr, S. (eds) *A Reader in Promoting Public Health.* Sage, London, pp. 235–245.

Labonté, R. and Laverack, G. (2008) *Health Promotion in Action.* Palgrave Macmillan, Basingstoke.

Labonte, T. and Laverack, G. (2010) Capacity building in health promotion, Part 1: For whom? And for what purpose? *Critical Public Health* 11, 111–127.

Lahtinen, E., Koskinen-Ollonqvist, P., Rouvinen-wilenius, P., Tuominen, P. and Mittelmark, M. (2005) The development of quality criteria for research: a Finnish approach. *Health Promotion International* 20, 306–315.

Lalonde, M. (1974) *A New Perspective on the Health of Canadians: A Working Document.* Ministry of National Health and Welfare, Ottawa.

Lambert, H. and McKevitt, C. (2002) Anthropology in health research: from qualitative methods to multidisciplinarity. *British Medical Journal* 325, 210–213.

Larkey, L.K. and Hecht, M. (2010) A model of effects of narrative as culture-centric health promotion. *Journal of Health Communication* 15, 114–135.

Larsen, E.L. and Manderson, L. (2009) 'A good spot': health promotion discourse, healthy cities and heterogeneity in contemporary Denmark. *Health and Place* 15, 606–613.

Lasswell, H.D. (1948) The structure and function of communication in society. In: Bryson L. (ed.) *The Communication of Ideas.* Harper, New York; cited in: McQuail, D. and Windahl, S. (1993) *Communication Models: for the Study of Mass Communication*, 2nd edition. Pearson Education Limited, Harlow, UK.

Latner, J.D. and Stunkard, A.J. (2003) Getting worse: the stigmatization of obese children. *Obesity Research* 11, 452–456.

Lave, J. and Wenger, E. (1998) *Communities of Practice: Learning, Meaning, and Identity.* Cambridge University Press, Cambridge.

Laverack, G. (2004) *Health Promotion Practice: Power and Empowerment.* Sage, London.

Laverack, G. (2005) *Public Health. Power, Empowerment and Professional Practice.* Palgrave, Basingstoke, UK.

Laverack, G. (2006) Improving health outcomes through community empowerment: a review of the literature. *Journal of Health, Population and Nutrition* 24, 113–120.

Laverack, G. (2007) *Health Promotion Practice.* Open University Press, Maidenhead, UK.

Laverack G. (2009) *Public Health, Power, Empowerment and Professional Practice*, 2nd edition. Palgrave Macmillan, Basingstoke, UK.

Laverack, G. (2010) Influencing public health policy: to what extent can public action defining the policy concerns of government? *Journal of Public Health* 18, 21–28.

Laverack, G. and Dap, D.H. (2003) Transforming information, education and communication in Vietnam. *Health Education* 103, 363–369.

Laverack, G. and Labonte, R. (2000) A planning framework for accommodation of empowerment goals within health promotion planning. *Health Policy and Planning* 15, 255–262.

Laverack, G. and Wallerstein, N. (2001) Measuring community empowerment: a fresh look at organizational domains. *Health Promotion International* 16, 179–185.

Laverack, G. and Whipple, A. (2010) The sirens' song of empowerment: a case study of health promotion and the New Zealand Prostitutes Collective. *Global Health Promotion* 17, 33–38.

Lawlor, D.A., Frankel, S., Shaw, M., Ebrahim, S. and Smith, G.D. *(*2003) Smoking and ill-health: does lay epidemiology explain the failure of smoking cessation programs among deprived populations? *American Journal of Public Health* 93, 266–270.

Lawton, J. (2003) Lay experiences of health and illness: past research and future agendas. *Sociology of Health and Illness* 25, 23–40.

Lawton, R., Connor, M. and McEachan, R. (2009) Desire or reason: predicting health behaviour from affective and cognitive attitudes. *Health Psychology* 28, 56–65.

Layard, R. (2006) Happiness and public policy: a challenge to the profession. *The Economic Journal* 116, 24–33.

Layard, R. (2011) *Happiness: Lessons from a New Science*. Penguin, London.

Lazarsfeld, P.F. and Merton, R.K. (1955) Mass communication, popular taste and organised social action. In: Schramm, W. (ed.) *Mass Communication*. University of Illinois Press, Urbana, Illinois.

Leach, B., Paluzzi, J. and Munderi, P. (2005) *Prescription for Healthy Development: Increasing Access to Medicines*. Earthscan, London.

Leach, R. (2002) *Political Ideology in Britain*. Palgrave, Basingstoke, UK.

Ledwith, M. (2005) *Community Development: A Critical Approach*. The Policy Press, Bristol, UK.

Lee, R.G. and Garvin, T. (2003) Moving from information transfer to information exchange in health and health care. *Social Science & Medicine* 56, 449–464.

Lefebvre, R.C. (1997) The social marketing imbroglio in health promotion. In: Sidell, M., Jones, L., Katz, J. and Peberdy, A. (eds) *Debates and Dilemmas in Promoting Health: A Reader*. Open University Press, Basingstoke, UK, pp. 108–113.

Lehman, U. and Sanders, D. (2007) *Community Health Workers: What do we know about them? The State of the Evidence on Programmes, Activities, Costs and Impact on Health Outcomes of using Community Health Workers*. Department of Human Resources for Health, Evidence and Information for Policy. WHO, Geneva.

Leininger, M. (1991) *Cultural Care Diversity and Universality*. National League for Nursing, New York.

Leonard, M. (2004) Bonding and bridging social capital: reflections from Belfast. *Sociology* 38, 927–944.

Lerer, L.B. (1999) Health impact assessment. *Health Policy and Planning* 14, 198–203.

Lessa, I. (2006) Discursive struggles within social welfare: restaging teen motherhood. *British Journal of Social Work* 36, 283–298.

Lester, R.T., Ritvo, P., Mills, E.J., Kariri, A., Kranja, S., Chung, M., Jack, W., Habyarimana, J., Sadatsafavi, M., Najafzadeh, M., Marra, C.A., Estambale, B., Ngugi, E., Ball, T.B., Thabane L., Gelmon L., Kimani, J., Ackers, M. and Plummer, F.A. (2010) Effects of a mobile phone short message service on antiretroviral treatment adherence in Kenya: a randomised trial. *Lancet* 376, 1838–1845.

Levitas, R., Pantazis, C., Fahmy, E., Gordon, D., Lloyd, E. and Patsios, D. (2007) The Multidimensional Analysis of Social Exclusion, A Research Report for the Social Exclusion Task Force. Available at: http://www.cabinetoffice.gov.uk/social_exclusion_task_force/publications/multidimen

Lewis, Y.R., Shain, L., Quinn, S.C., Turner, K. and Moore, T. (2002) Building community trust: lessons from an STD/HIV peer educator program with African American barbers and beauticians. *Health Promotion Practice* 3, 133–143.

Lievrouw, L. (2009) *Alternative and Activist New Media*. Polity Press, Oxford, UK.

Lightsey, D., McQueen, D. and Anderson, L. (2005) Health promotion in the USA: building a science-based health promotion policy. In: Scriven, A. and Garman, S. (eds) *Promoting Health: Global Perspectives*. Palgrave Macmillan, Basingstoke, UK.

Lin, P., Simoni, J.M. and Zemon, V. (2005) The health belief model, sexual behaviours and HIV risk among Taiwanese immigrants. *AIDS Education and Research* 17, 469–483.

Lindström, B. and Eriksson, M. (2006) Contextualizing salutogenesis and Antonovsky in public health development. *Health Promotion International* 21, 238–44.

Lindström, B. and Eriksson, M. (2009) The salutogenic approach to the making of HiAP/healthy public policy: illustrated by a case study. *Global Health Promotion* 16, 17–28.

Lindstrom, M., Hanson, B.S., Ostergren, P.O. and Berglund, G. (2000) Socio-economic differences in smoking cessation: the role of social participation. *Scandinavian Journal of Public Health* 28, 200–208.

Linhorst, D.M., Hamilton, G., Young, E. and Eckert, A. (2002) Opportunities and barriers to empowering people with severe mental illness through participation in treatment planning. *Social Work* 47, 425–434.

Linnan, L. and Ferguson, Y.O. (2007) Beauty salons: a promising health promotion setting for reaching and promoting health among African American women. *Health Education and Behavior* 34, 517–530.

Linney, B. (1995) *Pictures, People and Power*. Macmillan Education Ltd, London.

Lipsky, M. (1980) Street level bureaucracy: dilemmas of the individual in public services, Russell Sage. In: Hill, M. (eds) (1993) *The Policy Process. A Reader*. Prentice Hall, London.

Lock, K. (2000) Health impact assessment. *British Medical Journal* 320, 1395–1398.

London, L. and Bailie, R. (2001) Challenges for improving surveillance for pesticide poisoning: policy implications for developing countries. *International Journal of Epidemiology* 30, 564–570.

Luft, J. and Ingham, H. (1955) *The Johari Window: A Graphic Model for interpersonal relations*. University of California at Los Angeles, Extension Office, Western Training Laboratory in Group Development.

Lukes, S. (2005) *Power: a Radical View*. Palgrave Macmillan, Basingstoke, UK.

Lundahl, B.W., Kunz, C., Brownell, C., Tollefson, D. and Burke, B.L. (2010) Meta-analysis of motivational interviewing: twenty-five years of empirical students. *Research on Social Work Practice* 20, 137–160.

Lupton, D. (1992) Discourse analysis – a new methodology for understanding the ideologies of health and illness. *Australian Journal of Public Health* 16, 145–150.

Lyons, A.C. and Chamberlain, K. (2006) *Health Psychology*. Cambridge University Press, Cambridge.

Macdonald, G. and Davies, J.K. (1998) Reflection and vision: proving and improving the promotion of health. In: Davies, J.K. and Macdonald, G. (eds) *Quality, Evidence and Effectiveness in Health Promotion: Striving for certainties*. Routledge, London.

MacDonald, T. (2006) *Health, Trade and Human Rights*. Radcliffe Publishing, Oxford, UK.

Macdonald, T. (2007) *The Global Human Right to Health: Dream or Possibility?* Radcliffe Publishing, Oxford, UK.

MacDonald, T.H. (1998) *Rethinking Health Promotion, A Global Approach*. Routledge, London.

MacDowall, W., Boenll, C. and Davies, M. (2006) *Health Promotion Practice*. Open University Press, Maidenhead, UK.

MacGillivray, A. and Walker, P. (2000) Local social capital: making it work on the ground. In: Baron, S., Field, J. and Schuller, T. (eds) *Social Capital: Critical Perspectives*. Oxford University Press, Oxford, pp. 243–264.

MacGregor, A., Currie, C. and Wetton, N. (1998) Eliciting the views of children about health in schools through the draw and write technique. *Health Promotion International* 13, 307–318.

Macintyre, S. and Petticrew, M. (2000) Good intentions and received wisdom are not enough. *Journal of Epidemiology & Community Health* 54, 802–803.

Macintyre, S., McKay, L. and Ellaway, A. (2006) Lay concepts of the relative importance of different influences on health: are there major socio-demographic variations? *Health Education Research* 21, 73–739.

Maeve, M.K. (1999) Adjudicated health: incarcerated women and the social construction of health. *Crime, Law and Social Change* 31, 49–71.

Maibach, E. and Parrott, R. (1995) *Designing Health Messages: Approaches from Communication Theory and Public Health Practice*. Sage, London.

Maio, G.R., Haddock, G.G. and Jarman, H.L. (2007) Social psychological factors in tackling obesity, *Obesity Reviews* 8 (Supplement 1), 123–125.

Manandhar, M., Maimbolwa, M., Muulu, E., Mulenga, M.M. and O'Donovan, D. (2008) Intersectoral debate on social research strengthens alliances, advocacy and action for maternal survival in Zambia. *Health Promotion International* 24, 58–67.

Manji, F. (2006) Collaboration with the South: agents of aid or solidarity? In: Eade, D. (ed.) *Development, NGOs and Civil Society*. Oxfam, Oxford, UK.

Manoff, R. (1985) *Social Marketing: New Imperative for Public Health*. Praeger, New York.

Marks, D. (2004) Rights to health, freedom from illness: a life and death matter. In: Murray, M. (ed.) *Critical Health Psychology*. Palgrave Macmillan, Basingstoke, UK.

Marks, D.F. (2002a) Editorial essay: Freedom, responsibility and power: contrasting approaches to health psychology. *Journal of Health Psychology* 7, 5–19.

Marks, D.F. (2002b) *Perspectives on Evidence-based Practice*. Health Development Agency, London.

Marks, D.F., Murray, M., Evans, B., Willig, C., Woodall, C. and Sykes, C.M. (2005) *Health Psychology: Theory, Research and Practice*, 2nd edition. Sage, London.

Marks, N. (2011) *The Happiness Manifesto: How Nations and People can Nurture Well-being*. TED Books, New York.

Marmot, M. (2004) *Status Syndrome*. Bloomsbury, London.

Marmot M. (2010) *Fair Society, Healthy Lives: Strategic Review of Health Inequalities in England Post-2010*. London.

Marmot, M. and Wilkinson, R.G. (2001) Psychosocial and material pathways in the relation between income and health: a response to Lynch *et al*. *British Medical Journal* 322, 1233–367.

Marmot, M.G. (1988) Improvement of social environment to improve health. *Lancet* 351, 57–60.

Marsh, D. and Rhodes, R.A.W. (1992) *Policy Networks in British Government*. Clarendon Press, Oxford, UK.

Marteau, T.M., Ogilvie, D., Roland, M. and Suhrcke, M. (2011) Judging nudging: can nudging improve population health? *British Medical Journal* 342, 263–265.

Martell, L. (2010) *The Sociology of Globalization*. Polity, Cambridge, UK.

Matthewson, S.H. (2009) Man is the remedy of man: constructions of masculinity and health-related behaviours among young men in Dakar, Senegal. LSE International Development Working Paper 91. Available at: www2.lse.ac.uk/internationalDevelopment/pdf/WP91.pdf (accessed 3 November 2012).

Mayall, B. (1994) *Negotiating Health: Primary School Children at Home and School*. Cassell, London.

Maycock, B., Howat, P. and Levin, T. (2001) A decision-making model for health promotion advocacy: the case of drunk driving control measures. *Promotion and Education* 8, 59–64.

Mayo, M. (1994) *Communities and Caring: The Mixed Economy of Welfare*. Macmillan, Basingstoke, UK.

McClean, S. (2003) Globalization and health. In: Orme, J., Powell, J., Taylor, P., Harrison, T. and Grey, M. (eds) *Public Health for the 21st Century: New Perspectives on Policy, Participation and Practice*. Open University Press, Maidenhead, UK.

McElhone, S., Walker, J., Christie, D., Sahota, P., Dixey, R. and Rudolf, M.C.J. (2005) What sort of quality of life do obese children and adolescents in the UK have? *Obesity Reviews* 6 (Supplement 1), 133.

McGregor, C. (2004) Care(full) deliberation: a pedagogy for citizenship. *Journal of Transformative Education* 2, 90–106.

McGuire, W. (1989) Theoretical foundations of campaigns. In: Rice, R. and Atkin, C. (eds) *Public Communication Campaigns*. Sage, Newbury Park, California, pp. 43–65.

McKee, M., Sim, F. and Pomerleau, J. (2005) The emergence of public health and the centrality of values. In: Pomerleau, J. and McKee, M. (eds) *Issues in Public Health*. Open University Press, Maidenhead, UK.

McKeown, T. (1979) *The Role of Medicine: Dream, Mirage or Nemesis?* Blackwell, Oxford, UK.

McKinlay, J.B. (1979) A case for refocusing upstream: the political economy of illness. In: Jaco, E.G. (ed.) *Patients, Physicians and Illness*. The Free Press, New York.

McKnight, J.L. (1978) Politicizing health care. *Social Policy* 9, 36–39.

McKnight, J.L. (2003) Regenerating community: the recovery of a space for citizens. The IPR Distinguished Public Policy Research Lecture Series, Institute for Policy Research, Northwestern University. Available at: www.abcdinstitute.org/docs/abcd/regenerating.pdf (accessed 3 November 2012).

McLuhan, M. and Fiore, Q. (1967) *The Medium is the Message*. Penguin, Harmondsworth, UK.

McMichael, C., Waters, E. and Volmink, J. (2005) Evidence-based public health: what does it offer developing countries? *Journal of Public Health* 27, 215–221.

McQueen, D. (2000) Perspectives on health promotion: theory, evidence, practice and the emergence of complexity. *Health Promotion International* 15, 95–97.

McQueen, D.V. (2001) Strengthening the evidence base for health promotion. *Health Promotion International* 16, 261–268.

McQueen, D.V., Kickbusch, I., Potvin, L., Peliakn, J.M., Balbo, L. and Abel, T. (eds) (2007) *Health and Modernity: The Role of Theory in Health Promotion.* Springer, New York.

Mda, Z. (1993) *When People Play People: Development Communication through Theatre.* Zed Books, London.

Mehrotra, S. (2000) *Integrating Economic and Social Policy; Good Practices from High Achieving Countries.* Innocenti Working Paper No 80. UNICEF, Florence, Italy.

Mekonnen, Y. and Mekonnen, A. (2003), Factors influencing the use of maternal healthcare services in Ethiopia. *Journal of Health, Population and Nutrition* 21, 374–382.

Mendelsohn, H. (1968) Which shall it be: mass education or mass persuasion for health? *American Journal of Public Health* 58, 131–137.

Meyer, J. and Land, R. (2005) Threshold concepts and troublesome knowledge (2): epistemological considerations and a conceptual framework for teaching and learning. *Higher Education* 49, 373–388.

Meyer, J., Land, R. and Baille, C. (eds) (2010) *Threshold Concepts and Transformational Learning.* Sense Publishers, Boston, Massachusetts.

Mezirow, J. (1981) A critical theory of adult learning and education. *Adult Education* 32, 3–24.

Mezirow, J. (2003) Transformative learning as discourse. *Journal of Transformative Education* 1, 58–63.

Michael, J. (2008) *Healthcare for All: Report of the Independent Inquiry into Access to Healthcare for People with Learning Disabilities.* DOH, London.

Mielewczyk, F. and Willig, C. (2007) Old clothes and an older look: the case for a radical makeover in health behaviour research, *Theory and Psychology* 17, 811–837.

Milburn, K. (1995) A critical review of peer education with young people with special reference to sexual education. *Health Education Research* 10, 407–420.

Milio, N. (1988) Making healthy public policy; developing the science by leading the art: an ecological framework. *Health Promotion* 2, 263–274.

Miller, W.R. and Rollnick, S. (2002) *Motivational Interviewing: Preparing People for Change,* 2nd edition. The Guildford Press, London.

Minkler, M. (2000) Health promotion at the dawn of the 21st century. Challenges and dilemmas. In: Schneider Jamer, M. and Stokols, D. (eds) *Promoting Human Wellness. New Frontiers for Research, Practice, and Policy.* University of California Press, London.

Mistry, R. (1996) *A Fine Balance.* Faber and Faber, London.

Mittelmark, M. (2003) The role of professional education in building capacity for health promotion in the global South: a case study from Norway. *Ethnicity and Disease* 13, 35–39.

Mittelmark, M. (2005) Global health promotion: challenges and opportunities. In: Scriven, A. and Garman, S. (eds) (2005) *Promoting Health: Global Perspectives.* Palgrave Macmillan, Basingstoke, UK.

Mittelmark, M. (2009) Views of Health Promotion Online (VHPO) is alive and kicking, at www.vhpo.net! *Global Health Promotion* March 16, 3–4.

Mittelmark, M. (2010) Writing for the Global Health Promotion audience: Global Health Promotion's niche. *Global Health Promotion* 17, 3.

Mittlemark, M.B. (1999) Social ties and health promotion: suggestions for population based research. *Health Education Research* 14, 447–451.

Mock, J., McPhee, S.J., Nguyen, T., Wong, C., Doan, H., Lai, K.Q., Nguyen, K.H., Nguyen, T.T. and Bui-Tong, N. (2007) Effective lay health worker outreach and media-based education for promoting cervical cancer screening among Vietnamese American women. *American Journal of Public Health* 97, 1693–1700.

Moghadam, V. (2005) Globalizing Women: Transnational Feminist Networks. Johns Hopkins University Press, Baltimore, Maryland.

Mohindra, K.S. (2007) Healthy public policy in poor countries: tackling macro-economic policies. *Health Promotion International* 22, 163–169.

Monkman, K., Miles, R. and Easton, P. (2007) The transformatory potential of a village empowerment program: the Tostan Replication in Mali. *Women's Studies International Forum* 30, 451–464.

Moodie, R. (2011) Nanny knows best: why big tobacco's attack on Mary Poppins ought to backfire. The Conversation website. Available at: http://theconversation.edu.au/nanny-knows-best-why-big-tobaccos-attack-on-marypoppins-ought-to-backfire-1851 (accessed 3 November 2012).

Mooney, C.Z. (2000) Is travel distance a barrier to veterans use of VA hospitals for medical/surgical care? *Social Science & Medicine* 50, 1743–1755.

Moore, S. (2010) Is the healthy body gendered? Toward a feminist critique of the new paradigm of health. *Body & Society* 16, 95–118.

Moran, P., Coffey, C., Romaniuk, H., Olsson, C., Borschmann, R., Carlin, J. and Patton, G.C. (2011) The natural history of self-harm from adolescence to young adulthood: a population-based cohort study. *The Lancet* Early Online Publication, 17 November 2011, doi:10.1016/S0140-6736(11)61141-0.

Morgan, A. and Ziglio, E. (2007) Revitalising the evidence base for public health: an assets model. *IUHPE –Promotion and Education Supplement* 2, 16–22.

Morgan, L.M. (2001) Community participation in health: perpetual allure, persistent challenge. *Health Policy and Planning* 16, 221–230.

Morgen, S. (2002) *Into Our Own Hands: The Women's Health Movement in the United States, 1969–1990.* Rutgers University Press, New Brunswick, New Jersey.

Morris, M. and Bunjun, B. (2007) *Using Intersectional Feminist Frameworks in Research: A Resource for Embracing the Complexities of Women's Lives.* Canadian Research Institute for the Advancement of Women, Ottawa, 51 14.

Moyo, D. (2009) *Dead Aid: Why Aid is Not Working and How There is Another Way for Africa.* Penguin, London.

Muir Gray, J.M. (1997) *Evidence Based Healthcare.* Churchill Livingstone, London.

Mukangara, F. and Koda, B. (1997) *Beyond Inequalities: Women in Tanzania.* Tanzania Gender Networking Programme, Dar-es-Salaam.

Mullen, L. (1994) Control and responsibility: Moral and religious issues in lay health accounts. *Sociological Review* 42, 414–37.

Mullen, P.D., Evans, D., Forster, J., Gottlieb, N.H., Kreuter, M., Moon, R., O'Rourke, T. and Strecher, V.J. (1995) Settings as an important dimension in health education/promotion policy, programs, and research. *Health Education Quarterly* 22, 329–345.

Mungabareena Aboriginal Corporation and Women's Health Goulburn North East (2008) Using a Health Promotion Framework with an 'Aboriginal Lens'. WHNGE. Available at: www.whealth.com.au (accessed 3 November 2012).

Muntaner, C. and Lynch, J. (1999) Income inequality, social cohesion and class relations: a critique of Wilkinson's neo-Durkheimian research programme. *International Journal of Health Services* 29, 59–81.

Murray, M., Pullman, D. and Heath Rodgers, T. (2003) Social representations of health and illness among 'baby-boomers' in Eastern Canada. *Journal of Health Psychology* 8, 485–499.

Naidoo, J. and Wills, J. (1994) *Health Promotion: Foundations for Practice.* Bailliere Tindall, London.

Naidoo, J. and Wills, J. (2000) *Health Promotion: Foundations for Practice (Public Health and Health Promotion).* Elsevier, London.

Naidoo, J. and Wills, J. (2005) *Public Health and Health Promotion: Developing Practice*, 2nd edition. Bailliere Tindall, London.

Naidoo, J. and Wills, J. (2009) *Health Promotion: Foundations for Practice*, 3rd edition. Bailliere Tindall, London.

Naidoo, J., Orme, J. and Barrett, G. (2003) Capacity and capability in public health. In: Orme, J., Powell, J., Taylor, P., Harrison, T. and Grey, M. (2003) *Public Health for the 21st Century: New Perspectives on Policy, Participation and Practice.* Open University Press, Maidenhead, UK.

Naples, N. (2003) *Feminism and Method: Ethnography, Discourse Analysis, and Activist Research.* Routledge, New York.

Narayan, D. (1999) *Bonds and Bridges: Social Capital and Poverty.* World Bank, Washington, DC.

National Health and Medical Research Council (1996) *Promoting the Health of Indigenous Australians. A Review of Infrastructure Support for Aboriginal and Torres Strait Islander Health Advancement.* Final report and recommendations, NHMRC, Canberra, part 2, 4.

National Health Service Executive (1998) *Information for Health – An Information Strategy for the Modern NHS 1998–2005.* HMSO, London.

National Institute for Health and Clinical Excellence (2008) *Community Engagement.* NICE, London.

Navaneetham, K. and Dharmalingam, A. (2002) Utilisation of maternal health care services in Southern India. *Social Science & Medicine* 55, 1849–1869.

Navarro, V. (2009) What we mean by social determinants of health. *Global Health Promotion* 16, 5–16.

Nelson, G. and Prilleltensky, I. (2010) *Community Psychology: In Pursuit of Liberation and Wellbeing.* Palgrave Macmillan, Basingstoke, UK.

New, B. (1999) *Public Health and Public Values.* King's Fund, London.

Newell, C. and South, J. (2009) Participating in community research: exploring the experiences of lay researchers in Bradford. *Community, Work and Family* 12, 75–89.

Nichter, M. (1985) Drink boiled water: a cultural analysis of a health education message. *Social Science & Medicine* 21, 667–669.

Nkrumah, K. (1957) Broadcast to the Nation 24 December. Available at: http://www.panafrican perspective.com/nkrumahquotes.html (accessed 10 February 2012).

Nussbaum, M.C. (2000) *Women and Development: The Capabilities Approach.* Cambridge University Press, Cambridge.

Nutbeam, D. (1993) Advocacy and mediation in creating supportive environments for health. *Health Promotion International* 8, 165–166.

Nutbeam, D. (1998a) Evaluating health promotion: progress, problems and solutions. *Health Promotion International* 13, 27–44.

Nutbeam, D. (1998b) Health Promotion Glossary. *Health Promotion International* 13, 349–364.

Nutbeam, D. (1998c) *Health Promotion Glossary.* WHO, Geneva.

Nutbeam, D. (2000) Health literacy as a public health goal: a challenge for contemporary health education and communication strategies into the 21st century. *Health Promotion International* 15, 259–267.

Nutbeam, D. (2008) What would the Ottawa Charter look like if it was written today? *Critical Public Health* 18, 435–441.

Nutbeam, D. and Kickbush, I. (2000) Advancing health literacy: a global challenge for the 21st century. *Health Promotion International* 15, 183–184.

Nyamwaya, D. (2003) Health Promotion in Africa: strategies, players, challenges and prospects. *Health Promotion International* 18, 85–87.

Nyamwaya, D. (2005) Trends and factors in the development of health promotion in Africa 1973–2003. In: Scriven, A. and Garman, S. (eds) *Promoting Health: Global Perspectives.* Palgrave Macmillan, Basingstoke, UK.

O'Donnell, M.P. (2009) Definition of health promotion 2.0: embracing passion, enhancing motivation, recognizing dynamic balance, and creating opportunities. *American Journal of Health Promotion* 24, iv.

O'Hara, L. and Gregg, J. (2006) The war on obesity: a social determinant of health. *Health Journal of Australia* 17, 260–263.

Obermeyer, C.M. and Potter, J.E. (1991) Maternal health care utilisation in Jordan: a study of patterns and determinants. *Studies in Family Planning* 22, 177–187.

Obrist, H.U. (2011) *Ai Weiwei speaks with Han Ulrich Obrist.* Penguin, Harmondsworth, UK.

Office for National Statistics (ONS) (2003) *Social Trends No. 33.* The Stationery Office, London.

Ogden, C.L., Flegal, K.M., Carroll, M.D. and Johnson, C.L. (2002) Prevalence and trends in overweight among US children and adolescents, 1999–2000. *Journal of the American Medical Association* 288, 1728–1732.

Oliver, M. (1983) *Social Work and Disabled People.* Macmillan, Basingstoke, UK.

Oliver, M. (1990) *The Politics of Disablement.* Macmillan, Basingstoke, UK.

Ollilia, E. (2005) Global health priorities – priorities of the wealthy? *Globalisation and Health* 1, 1–6.

Omonzejele, P.F. (2008) African concepts of health, disease and treatment: an ethical inquiry. *Explore* 4, 120–26.

Onya, H. (2009) Health promotion capacity building in Africa: a call for action. *Global Health Promotion* 16, 47–50.

Orme, J. and Dooris, M. (2010) Integrating health and sustainability: the higher education sector as a timely catalyst. *Health Education Research* 25, 425–437.

Orme, J., Powell, J., Taylor, P., Harrison, T. and Grey, M. (2003) *Public Health for the 21st century.* Open University Press, Buckingham, UK.

Osaghae, E.E. (1995) The study of political transitions in Africa. *Review of African Political Economy* 64, 183–197.

Ostlin, P., Eckermann, E., Mishra, U., Nkowane, M. and Wallstam, E. (2007) Gender and health promotion: a multisectoral policy approach. *Health Promotion International* 21(S1), doi:10.1093/heapro/dal048.

Outram, D. (2006) *The Enlightenment,* 2nd edition. Cambridge University Press, Cambridge.

Ozgediz, D. and Riviello, R. (2008) The 'other' neglected diseases in global public health: surgical conditions in sub-Saharan Africa. *PLoS Med* 5(6):e121.

Palmer, S., Tubbs, I. and Whybrow, A. (2003) Health coaching to facilitate the promotion of healthy behaviour and achievement of health-related goals. *International Journal of Health Promotion and Education* 41, 91–93.

Papacharissi, Z.A. (2010) *A Private Sphere: Democracy in a Digital Age.* Polity Press, Oxford, UK.

Pappaioanou, M., Malison, M., Wilkins, K., Otto, B., Goodman, R.A., Elliott Churchill, R., White, M. and Thacker, S.B. (2003) Strengthening capacity in developing countries for evidence-based public health: the data for decision-making project. *Social Science & Medicine* 57, 1925–1937.

Parkin, D.M., Boyd, L. and Walker, L.C. (2011) The fraction of cancer attributable to lifestyle and environmental factors in the UK in 2010: summary and conclusions. *British Journal of Cancer* 105(S2), S77–S81.

Parry, G., Moyser, G. and Day, N. (1992*) Political Participation and Democracy in Britain*. Cambridge University Press, Cambridge.

Parsons, T.J., Power, C., Logan, S. and Summerbell, C.D. (1999) Childhood predictors of adult obesity: a systematic review. *International Journal of Obesity and Related Metabolic Disorders* 23 (Supplement 8), S1–107.

Parsons, W. (1995) *Public Policy: An Introduction to the Theory and practice of Policy Analysis*. Edward Elgar, London.

Paton, K., Sengupta, S. and Hassan, L. (2005) Settings, systems and organization development: the healthy living and working model. *Health Promotion International* 20, 81–89.

Pawson, R. and Tilley, N. (1997) *Realistic Evaluation*. Sage, London.

Pearce, J. (2006) Development, NGOs, and civil society: the debate and its future. In: Eade, D. (ed.) *Development, NGOs and Civil Society*. Oxfam, Oxford, UK.

Pearce, N. and Davey Smith, G. (2003) Is social capital the key to inequalities in health? *American Journal of Public Health* 93, 122–129.

Pearson, S., Batty, E., Cook, B., Foden, M., Knight-Fordham, R. and Peters, J. (2010) *Improving health outcomes in deprived communities*. Evidence from the New Deal for Communities Programme, a report commissioned by Communities and Local Government.

Pederson, A., Rootman, I. and O'Neill, M. (2005) Health promotion in Canada: back to the past or towards a promising future? In: Scriven, A. and Garman, S. (eds) *Promoting Health: Global Perspectives*. Palgrave Macmillan, Basingstoke, UK.

Pederson, A., Ponic, P., Greaves, L., Mills, S., Christilaw, J., Frisby, W., Humphries, K., Poole, N. and Young, L. (2010) Igniting an agenda for health promotion for women: critical perspectives, evidence-based practice, and innovative knowledge translation. *Canadian Journal of Public Health* May/June, 259–261.

Pedler, M., Burgoyne, J. and Boydell, T. (1991) *The Learning Company: a Strategy for Sustainable Development*. McGraw-Hill, Maidenhead, UK.

Peerson, A. and Saunders, M. (2009) Health literacy revisited: what do we mean and why does it matter? *Health Promotion International* 24, 285–296.

Peltzer, K.M., Mosala, T., Shisana, O., Nqueko, A. and Mngqundaniso, N. (2007) Barriers to prevention of HIV transmission from mother to child (PMTCT) in a resource poor setting in the Eastern Cape, South Africa. *African Journal of Reproductive Health*, 11, 57–66.

People's Health Movement (2012) Available at: http://www.phmovement.org/ (accessed 30 January 2012).

Perkmann, M. (2002) Policy entrepreneurs, multi-level governance and policy networks in the European Polity: The case of the EUREGIO. Department of Sociology, Lancaster University. Available at: http://www.lancs.ac.uk/fass/sociology/papers/perkmann-policy-entrepreneurs.pdf (accessed 3 November 2012).

Petersen, P.E. and Kwan, S. (2010) The 7th WHO Global Conference on Health Promotion-towards integration of oral health (Nairobi, Kenya 2009). *Community Dental Health* 27 (Supplement 1), 129–136.

Peterson, C. (2007) *Hearing from Students: How Transformative Education Really Changes Lives*. NAFSA, Seattle, Washington.

Peto, R. (2011) The fraction of cancer attributable to lifestyle and environmental factors in the UK in 2010. *British Journal of Cancer* 105(S2), Si–S81.

Petticrew, M. and Roberts, H. (2003) Evidence, hierarchies, and typologies: horses for courses. *Journal of Epidemiology Community Health* 57, 527–529.

Petticrew, M., Whitehead, M., Macintyre, S., Graham, H. and Egan, M. (2004) Evidence for public health policy on inequalities: 1: The reality according to policymakers. *Journal of Epidemiology Community Health* 58, 811–816.

PEW (2000) Pew Internet and American Life Report: The Online Health Care Revolution: How the Web Helps Americans Take Better Care of Themselves. Available at: http://www.pewinternet.org/reports/reports.asp?Report=26&Section=ReportLevel2&Field=Level2ID&ID=134 (accessed 26 April 2011).

Pierret, J. (1993) Constructing discourses about health and their social determinants. In: Radley, A. (ed.) *Worlds of Illness: Biographical and Cultural Perspectives on Health and Disease.* Routledge, London, pp. 9–26.

Pill, R. and Stott, N. (1982) Concepts of illness causation and responsibility: some preliminary data from a sample of working class mothers. *Social Science & Medicine* 16, 43–52.

Pill, R. and Stott, N. (1987) The stereotype of 'working class fatalism' and the challenge for primary care health promotion. *Health Education Research* 2, 105–114.

Piper, S. (2009) *Health Promotion for Nurses. Theory and Practice.* Routledge, Oxford, UK.

Pisek, P.E. and Greenhalgh, T. (2001) The challenge of complexity in health care. *British Medical Journal* 323, 625–628.

Pleasant, A. and Kuruvilla, S. (2008) A tale of two health literacies: public health and clinical approaches to health literacy. *Health Promotion International* 23, 152–159.

Pogge, T. (2007) *World Poverty and Human Rights*, 2nd edition. Polity Press, Cambridge, UK.

Poland, B., Krupa, G. and McCall, D. (2009) Settings for health promotion: an analytic framework to guide intervention in design and implementation. *Health Promotion Practice* 10, 505–516.

Poland, B.D., Green, L.W. and Rootman, I. (2000) Reflections on settings for health promotion. In: Poland, B.D., Green, L.W. and Rootman, I. (eds) *Settings for Health Promotion. Linking Theory and Practice.* Sage, Thousand Oaks, California.

Poortinga, W. (2006) Social relations or social capital? Individual and community health effects of bonding social capital. *Social Science & Medicine* 63, 255–270.

Popay, J. and Dhooge, Y. (1989) Unemployment, cod's head soup and radical social work. In: Langan, M. and Lee, P. (eds) *Radical Social Work Today*. Routledge, London, pp. 140–164.

Popay, J., Williams, G., Thomas, C. and Gatrell, A. (1998) Theorising inequalities in health: the place of lay knowledge. *Sociology of Health and Illness* 20, 619–644.

Popay, J., Bennett, S., Thomas, C., Williams, G., Gatrell, A. and Bostock, L. (2003) Beyond 'beer, fags, egg and chips'? Exploring lay understandings of social inequalities in health. *Sociology of Health and Illness* 25, 1–23.

Pope, V. (2008) Met Office's bleak forecast on climate change. The head of the Met Office centre for climate change research explains why the momentum on emissions targets must not be lost. *The Guardian*. Available at: http://www.guardian.co.uk/environment/2008/oct/01/climatechange.carbonemissions (accessed 13 January 2010).

Popple, K. and Shaw, M. (1997) Editorial introduction. Social movements: re-asserting 'community'. *Community Development Journal* 32, 191–198.

Porter, C. (2006) Ottawa to Bangkok: changing health promotion discourse. *Health Promotion International* 22, 72–79.

Portes, A. and Landolt, P. (1996) Unsolved mysteries; the Tocqueville files II. The downside of social capital. *The American Prospect* 7, 18–21.

Post, S.G. (2005) Altruism, happiness, and health: it's good to be good. *International Journal of Behavioural Medicine* 12, 66–77.

Postman, N. (1995) *The End of Education.* Knopf, New York.

Potter, I. (1997) Looking back, looking ahead – health promotion: a global challenge. *Health Promotion International* 12, 273–277.

Potts, L. (ed.) (2000) *Ideologies of Breast Cancer, Feminist Perspectives.* Macmillan Press, Basingstoke, UK.

Potts, L., Dixey, R. and Nettleton, S. (2007) Bridging differential understanding of environmental risk of breast cancer: why so hard? *Critical Public Health* 17, 337–350.

Potts, L., Dixey, R. and Nettleton, S. (2008) Precautionary tales: Exploring the obstacles to debating the primary prevention of breast cancer. *Critical Social Policy* 28, 115–135.

Pratt, D.D. and Associates (2005) *Five perspectives on teaching in adult and higher education – reprint of the 1998 edition with corrections.* Krieger Publishing Company, Malabar, Florida.

Prentice, A.M. (2006) The emerging epidemic of obesity in developing countries. *International Journal of Epidemiology* 35, 93–99.

Pridmore, P. (1999) *Participatory Approaches to Promoting Health in Schools: A Child to Child Training Manual.* Institute of Education/CTC, London.

Prior, L. (2003) Belief, knowledge and expertise: the emergence of the lay expert in medical sociology. *Sociology of Health and Illness* 25, 41–57.

Prochaska, J.O. and DiClemente, C.C. (1983) Stages and processes of self-change of smoking: toward an integrative model of change. *Journal of Consulting and Clinical Psychology* 51, 390–395.

Public Health Resource Unit (2008) Public Health Skills and Career Framework. PHRU, London. Available at: http://www.sph.nhs.uk/sph-files/PHSkills-CareerFramework_Launchdoc_April08.pdf (accessed 10 February 2012).

Purdue, D. (2001) Neighbourhood governance: leadership, trust and social capital. *Urban Studies* 38, 2211–2224.

Purdy, M. (1997) Humanist ideology and nurse education – humanistic education theory. *Nurse Education Today* 17, 192–195.

Putnam, R.D. (1993a) *Making Democracy Work. Civic Traditions in Modern Italy*. Princeton University Press, Princeton, New Jersey.

Putnam, R.D. (1993b) The prosperous community. *The American Prospect* 4, 35–42.

Putnam, R.D. (2000) *Bowling Alone. The Collapse and Revival of American Community*. Simon and Schuster, New York.

Rada, J., Ratima, M. and Howden-Chapman, P. (1999) Evidence based purchasing of health promotion: methodology for reviewing evidence. *Health Promotion International* 14, 177–187.

Radley, A. and Billig, M. (1996) Accounts of health and illness: dilemmas and representations. *Sociology of Health and Illness* 18, 220–240.

Raeburn, J.M. and Rootman, I. (1998) *People Centred Health Promotion*. John Wiley & Sons, Chichester, UK.

Ramaswamy, M. and Freudenberg, N. (2007) Health promotion in jails and prisons: an alternative paradigm for correctional health services. In: Greifinger, R.B., Bick, J. and Goldenson, J. (eds) *Public Health Behind Bars. From Prisons to Communities*. Springer, New York.

Ramos, D. and Perkins, D. (2006) Goodness of fit assessment of an alcohol intervention program and underlying theories of change. *Journal of American College Health* 55, 57–64.

Raphael, D. (2000) The question of evidence in health promotion. *Health Promotion International* 15, 355–367.

Raphael, D. (2003) Barriers to addressing the societal determinants of health: public health units and poverty in Ontario, Canada. *Health Promotion International* 18, 397–405.

Raphael, D. (2011) A discourse analysis of the social determinants of health. *Critical Public Health* 21, 221–236.

Rappaport, J. (1985) The power of empowerment language. *Social Policy* 15, 15–21.

Rawls, J. (1971) *A Theory of Justice*. Harvard University Press, Cambridge, Massachusetts.

Reilly, J.J., Montgomery, C., Jackson, D., MacRitchie, J. and Armstrong, J. (2001) Energy intake by multiple pass 24 hr recall and total energy expenditure: a comparison in a representative sample of 3–4 year-olds. *British Journal of Nutrition* 86, 601–605.

Renfrew, M.J., Dyson, L., Herbert, J., McFadden, A., McCormick, F., Thomas, J. and Spiby, H. (2008) Developing evidence-based recommendations in public health – incorporating the views of practitioners, service users and user representatives. *Health Expectations* 11, 3–15.

Reynolds, L. and Thorpe, A. (2009) How to help people to change behaviour. In: Griffiths, J., Rao, M., Adshead, F. and Thorpe, A. (2009) *The Health Practitioner's Guide to Climate Change: Diagnosis and Cure*. Earthscan, London.

Richmond, K.M. (2009) Factories with Fences: the Effect of Prison Industries on Female Inmates. Unpublished PhD thesis, University of Maryland.

Riddell, R.C. (2008) *Does Foreign Aid Really Work?* Oxford University Press, Oxford.

Rifkin, S.B. (1996) Paradigms lost: toward a new understanding of community participation in health programmes. *Acta Tropica* 61, 79–92.

Rifkin, S.B. (2009) Lessons from community participation in health programmes: a review of post Alma-Ata experience. *International Health* 1, 31–36.

Rifkin, S.B., Lewando-Hunt., G. and Draper, A.K. (2000) *Participatory Approaches in Health Promotion and Health Planning: a Literature Review*. Health Development Agency, London.

Riger, S. (2002) What's wrong with empowerment? In: Revenson, T.A., D'Augelli, A.R., French, S.E., Hughes, D., Livert, D.E., Seidman, E., Shinn, M. and Yoshikawa, H. (eds) *Quarter Century of Community Psychology: Readings from the American Journal of Community Psychology*. Kluwer Academic/Plenum, New York.

Rissel, C. (1994) Empowerment: the holy grail of health promotion? *Health Promotion International* 9, 39–47.

Roberts, I. with Edwards, P. (2010) *The Energy Glut. The Politics of Fatness in an Overheating World*. Zed Books, London and New York.

Roberts, N.C. and King, P.J. (1991) Policy entrepreneurs: Their activity structure and function in the policy process. *Journal of Public Administration Research and Theory* 2, 147–175.

Roberts, R., Towell, T. and Golding, J.F. (2001) *Foundations of Health Psychology*. Palgrave, Basingstoke, UK.

Robertson, A. (1998) Shifting discourses on health in Canada: from health promotion to population health. *Health Promotion International* 13, 155–166.

Robertson, S. (2006) Not living life in too much of an excess: lay men understanding health and well-being. *Health: An Interdisciplinary Journal for the Social Study of Health, Illness and Medicine* 10, 175–189.

Robins, S. (2004) Long live Zackie, long live: AIDS activism, science and citizenship after apartheid. *Journal of Southern African Studies* 30, 651–672.

Robinson, M. and Robertson, S. (2010) Young men's health promotion and new information communication technologies: illuminating the issues and research agendas. *Health Promotion International* 25, 363–370.

Rodwell, C.M. (1996) An analysis of the concept of empowerment. *Journal of Advanced Nursing* 23, 305–313.

Rogers, C.R. (1969) *Freedom to Learn*. Merrill, New York.

Rogers, E. (1976) Communication and development: the passing of a paradigm. *Communication Research* 3, 213–240.

Rogers, E.M. (1986) *Communication Technology: The New Media in Society*. The Free Press, New York.

Rogers, E.M. (1995) *The Diffusion of Innovations*, 4th edition. The Free Press, New York.

Rogers, E.M. (2003) *Diffusion of Innovations*, 5th edition. The Free Press, New York.

Rogers, E.M. and Shoemaker, F. (1971) *The Communication of Innovations*. The Free Press, New York.

Rogers, R.W. (1975) A protection motivation theory of fear appeals and attitude change. *Journal of Psychology* 91, 93–114.

Rogers, R.W. (1983) Cognitive and physiological processes in fear appeals and attitude change: a revised theory of protection motivation. In: Cacippo, J.R. and Petty, R.E. (eds) *Social Psychology: A Source Book*. Guilford Press, New York, pp. 153–176.

Rogoff, B. (1993) Observing sociocultural activity on three planes. In: Wertsch, J.V., del Rio, P. and Alvarez, A. (eds) *Sociocultural Studies of Mind*. Cambridge University Press, New York, pp. 139–163.

Rohleder, P., Bozalek, V., Carolissen, R., Leibowitz, B. and Swartz, L. (2008) Students' evaluations of the use of e-learning in a collaborative project between two South African universities. *Higher Education* 56, 95–107.

Rootman, I., Goodstadt, M., Hyndman, B., McQueen, D.V., Potvin, L., Springett, J. and Ziglio, E. (eds) (2001) *Evaluation in Health Promotion. Principles and Perspectives*. WHO, Geneva.

Rose, R. (2000a) How much does social capital add to individual health? A survey study of Russians. *Social Science & Medicine* 51, 1421–1435.

Rose, R. (2000b) Citizenship and the third way. *American Behavioural Scientist* 43, 1395–1411.

Rosenstock, I.M., Strecher, V.J. and Becker, M.H. (1988) Social learning theory and the health belief model. *Health Education Quarterly* 15, 175–183.

Roysamb, E., Tambs, K., Reichborn-Kjennerud, T., Neale, M.C. and Harris, J. (2006) Happiness and health: environmental and genetic contributions to the relationship between subjective well-being, perceived health, and somatic illness. *Journal of Personality and Social Psychology* 85, 1136–1146.

Rubak, S., Sandboek, A., Lauritzen, T. and Christensen, B. (2005) Motivational Interviewing: a systematic review and meta-analysis. *British Journal of General Practice* 55, 305–312.

Rutherford, J. (2007) *After Identity*. Lawrence and Wishart, London.

Rutten, A., Gelius, P. and Abu-Omar, K. (2011) Policy development and implementation in health promotion – from theory to practice: the ADEPT model. *Health Promotion International* 26, 322–329.

Rychetnik, L., Frommer, M., Hawe, P., Shiell, A. (2002) Criteria for evaluating evidence on public health interventions. *Journal of Epidemiology Community Health* 56, 119–127.

Sackett, D.L., Rosenberg, W.M.C., Gray, J.A.M., Haynes, R.B. and Richardson, W.S. (1996) Evidence-based medicine: what it is and what it isn't. *British Medical Journal* 312, 71–72.

Salamon, L.M. (1993) *The Global Associational Revolution: the Rise of the Third Sector on the*

World Scene. Occasional paper 15, Institute of Policy Studies, Johns Hopkins University, Baltimore, MD.

Salant, T. and Gehlert, S. (2008) Collective memory, candidacy and victimisation: community epidemiologies of breast cancer risk. *Sociology of Health and Illness* 30, 599–615.

Saltonstall, R. (1993) Healthy bodies, social bodies: men's and women's concepts and practices of health in everyday life. *Social Science & Medicine* 36, 7–14.

Sanders, D. with Carver, R. (1985) *The Struggle for Health: Medicine and the Politics of Underdevelopment.* Macmillan Educational, Basingstoke, UK.

Sanders, D., Stern, R., Struthers, P., Ngulube, T.J. and Onya, H. (2008) What is needed for health promotion in Africa: band-aid, live aid or real change? *Critical Public Health* 18, 509–519.

Saracci, R. (1997) The World Health Organization needs to reconsider its definition of Health. *British Medical Journal* 314, 1409–1410.

Sarafino, E. (2002) *Health Psychology: Biopsychosocial Interactions*, 4th edition. John Wiley & Sons, Chichester, UK.

Saskatchewan Health (2002) A population health promotion framework for Saskatchewan regional health authorities. Regina, Canada.

Sawyerr, A. (2002) *Challenges Facing African Universities: Selected Issues.* Paper presented to the 45th Annual Meeting of the African Studies Association, 5–8 December, Washington, DC.

Scholte, J.A. (2000) *Globalization: a Critical Introduction.* Macmillan, Basingstoke, UK.

Schramm, W. (1954) How communication works. In: McQuail, D. and Windahl, S. (eds) (1993) *Communication Models: for the Study of Mass Communications*, 2nd edition. Longman, London.

Schuller, T., Baron, S. and Field, J. (2000) Social capital: a review and a critique. In: Baron, S., Field, J. and Schuller, T. (eds) *Social Capital. Critical Perspectives.* Oxford University Press, Oxford, pp. 1–38.

Schwartz, R., Goodman, R. and Steckler, A. (1995) Policy advocacy interventions for health promotion and education: advancing the state of practice. *Health Education Quarterly* 22, 421–426.

Scott-Samuel, A. and Springett, J. (2007) Hegemony or health promotion? Prospects for reviving England's lost discipline. *Journal of the Royal Society of Health* 127, 211–214.

Scott-Samuel, A. and Wills, J. (2007) Health promotion in England: sleeping beauty or corpse? *Health Education Journal* 66, 115–119.

Seedhouse, D. (1997) *Health Promotion: Philosophy, Prejudice and Practice.* John Wiley & Sons, Chichester, UK.

Seedhouse, D. (2001a) Health promotion's ethical challenge. *Health Promotion Journal of Australia* 12, 135–138.

Seedhouse, D. (2001b) *Health: The Foundations for Achievement*, 2nd edition. John Wiley & Sons, Chichester, UK.

Seidell, J.C. (2000) Obesity, insulin resistance and diabetes – A worldwide epidemic. *British Journal of Nutrition* 83, S5–8.

Sen, A. (1980) Equality of what? In: McMurrin, S.M. (ed.) *Tanner Lectures on Human Values.* Ed. I. University of Utah Press, Salt Lake City, Utah. Reprinted in Sen, A. (1982) *Choice, Welfare and Measurement.* Blackwell, Oxford, UK, pp. 353–369.

Sen, A. (1993) Capability and well-being. In: Nussbaum, M. and Sen, A. (eds) *The Quality of Life.* Oxford University Press, Oxford.

Sen, A. (1999) *Development as Freedom.* Taylor and Francis, New York.

Senge, P. (1994) *The Fifth Discipline Field Book: Strategies and Tools for Building a Learning Organization.* Nicholas Brealey Publishing, London.

Senge, P.M. (1990) *The Fifth Discipline: The Art and Practice of the Learning Organization.* Doubleday Currency, New York.

Serdula, M.K., Ivery, D., Coates, R.J., Freeman, D.S., Williamson, D.F. and Byers, T. (1993) Do obese children become obese adults? A review of the literature. *Preventive Medicine* 22, 167–177.

Serpell, R., Mumba, P. and Chansa-Kabali, T. (2011) Early educational foundations for the development of civic responsibility: an African experience. In: Flanagan, C.A. and Christens, B.D. (eds) *Youth Civic Development: Work at the Cutting Edge. New Directions for Child and Adolescent Development* 134, 77–93.

Serrat, O. (2009) A primer on organisational learning, knowledge solutions. *Asian Development Bank* 6, 1–6.

Sfard, A. (1998) On two metaphors for learning and the dangers of choosing just one. *Educational Researcher* 27, 4–13.

Shannon, C. and Weaver, W. (1949) *The Mathematical Theory of Communication.* University

of Illinois Press, Urbana, Illinois. In: McQuail,
D. and Windahl, S. (1993) *Communication
Models: for the Study of Mass Communication*,
2nd edition. Longman, London.

Shapiro, J. (1993) *No Pity: People with Disabilities
Forging a New Civil Rights Movement*. Random,
New York.

Sharma, R. (no date) *An Introduction to Advocacy:
A Training Guide*. USAID, Africa Bureau, Office
of Sustainable Development.

Sharp, J. (2008) *Geographies of Post-colonialism*.
Sage, London.

Shaw, M. (2004) Community work: policy,
politics and practice. Working Papers in Social
Science and Policy, The University of Hull,
Hull, UK.

Shepherd, J., Garcia, J., Oliver, S., Harden, A.,
Rees, R., Brunton, G. and Oakley, A. (2001)
*Young People and Healthy Eating: a Systematic
Review of Barriers and Facilitators*. EPPI-Cen-
tre, Social Science Research Unit, London.

SHEPS (no date) Vision, Principles and Practice
Document. Faculty of Health, University of
Central England, Birmingham, UK. Available at:
www.health.bcu.ac.uk/./sheps%20vision,
principles&practice.doc

Shircore, R. (2009) *Guide for World Class Commis-
sioners. Promoting Health and Well-Being:
Reducing Inequalities*. Royal Society for Public
Health, London.

Shove, E. (2010) Submission to the House of Lords
Science and Technology Select Committee call
for evidence on behavior change.

Shuklenk, U. (2003) AIDS: bioethics and public
policy. *New Review of Bioethics* 1, 127–144.

Siahpush, M. (2000) A critical review of the sociology of alternative medicine: research on users,
practitioners and the orthodoxy. *Health: An
Interdisciplinary Journal for the Social Study of
Health, Illness and Medicine* 4, 159–178.

Sidell, M. (2010) Older people's health: applying
Antonovsky's salutogenic paradigm. In: Doug-
las, J., Earle, S., Handsley, S., Jones, L., Lloyd,
C. and Spurr, S. (eds) *A Reader Promoting
Public Health, Challenge and Controversy*, 2nd
edition. Sage, London, pp. 27–32.

Sidell, M., Jones, L., Katz, J. and Peberdy, A. (1997)
Debates and Dilemmas in Promoting Health.
Macmillan Press, Basingstoke, UK.

Sindall, C. (2002) Does health promotion need a
code of ethics? *Health Promotion International*
17, 201–203.

Singh, B. (2011) The Power of New Media, The
Youth Effect. Available at: http://www.youth
effect.org/bhavneetsingh/ (accessed 30 January
2012).

Skinner, D., Mfecane, S., Gumede, T., Henda, N.
and Davids, A. (2005) Barriers to accessing
PMTCT services in a rural area of South Africa.
African Journal of AIDS Research 4, 115–123.

Smedley, B. and Syme, L. (2000) *Promoting
Health: Intervention Strategies from Social
and Behavioural Research*. National Academic Press, Washington, DC.

Smith, B., Tang, K.C. and Nutbeam, D. (2006)
WHO Health Promotion Glossary: new terms.
Health Promotion International 21, 340–345.

Smith, C. (2000) Healthy prisons: a contradiction
in terms? *The Howard Journal of Criminal
Justice* 39, 339–353.

Smith, K.E, Bambra, C. and Joyce, K.E. (2009)
Partners in health? A systematic review of the
effects on health and health inequalities of partnership working. *Journal of Public Health* 31,
210–221.

Smithies, J. and Webster, G. (1998) *Community
Involvement in Health. From Passive Recipients
to Active Participants*. Ashgate Publishing,
Aldershot, UK.

Social Exclusion Unit (2002) *Reducing Re-offending
by Ex-prisoners*. Crown, London.

Solomon, B.B. (1976) *Black Empowerment: Social
Work in Oppressed Communities*. Columbia
University Press, New York.

South, J. (2005) Community Arts for Health: an
Evaluation of a District Programme. *Health
Education* 106, 155–168.

South, J. and Woodall, J. (2010) *Empowerment
and Health & Well-being: Evidence Summary*.
Centre for Health Promotion Research, Leeds
Metropolitan University, Leeds, UK.

South, J. and Woodall, J. (2011) Planning and evaluating health promotion in settings. In: Scriven,
A. and Hodgins, M. (eds) *Health Promotion
Settings: Principles and Practice*. Sage, London,
pp. 69–86.

South, J., Woodward, J., Lowcock, D. and
Woodall, J. (2006) *An Evaluation of the Brad-
ford District Health Trainers Programme – an
Early Adopter Site*. Centre for Health Promo-
tion Research, Leeds Metropolitan University,
Leeds, UK.

South, J., Meah, A., Bagnall, A.-M., Kinsella, K.,
Branney, P., White, J. and Gamsu, M. (2010a)

People in Public Health – a study of approaches to develop and support people in public health roles. Final report. NIHR Service Delivery and Organisation programme. Available at: http://www.sdo.nihr.ac.uk/files/project/206-final-report.pdf

South, J., Raine, G. and White, J. (2010b) *Community Health Champions: Evidence Review.* Centre for Health Promotion Research, Leeds Metropolitan University, Leeds, UK.

South, J., Meah, A. and Branney, P. (2011) 'Think differently and be prepared to demonstrate trust': findings from public hearings, England on supporting lay people in public health roles. *Health Promotion International* doi:10.1093/heapro/dar022.

South, J., White, J. and Gamsu, M. (2012) *People Centred Public Health.* The Policy Press, Bristol, UK.

Sparks, M. (2011) Building healthy public policy: don't believe the misdirection. *Health Promotion International* 26, 259–262.

Speller, V. (2006) Developing healthy settings. In: Macdowall, W., Bonell, C. and Davis, M. (eds) *Health Promotion Practice.* Open University Press, Maidenhead, UK.

Speller, V., Wimbush, E. and Morgan, A. (2005) Evidence-based health promotion practice: how to make it work, *Promotion & Education* 12, 15–20.

Spicker, P. (2006) *Policy Analysis for Practice. Applying Social Policy.* The Policy Press, Bristol, UK.

Springett, J., Owens, C. and Callaghan, J. (2007) The challenge of combining 'lay' knowledge with 'evidence-based' practice in health promotion: Fag Ends Smoking Cessation. *Service Critical Public Health* 17, 243–256.

Sproston, K. and Primatesta, P. (eds) (2003) *Health Survey for England 2002: The Health of Children and Young People.* Joint Health Surveys Unit, National Centre for Social Research, Department of Epidemiology and Public Health at the Royal Free and University College Medical School, London.

St Leger, L. (1997) Health promoting settings: from Ottawa to Jakarta. *Health Promotion International* 12, 99–101.

St Leger, L. (2001) Building and finding the new leaders in health promotion: where is the next wave of health promotion leaders and thinkers? Are they emerging from particular regions, and

are they less than 40 years old? *Health Promotion International* 16, 301–303.

Stacey, M. (1976) The health service consumer: a sociological misconception, sociology of the health service. *Sociological Review Monograph,* no. 22, University of Keele, Keele, UK.

Stainton-Rogers, W. (1991) *Explaining Health and Illness: An Exploration of Diversity.* Harvester/Wheatsheaf, London.

Standing Conference for Community Development (2001) *Strategic Framework for Community Development.* SCCD, Sheffield, UK.

Standing, H., Mushtaque, A. and Chowdhury, R. (2008) Producing effective knowledge agents in a pluralistic environment: what future for community health workers? *Social Science & Medicine* 66, 2096–2107.

Staples, L.H. (1990) Powerful ideas about empowerment. *Administration in Social Work* 14, 29–42.

Steinberg, S. (2006) *Introduction to Communication.* Juta and Co., Cape Town.

Steingraber, S. (1997) *Living Downstream: an Ecologist looks at Cancer and the Environment.* Addison Wesley, Boston, Massachusetts.

Stephenson, R. and Hennink, M. (2004) Barriers to family planning service use among the urban poor in Pakistan. *Asia-Pacific Population Journal* 19, 5–26.

Steptoe, A., Prekins-Porras, L., McKay, C., Rink, E., Hilton, S. and Cappuccio, F. (2003) Behavioural counselling to increase consumption of fruit and vegetables in low income adults: randomised trial. *British Medical Journal* 326, 855–858.

Stern, R. (1990) Healthy communities: reflections on building alliances in Canada. A view from the middle. *Health Promotion International* 5, 225–231.

Stevens, A. (2007) Survival of the ideas that fit: an evolutionary analogy for the use of evidence in policy. *Social Policy and Society* 6, 25–35.

Stevens, C. (2008) Social capital in its place: using social theory to understand social capital and inequalities in health. *Social Science & Medicine* 66, 1174–1184.

Stiglitz, J. (2006) *Making Globalisation Work. The Next Steps to Global Justice.* Allen Lane, London.

Stock, C., Milz, S. and Meier, S. (2010) Network evaluation: principles, structures and outcomes of the German working group of health promoting universities. *Global Health Promotion* 17, 25–32.

Stout, C., Morrow, J., Brandt, E.N. and Wolf, S. (1964) Study of an Italian–American community in PA; unusually low incidence of death from myocardial infarction. *Journal of the American Medical Association* 188, 845.

Straub, R.O. (2007) *Health Psychology: A Biopsychosocial Approach*, 2nd edition. Worth Publishers, New York.

Sutton, R. (1999) *The Policy Process: An Overview*. Working paper 118. Overseas Development Agency, London.

Sutton, S. (2005) Stage theories of health behaviour. In: Conner, M. and Norman, P. (eds) *Predicting Health Behaviours*, 2nd edition. Open University Press, Buckingham, UK, pp. 223–275.

Svenson, G. (1998) *European Guidelines for Youth AIDS Peer Education*. European Commission, Luxembourg.

Swami, V., Arteche, A., Chamorro-Premuzic, T., Maakip, I., Stanistreet, D. and Furnham, A. (2009) Lay perceptions of current and future health, the causes of illness, and the nature of recovery: explaining health and illness in Malaysia. *British Journal of Health Psychology* 14, 519–540.

Syme, S.L. (2004) Social determinants of health: the community as an empowered partner. *Preventing Chronic Disease*, 1(1). Available at: http://www.cdc.gov/pcd/issues/2004/jan/ 03_0001.htm (accessed 3 November 2012).

Szreter, S. and Woolcock, M. (2002) *Health by Association? Social Capital, Social Theory and the Political Economy of Public Health*. Von Hugel Institute Working Paper, Cambridge, UK.

Tavares, M.F.L., Barros, C.M.S., Marcondes, W.B., Bodstein, R., Cohen, S.C., Kligerman, D.C., Comarú, F., Carlos Santos Silva, C.S., Bógus, C.M., da Rocha, R.M., de Mello, R.M., Adesse, L., Edmundo, K. and Mendes, R. (2005) Theory and practice in the context of health promotion evaluation. *Promotion and Education*, Special Edition 1, 27–30.

Taylor, M. (2000a) Communities in the lead: power, organisational capacity and social capital. *Urban Studies* 37, 1019–1035.

Taylor, M. (2000b) Maintaining community involvement in regeneration: what are the issues? *Local Economy* 15, 251–267.

Taylor, P. (2003) The lay contribution to public health. In: Orme, J., Powell, J., Taylor, P., Harrison, T. and Grey, M. (eds) *Public Health for the 21st Century. New Perspectives on Policy, Participation and Practice*. Open University Press, Maidenhead, UK, pp. 128–144.

Taylor, P. (2007) The lay contribution to public health. In: Orme, J., Powell, J., Taylor, P., Harrison, T. and Grey, M. (eds) *Public Health for the 21st Century. New Perspectives on Policy, Participation and Practice*, 2nd edition. Open University Press, Maidenhead, UK, pp. 98–117.

Tesh, S. (1988) *Hidden Arguments: Political Ideology and Disease Prevention Policy*. Rutgers University Press, New Brunswick, New Jersey.

Thaler, R.H. and Sunstein, C.R. (2008) *Nudge: Improving Decisions about Health, Wealth and Happiness*. Penguin, London.

The Aldridge Foundation and Johnson, M. (2008) *The User Voice of the Criminal Justice System*. The Aldridge Foundation, London.

Thirlaway, K. and Upton, D. (2009) *The Psychology of Lifestyle: Promoting Healthy Behaviours*. Routledge, London.

Thomas, B., Dorling, D. and Davey Smith, G. (2010) Inequalities in premature mortality in britain: observational study from 1921 to 2007. *British Medical Journal* 341, 3639.

Thurston, W.E. and Blundell-Gosselin, H.J. (2005) The farm as a setting for health promotion: results of a needs assessment in South Central Alberta. *Health & Place* 11, 31–43.

Tian, X., Zhou, L., Mao, X., Zhao, T., Song, Y. and Jagusztyn, M. (2003) Beijing health promoting universities: practice and evaluation. *Health Promotion International* 18, 107–113.

Tilford, S. and Tones, K. (2001) *Health Promotion: Effectiveness, Efficiency and Equity* 3rd edition. Nelson Thornes, Cheltenham, UK.

Tillinghast, S.J. and Tchernjavskii, V.E. (1996) Building health promotion into health care reform in Russia. *Journal of Public Health Medicine* 18, 473–477.

Tobiasz-Adamcyzk, B., Brzyska, M., Wozniak, B. and Kopacz, M.S. (2009) The current state and challenges for the future of health promotion in Polish older people. *International Journal of Public Health* 54, 341–348.

Tones, K. (1997) Health promotion as Empowerment. In: Sidell, M., Jones, L., Katz, J. and Peberdy, A. (eds) *Debates and Dilemmas in Promoting Health: A Reader*. The Open University, Milton Keynes, UK, pp. 33–42.

Tones, K. (2001) Health promotion: the empowerment imperative. In: Scriven, A. and Orme, J. (eds) *Health Promotion: Professional Perspectives*, 2nd edition. Palgrave, London.

Tones, K. (2002) Health literacy: old wine in new bottles? *Health Education Research* 17, 287–290.

Tones, K. and Green, J. (2004) *Health Promotion: Planning and Strategies*. Sage, London.

Tones, K. and Tilford, S. (2001) *Health Promotion, Effectiveness, Efficiency and Equity*. Nelson Thornes, Cheltenham, UK.

Trenberth, L. (2005) The role, nature and purpose of leisure and its contribution to individual development and well-being. *British Journal of Guidance and Counselling* 33, 7–26.

Tritter, J.Q. and McCallum, A. (2006) The snakes and ladders of user involvement: moving beyond Arnstein. *Health Policy* 76, 156–168.

Tsouros, A., Dowding, G., Thompson, J. and Dooris, M. (1998) (eds) *Health Promoting Universities: Concept, Experience and Framework for Action*. WHO, Copenhagen.

Tuckett, D., Boulton, M., Olson, C. and Williams, A. (1985) *Meetings Between Experts*. Tavistock, London.

Tukahirwa, J.T. (2011) Civil society in urban sanitation and solid waste management: the role of NGOs and CBOs in metropolises of East Africa. PhD Thesis, University of Wageningen, Netherlands.

Tumwine, J. (2011) Implementation of the Framework Convention on Tobacco Control in Africa: current status of legislation. *International Journal of Environmental Research and Public Health* 8, 4312–4331, doi:10.3390/ijerph8114312.

UN (1948) Universal Declaration of Human Rights. Available at: http://www.un.org/events/human rights/2007/hrphotos/declaration%20_eng.pdf (accessed 24 January 2012).

UN (1986) Declaration on the Right to Development. Available at: http://www2.ohchr.org/english/law/rtd.htm (accessed 3 November 2012).

UN (2006) Breaking Barriers: Gender Perspectives and the Empowerment of Women in Least Developed Countries. Available at: http://www.unohrlls.org/UserFiles/File/Publications/Gender perspectives.pdf (accessed 3 November 2012).

UN (2009) The Millennium Development Goals Report 2009. Available at: http://www.un.org/millenniumgoals (accessed 3 November 2012).

UN (2011) *Prevention and Control of Non-communicable Diseases: Report of the Secretary-General*. General Assembly, UN, 19 May 2011, A/66/83.

UNAIDS (1999) *Peer education and HIV/AIDS: Concepts, uses and challenges*. Joint United Nations Programme on HIV/AIDS (UNAIDS), Geneva.

UNAIDS (2007) *AIDS Epidemic Update: December 2007*. UNAIDS and WHO, Geneva.

UNAIDS (2009) *09 AIDS Epidemic Update: November 2009*. UNAIDS and WHO, Geneva.

UNDP (2003) *Human Development Report 2003*. United Nations Development Programme, New York.

UNICEF (2009) The State of the World's Children. Available at: http:// www.unicef.org (accessed 3 November 2012).

Vader, J-P. (2006) Spiritual health: the next frontier. *European Journal of Public Health* 16, 457.

van der Zee, B. (2011) *The Protester's Handbook*. Guardian Books, London.

Venkatapuram, S. (2011) *Health Justice*. Polity Press, Cambridge, UK.

Vivian, J. (1994) NGOs and sustainable development in Zimbabwe: no magic bullets. *Development and Change* 25, 181–209.

Wainwright, S. (2003) *Measuring Impact. A Guide to Resources*. National Council for Voluntary Organisations, London.

Wakefield, M.A., Loken, B. and Hornik R.C. (2010) Use of mass media campaigns to change health behaviour. *Lancet* 376, 1261–1271.

Wakefield, S.E.L. and Poland, B. (2005) Family, friend or foe? Critical reflections on the relevance and role of social capital in health promotion and community development. *Social Science & Medicine* 60, 2819–2832.

Walby, S. (2007) Complexity theory, systems theory, and multiple intersecting social inequalities. *Philosophy of the Social Sciences* 37, 449–70.

Walker, A. and Wigfield, A. (2003) *Social Quality, Social Capital and Quality of Life*. Discussion Paper for ENIQ, February 2003.

Wall, E., Ferrazzi, G. and Schryer, F. (1998) Getting the goods on social capital. *Rural Sociology* 63, 300–322.

Wallack, L. and Dorfman, L. (1996) Media advocacy: a strategy for advancing policy and promoting health. *Health Education Quarterly* 23, 293–317.

Wallerstein, N. (1992) Powerlessness, empowerment, and health: implications for health promotion programs. *American Journal of Health Promotion* 6, 197–205.

Wallerstein, N. (2002) Empowerment to reduce health disparities. *Scandinavian Journal of Public Health* 30, 72–77.

Wallerstein, N. (2006) What is the evidence on effectiveness of empowerment to improve health? *Report for the Health Evidence Network (HEN)*.

Walt, G. (1994) *Health Policy. An Introduction to Process and Power*. Zed Books, London.

Walt, G. and Buse, K. (2006) Global cooperation in international public health. In: Merson, M.H., Black, R.E. and Mills, A.J. (eds) *International Public Health: Diseases, Programs, Systems and Policies*. Jones and Bartlett Publishers, Boston, Massachusetts, pp. 649–680.

Walt, G. and Gilson, L. (1994) Reforming the health sector in developing countries: the central role of policy analysis. *Health Policy and Planning* 9, 353–370.

Walt, G., Shiffman, J., Schneider, H., Murray, S.F., Brugha, R. and Gilson, L. (2002) Doing health policy analysis: methodological and conceptual reflections and challenges. *Health Policy Planning* 23, 300–317.

Wang, S., Ross, J.R. and Hiller, J.E. (2005) Applicability and transferability of interventions in evidence-based public health. *Health Promotion International* 21, 76–83.

Wang, Y., Ge, K. and Popkin, B.M. (2000) Tracking of body mass index from childhood to adolescence: a 6-year follow-up study in China. *American Journal of Clinical Nutrition* 72, 1018–1024.

Ward, D. and Mullender, A. (1991) Empowerment and oppression: an indissoluble pairing for contemporary social work. *Critical Social Policy* 11, 21–29.

Warwick-Booth, L., Cross, R. and Lowcock, D. (2012) *Health Studies: An Overview Of Contemporary Perspectives*. Polity Press, Cambridge, UK.

Watson, J. (2000) *Researching Health Promotion*. Psychology Press, London.

Watson, M. (2008) Going for gold: the health promoting general practice. *Quality in Primary Care* 16, 177–185.

Webb, D. and Wright, D. (2000) Postmodernism and health promotion: implications for the debate on effectiveness. In: Watson, J. and Platt, S. (eds) *Researching Health Promotion*. Routledge, London.

Weeks, J., Scriven, A. and Sayer, L. (2005) The health promoting role of health visitors: adjunct or synergy. In: Scriven, A. (ed.) (2005) *Health Promoting Practice: The Contribution of Nurses and Allied Health Professionals*. Palgrave Macmillan, Basingstoke, UK, pp. 31–44.

Weitzman, E.R. and Kawachi, I. (2000) Giving means receiving: the protective effect of social capital on binge drinking on college campuses. *American Journal of Public Health* 90, 1936–1939.

Wells, J.S.G. (2007) Priorities, 'street level bureaucracy' and the community mental health team. *Health and Social Care in the Community* 5, 333–342.

Wenzel, E. (1997) A comment on settings in health promotion. *Internet Journal of Health Promotion*. Available at: http://www.rhpeo.net/ijhp-articles/1997/1/index.htm (accessed 3 November 2012).

Wenzel, E. (1999) Health policy formation and community participation. Available at: http://www.ldb.org/pbh7115/; cited in Carlise, S. (2000) Health promotion, advocacy and health inequalities. *Health Promotion International* 15, 369–376.

Werner, D. and Sanders, D. (1997) *Questioning the Solution: The Politics of Primary Health Care and Child Survival*. HealthWrights, Palo Alto, California.

White, A. and Johnson, M. (2000) Men making sense of their chest pain: niggles, doubts and denials. *Journal of Clinical Nursing* 9, 534–42.

White, A. and Richardson, N. (2011) Gendered epidemiology: making men's health visible in epidemiological research. *Public Health* 125, 407–410.

White, A., McKee, M., Richardson, N., Madsen S.A., de Sousa, B., de Visser, R., Hogston, R., Makara, P. and Zatoñski, W. (2011) Europe's men need their own health strategy. *British Medical Journal* 343, d7397.

White, A.K. and Pettifer, M. (2007) *Hazardous Waist: Tackling Male Weight Problems*. Radcliffe Publishing, Oxford, UK.

White, J., South, J. and Kinsella, K. (2010a) *An Evaluation of Social Prescribing Health Trainers in South and West Bradford*. Leeds Metropolitan University, Leeds, UK.

White, J., South, J. and Kinsella, K. (2010b) *The North Lincolnshire Health Trainer Service: an Evaluation*. Leeds Metropolitan University, Leeds, UK.

White, J., South, J., Woodall, J. and Kinsella, K. (2010c) *Altogether Better Thematic Evaluation – Community Health Champions and Empowerment*. Centre for Health Promotion Research, Leeds Metropolitan University, Leeds, UK.

Whitehead, D. (2004) The health promoting university (HPU): the role and function of nursing. *Nurse Education Today* 24, 466–472.

Whitehead, D. (2006) The health promoting prison (HPP) and its imperative for nursing. *International Journal of Nursing Studies* 43, 123–131.

Whitehead, M. (1992) The concepts and principles of equity and health. *International Journal of Health Services* 22, 429–445.

Whitehead, M. (1995) Tackling inequalities a review of policy initiatives. In: Benzeval, M.,

Judge, K. and Whitehead, M. (eds) *Tackling Inequalities in Health*. Kings Fund, London.

Whitehead, M. and Dahlgren, G. (2007) *Concepts and Principles for tackling social inequities in health. Levelling Up Part 1*. Studies on Social and Economic Determinants of Health, No. 2. WHO Collaborating Centre for Social Determinants of Health, University of Liverpool, UK.

Whitelaw, S., Baxendale, A., Bryce, C., Machardy, L., Young, I. and Witney, E. (2001) 'Settings' based health promotion: a review. *Health Promotion International* 16, 339–352.

WHO (World Health Organization) (1978) Declaration of Alma-Ata, International Conference on Primary Health Care, Alma-Ata, USSR, 6–12 September 1978. WHO, Geneva. Available at: http://www.who.int/publications/almaata_declaration_en.pdf (accessed 3 November 2012).

WHO (1985) *Targets for Health for All: Targets in Support of the European Regional Strategy for Health for All*. WHO Regional Office for Europe, Copenhagen.

WHO (1986a) *Healthy Cities: Promoting Health in the Urban Context*. WHO, Copenhagen. Available at: http://www.who.dk/healthy-cities/ (accessed 18 July 2011).

WHO (1986b) Ottawa Charter for health promotion. *Health Promotion* 1, iii–v.

WHO (1986c) *Ottawa Charter for Health Promotion. First International Conference on Health Promotion*, Ottawa, 17–21 November. WHO Regional Office for Europe, Copenhagen.

WHO (1988) *The Adelaide Recommendations: Healthy Public Policy*. WHO, Geneva, and the Commonwealth of Australia.

WHO (1991) *Third International Conference on Health Promotion*. Sundsvall, Sweden. WHO, Geneva.

WHO (1995) *Health in Prisons. Health Promotion in the Prison Setting. Summary Report on a WHO meeting*, London, 15–17 October 1995. WHO, Copenhagen.

WHO (1997a) *Obesity – Preventing and Managing the Global Epidemic*. Rep. WHO consult. Obes. WHO/NUT/NCD/98.1., WHO, Geneva.

WHO (1997b) *Jakarta Declaration on Leading Health Promotion into the 21st Century*. WHO, Geneva. Available at: http://www.who.int/healthpromotion/conferences/previous/jakarta/declaration/en/index1.html (accessed 12 October 2012).

WHO (1998a) *Health 21 – The Health for All Policy for the WHO European Region – 21 Targets for the 21st Century*. WHO, Copenhagen.

WHO (1998b) *Health Promotion Glossary*. WHO, Geneva.

WHO (2000) *Mexico Ministerial Statement for the Promotion of Health: From Ideas to Action*. Fifth Global Conference on Health Promotion: Bridging the Equity Gap, Mexico, 5–9 June. WHO, Geneva.

WHO (2002) *WHO Programme to Eliminate Sleeping Sickness: Building a Global Alliance*. WHO, Geneva.

WHO (2004) *Healthy Marketplaces in the Western Pacific: Guiding Future Action*. WHO, Geneva.

WHO (2005a) *The Bangkok Charter for Health Promotion in a Globalised World*. WHO, Geneva. Available at: www.who.int/healthpromotion/conferences/6gchp/bangkok_charter/en/index.html (accessed 12 October 2012).

WHO (2005b) *Climate and Health, Fact Sheet*. Available at: www.who.int/globalchange/news/fsclimandhealth/en/print.html (accessed 13 January 2010).

WHO (2006) *Working Together for Health*. WHO, Geneva.

WHO (2009a) Milestones in Health Promotion: Statements from Global Conferences. WHO, Geneva.

WHO (2009b) *The Relevance of Noncommunicable Diseases to the ECOSOC High-Level Segment, 2009*. Available at: http://www.esango.un.org/innovationfair/notes/Janet%20Voute%20WHO.ppt> (accessed 1 October 2011).

WHO (2011) *What is a Healthy City?* Available at: http://www.euro.who.int/en/what-we-do/health-topics/environment-and-health/urban-health/activities/healthy-cities/who-european-healthy-cities-network/what-is-a-healthy-city (accessed 18 July 2011).

Wiggers, J. and Sanson-Fisher, R. (1998) Evidence-based health promotion. In: Scott, R. and Weston, R. (eds) *Evaluating Health Promotion*. Stanley Thornes, Cheltenham, UK.

Wilkinson, R. (1996) *Unhealthy Societies: The Afflictions of Inequality*. Routledge, London.

Wilkinson, R. and Marmot, M. (2003) *The Solid Facts*. WHO, Copenhagen.

Wilkinson, R. and Pickett, K. (2009) *The Spirit Level. Why More Equal Societies Almost Always Do Better*. Allen Lane, London.

Wilkinson, R.G. and Pickett, K. (2010) *The Spirit Level: Why Equality is Better for Everyone*. Allen Lane, London.

Wilkinson, S. and Kitzinger, C. (1994) *Women's Health – Feminist Perspectives*. Taylor & Francis, London.

Williams, G.H. (2003) The determinants of health: structure, context and agency. *Sociology of Health and Illness* 25 (Silver Anniversary Issue), 131–154.

Williams, R. (1983) Concepts of health: an analysis of lay logic. *Sociology* 17, 185–204.

Wills, J. and Cook, T. (2011) Engaging with marginalised communities: the experience of London health trainers, *Perspectives in Public Health* (published on line 7 April 2011).

Wills, J. and Earle, S. (2007) Theoretical perspectives on promoting public health. In: Earle, S., Lloyd, C.E., Sidell, M. and Spurr, S. (eds) *Theory and Research in Promoting Public Health*. Sage, London, pp. 129–162.

Wills, J. and Woodhead, D. (2004) The glue that binds: articulating values in multidisciplinary public health. *Critical Public Health* 14, 7–15.

Wilson-Clay, B., Rourke, J.W., Bolduc, M.B., Stagg, J.D., Flatau, G. and Vagh, B. (2005) Learning to lobby for probreastfeeding legislation: the story of a Texas Bill to create a breastfeeding-friendly physician designation. *Journal of Human Lactation* 21, 191–198.

Wimbush, E. and Watson, J. (2000) An evaluation framework for health promotion: theory, quality and effectiveness. *Evaluation* 6, 301–321.

Windahl, S. and Signitzer, B. with Olson, J. (2009) *Using Communication Theory: An Introduction to Planned Communication*, 2nd edition. Sage, London.

Wise, S. (1995) Feminist ethics in practice. In: Hugman, R. and Smith, D. (eds) *Ethical Issues in Social Work*. Routledge, London.

Witte, K. and Allen, M. (2000) A meta analysis of fear appeals: implications for effective public health campaigns. *Health Education and Behavior* 27, 591–615.

Wolf, M. (2004) *Why Globalization Works: the Case for the Global Market Economy*. Yale University Press, New Haven, Connecticut.

Woodall, J. (2010) Control and choice in three category-C English prisons: implications for the concept and practice of the health promoting prison.

Unpublished PhD thesis, Faculty of Health, Leeds Metropolitan University, Leeds, UK.

Woodall, J. and South, J. (2011) Health promoting prisons: dilemmas and challenges. In: Scriven, A. and Hodgins, M. (eds) *Health Promotion Settings: Principles and Practice*. Sage, London, pp. 170–186.

Woodall, J., Raine, G., South, J. and Warwick-Booth, L. (2010) *Empowerment & Health and Well-being: Evidence Review*. Centre for Health Promotion Research, Leeds Metropolitan University, Leeds, UK.

World Bank (2002) World Development Indicators CD-ROM. World Bank, Washington, DC.

World Commission on Environment and Development (1987) *From One Earth to One World: An Overview*. Oxford University Press, Oxford.

Wrigley, T. (2000) Misunderstanding school improvement. *Improving Schools* 3, 23–29.

Wrigley, T., Thomson, P. and Lingard, R. (2011) *Changing Schools: Alternative Approaches to Making a World of Difference*. Routledge, London.

Yamey, G. (2002) Why does the world still need WHO? *British Medical Journal* 325, 1294–1298.

Yamey, G. and Feachem, R. (2011) Evidence-based policymaking in global health – the payoffs and pitfalls. *Evidence-Based Medicine* 16, 97–99.

Yorkshire and Humber Public Health Observatory (2008) Infant Mortality in Yorkshire and the Humber: Data Summary. Available at: http://www.yhpho.org.uk (accessed 3 November 2012).

Yuill, C., Crinson, I. and Duncan, E. (2010) *Key Concepts in Health Studies*. Sage, London.

Zarcadoolas, C., Pleasant, A. and Greer, D.S. (2005) Understanding health literacy: an expanded model. *Health Promotion International* 20, 195–203.

Ziglio, E., Hagard, S. and Brown, C. (2005) Health promotion development in Europe: barriers and opportunities. In: Scriven, A. and Garman, S. (2005) *Promoting Health: Global Perspectives*. Palgrave Macmillan, Basingstoke, UK.

Zoller, H.M. (2005) Health activism: communication theory and action for social change. *Communication Theory* 15, 341–364.

Zuo, Y., Norberg, M., Wen, M. and Rissel, C. (2006) Estimates of overweight and obesity among samples of preschool-aged children in Melbourne and Sydney. *Nutrition and Dietetics* 63, 179–183.

Index

Page numbers in **bold** type refer to figures, tables and boxes.

academic community, roles 144, 152, 153–154, 159
accountability 3, 38, **41**, 72, 133
activism
    achievement of social change 71, 128
    defined 52
    digital communication impacts 94
    ethics and dangers of 124
Adelaide conference (1988) 11
adult learning 83–84
advertising **56**, 90, 97, 98, 125
advocacy
    definition and types 68–69, **69**
    for health, by health promoters **10**, 71
    lobby and interest groups 70–71
    roles in policy making 69–70
    in social marketing 97
Africa
    common health problems 162
    community empowerment strategies 22
    foreign aid to 4–5
    formal and informal workplace settings 112, **113**
    health promotion **145**, 147–149, 152–153
    health service provision 140, 148
    importance of NGOs 74, 132
age, and attitudes to health 20, 155–157
    see also old people
agency concept 23
agenda setting 2, 63, 69
agricultural policy 60, 159
aid
    benefits and problems 4–5
    global agencies **75**
    overseas student funding 165
alcohol
    dependency, settings 111
    producers and lobby groups 70
    public policies on 11
    reducing use, motivational interviewing 102–103
alliances *see* partnerships
Alma-Ata conference (1978) 9, 143
    Alma-Ata Declaration **14**, 31, 148
Altogether Better programme (UK) 22, 26, **26**, 129
Arnstein's ladder of participation 44, **44**
asbestos health hazard 126–127
Asia
    Health Promotion Boards 147
    workplace health promotion 112
assets/resources, of communities 39, 49, **51**
asylum seekers 13, 22, 140, 167
Australia, Aboriginal people
    health inequalities 13, 52

health promotion guideline 28
    spiritual health 173

balance, in lay concepts of health 19, 21
Bangkok conference (2005) **2**, 12, 54, 115, 146
Bantaba approach (The Gambia) 94
Beattie's model of health promotion 134, **134**
behaviour
    change, related to health messages
        background factors 105–106
        effectiveness of linear model 79, 81, **82**, 174
        intention 104–105
        motivation **101**, 101–103, 104, 127
        stages of change 104, 115
    change theory, psychosocial models 102, 103–106, **105**
    consumer, in social marketing 97
    impacts of mass media 90–92
    manipulation
        nudging and persuasion 97–98
        role of state 5
        shock and shaming tactics 127–128
    and modifiable risk factors, NCDs 6
beliefs
    and behaviour change 103–104, 125
    in social constructionism 119
'Big Society' (UK) 51, 128
Bill & Melinda Gates Foundation 4, 68–69, **75**
biomedical model of health 7–8, **8**, 16, 28, 151
Black Report (UK, 1980) 4, 150
blindness 162
bonding networks, social capital 34
bottom-up processes
    characteristics **135**, 156
    policy implementation approaches 67–68,
          135–136, **137**
    self-help groups **43**
Brazil
    education and literacy 83
    health promotion and inequalities 147, 157, 161
    Porto Alegre participatory budgeting 45–46
breast cancer 6, 62, 153, 154–155
bridging networks, social capital 34, 38
Bristol Social Exclusion Matrix 158, **159**
British Medical Association 70, **76**

Canada, health promotion ideas 9, 69, 126, 146–147, 166–167
cancer
    care in developing countries 162
    lifestyle and environmental risk factors 6, 154–155

capacity development 122, 138, 149, 164–167
capitalism 70, 117
carers, unpaid 40
celebrities, and issue awareness 87–89
channels, communication 87–89, 90–95
charities, aims and funding **75**
Chicago, community health actions **45**
child health
    involvement of grandmothers (Senegal) **40**
    obesity 124, 136, 161
    pedestrian traffic accidents 7, 60
    perception of issues 155–156, 173
    survival of malaria (Tanzania) **97**
Child-to-Child initiative 130–131
childbearing *see* maternal mortality; women's health
China
    effects of global influences 94
    government policies 41, 56
    health of Chinese people 19, 145, 161
choice architects 98
cigarettes *see* smoking; tobacco
citizens
    democratic influence on policy 63, 73
    as 'fourth sector' 132
    power of, compared with 'clients' 44
    rights and duties 31, 128–131
class (socio-economic status)
    correlation with health 4, 157
    lay concepts of health, class variation 20
    related to health services use 140
climate change 55, 61, 70, 96, 160–161
coaching, health 102
collaboration between policy sectors 65–66
Commission on Social Determinants of Health
    (CSDH) 2–3, 57, 138, 157, 179
communication
    importance for health promotion 78–79,
        95–96
    methods and channels 87–89
        electronic/digital **94**, 94–95, **95**
        mass media 90–91
        motivational interviewing **101**, 101–103
        'nudge' concept 97–98
        peer education 92
        social marketing 96–97, **97**
        traditional and popular media 93–94
    misunderstanding of health messages 39, 80
    one-way knowledge transfer 81–82, **82**
    process components **79**, 84–90, **85**
    theories and models 79–81, **80**, **81**, 91–92
    two-way transformational exchange 79, 82–84
communities
    adoption of new ideas 136
    benefits of active involvement in 129
    cultural outlook and local knowledge 27–28
    definitions of term 30
    exclusion of outsiders 38
    level of social capital 32–36, **37**, 37–39, 93
    partnerships with universities 167
    representatives 73
    strength, importance for health 10, 30–32, **33**
community empowerment
    definition and terminology 23–24, **24**

encouragement, role of health promoters 25–26,
    94, 136, **137**
    evaluation 118
    importance in community development 43–46
    process continuum 24–25, **25**, 47–48, 49
community health workers (CHWs) 40–42, **41**, 43, 50
Community-Led Total Sanitation 127
computer (digital) literacy 87, 95, 100
conferences, international 2, 9, 11–13, **14**, 143
conservatism **64**, 71, 147
Copenhagen discussion paper (WHO, 2009) 9, 27
cost–benefit (value–expectancy) analysis 97, 103–104
costs
    cost-cutting measures 44–45, **62**
    of social capital development 37
    and trade-offs, healthy public policies 56, 57
critical race theory (CRT) 154
Cuba, health improvement 4, 13
cultural differences
    appropriate health promotion materials 89, 93–94
    customs, legality and morality 124, 125
    Eurocentric bias of research **105**, 106, 152–153
    lay concepts of health 18–21, 39

data collection, excluded groups 13–14
databases, social and health data 121
deaths, causes of 6, 13, 70, 162
decision making
    ethical considerations 123–128
    evidence-based
        for health promotion professionals 117–118,
            120–122, **121**
        for policy makers 57, 61–62, 122
    personal health choices 23, 96
    'private' matters and state policies 56, 58
    shared, professional–patient 39–40
    stages of process 92
democracy
    effect on autonomy, ethics of 125
    effects of electronic communication 94–95
    role of education 83
demographic trends, emerging health issues 11–12, 156
depression, causes 23
developing countries
    demographic and disease transitions 161–162
    focus of health promotion 147
    health care access 145, 149
development strategies
    aid versus self-reliance 4–5
    enhancing social capital in communities **37**
    global ideas, North/South differences 172–173
    involvement of NGOs 74, 131–132
    participatory, for communities 44–51, **50**
    sustainability 160–161
diabetes 12, 145, 162
diarrhoea, treatment and causes 7, 39, 127, 149
diet
    community fruit and vegetable growing **34**, **45**,
        49, 136
    effect of behavioural counselling 102
    global changes **59**
    healthy eating guidelines 70, 88–89

digital divide (media access) 95
disability
    anti-discrimination legislation 132
    exclusion from policy making 65, 157–158
    social networking 94
discourse analysis 146–147
diseases
    neglected, raising awareness of 12, 68–69, 162–163
    preventable, as causes of death 13
    specific policy actions 59
doctors *see* health practitioners; professionals
'double burden' (new and established diseases) 161–162
drugs, illegal use 127

economic growth
    assumption of resulting benefits 3, 170
    of poorer countries 56, 147, 159–160
education
    among peers (social learning) 92, 116
    institutions, roles in health promotion 144, 149,
        164–167
    levels and types of literacy 99–100
    online (distance learning) 165
    settings 110
        rural community programmes **47**
    top-down advice giving, effectiveness 81–82, 91
    training in health promotion competence 138–140
    transformative dialogue approaches 82–84
    see also schools
electronic (digital) communications 30, 87, 94–95, 100–101
employment, informal 112
empowerment
    of communities, implications 10, 23–24, **24**
    importance of literacy 99–101
    individual 23, 42, 84
    participation, degrees of 25–26, **26**, 44, **44**, 73
    understanding of concept 21–22
    see also community empowerment
enabling, scope in health promotion **10**
England
    community development (New Deal) 31
    current decline of health promotion 143, 150–151
    health trainer/champion programmes 42, 129, **129**, 140
    infant mortality variation **15**
Enlightenment, rational outlook 170
entrepreneurs, policy/social 68, 74–75
environment
    health risks in 6
    natural, importance for health 10, 160
environmentalism (green ideology) **64**, 70
epidemiology
    lay views 89–90, 100, 153
    role of gender 155
equity
    achievable policy aims 56, 57, 179–180
    health and wealth distribution 1–2, 4, 56, 157,
        180–181
    political viewpoints 58, **64**
    see also social justice
ethics
    behaviour manipulation 127–128
    equity principles 178, **179**

health intervention pros and cons 4–5, 124–126
    of paternalism 98
    resource rationing and doing nothing 126–127
    value base of health promotion 26–29, **27**,
        123–124, **176–177**
ethnic groups *see* marginalized groups; racism
evaluation
    appraisal of evidence 121
    of communication process 79
    of health promotion activities 103, 113–115, 118
        constructionist and pluralist 119–120, 168
        evaluative culture 122–123
        positivist 118–119
    spidergrams, participation studies **46**, 46–47
evidence
    basis for health promotion practice 26, 27,
        117–118
    collection difficulties 13–14, 113–115
    importance in policy making 61–62, 76, 122, 144
    nature of, epistomology 118
        hierarchical grading 118–119, **119**
        pluralistic typologies 120, **120**
    sources 121
    use in decision making, skills required 120–122,
        121, 123
Evidence to Policy initiative (E2Pi) 122
exclusion
    minority and 'invisible' groups 153–158
    of outsiders by tight-knit communities 38
    from policy-making process 65
    from settings-based work 112–113, **114**

Fag Ends Smoking Cessation Service (UK) **43**
families, cohesion as social capital 33, **33**, 35
family planning 56, 93, 124–125
Fankanta initiative (The Gambia) 93–94
fatalism 19–20, 125
female genital cutting (FGC) **47**, 125
feminism **64**, 154–155, 158
'fifth wave' thinking 174
financial systems (banking) crisis 2, 52, 128
Finnish approach, research 163–164
fitness, physical 18–19
food
    industry regulation 59
    security and hunger 11, 88, 161
foreign aid *see* aid
Framework Convention on Global Health 160

Galway consensus 138–140
gay rights 124, 154, 158
gender differences
    attitudes to health 20
    effect of globalization on equality 160
    health issue inequalities 155
    see also men; women's health
global warming *see* climate change
globalization 71, 73–74, 91, 159–160, 178
governments
    policy costs and trade-offs 56, **57**
    regulation of lobbyists 65, 70

governments (*continued*)
    responsibility for citizens' health 5, 10, 65,
        125–127, **126**
    support for partnerships 72
    tokenism and real achievements 50, 51, 57–58, 150
grassroots action
    effectiveness for sustainable change 135, 166
    reduction of health inequalities, strategies 58
Greenpeace 63, 70

Hamara Centre (Leeds) 167
happiness
    indices of 15, 16–17, 170, 172
    linked to community social capital 38, 171
health
    lay people's views and behaviour 17–21, 81, 153, 168–170
    measurement and indices 8, 15, **15**, 115
    philosophical domain **178**
    professional definitions 14–17
Health Action Model 101, 104, 105
Health and Lifestyle studies (UK, Blaxter) 18, 169
Health Belief Model 103, 104
health practitioners
    decision making, use of evidence 120–122
    as policy entrepreneurs 68
    primary health care, lay workers 40–43, **41**, 129, 136, 138
    staff shortage in Africa 148, 165
    upstream thinking and scope of action 7, 77, 118,
        139–140
    visiting, relevance for local people 5, 136
    see also professionals
health promotion
    compared with social marketing 96–97
    global vision and goals 2–3, 9, 107, **108**, 144–147
    planning cycle 118, 123, 175
    processes and actions 9–11, **10**, 58, 107–108, 180
    settings approach 108–113, **109**, **111**
    theoretical basis, revision and research 151–153,
        163–164
    value principles 26–29, **27**, 84, 123–128, **176–177**
health social movements (HSMs) 52
health care systems
    ethics 123–124
    orientation and focus 11, 41, 139, 145, 151
    positive and negative approaches to health 7–8, **8**
    restructuring **62**, 62–63
    service uptake rate 140, 145–146
healthworlds concept 168–170
Healthy Cities programme 22, 31, 113
'healthy public policy', *definition* 54–55, **55**, 59
heart disease 33, 99–100, 133, 157
HELP (health empowerment leverage project), UK 50, **52**
HIV/AIDS
    communication initiatives 93–94
    expert advisory groups and activists 65, 71, 132
    incidence 13, 149, 160
holding frameworks 141
hospitals **45**, 110
human rights
    individual rights and public interest 125–126
    nudging as infringement 98
    UN declaration 1, 171

humanistic education approach 21, 83–84, 85
hunger *see* food

ideology 63, **64**, 71, 150
illness
    absence of, as definition of health 16, 18
    and receptivity to health messages 89
immunization 59, 90, 145
impact assessment 73
implementation
    of evidence-based decisions 121–122
    gaps between intentions and progress 143, 149, 166
    of policies 66–68, 70, 122, 135
incremental policy development 60, **61**
indicators
    health 8, 136
    tracking, for capacity building 164, **164**
    well-being/happiness 15, 16–17, 170, 172
indigenous people
    life expectancy 13
    relevance of health promotion 27–28
    see also Australia, Aboriginal people
individuals
    assets of **51**, 99–101
    connections with different settings 111
    empowerment 23, 25, 115
    interpersonal communication 86–87, **87**, 91–92
    participation in policy making 73, **76**
    relationships, in communities 34–35
    responsibility and control of health 19–20, 21, 98,
        103–106
industrialized (developed) countries 145, 147
inequality
    effects of globalization 159–160
    infant mortality as indicator **15**
    in society, effects on health 1–2, 4, 33, 157
    statistics and data collection 13–14, 57
infant mortality **15**
infections *see* diseases
information access *see* knowledge
innovations, diffusion theories 92, 136
insecticide-treated nets (ITNs) 81, **97**
intention and behaviour change 104–105
interest groups 70–71
International Monetary Fund (IMF) 74, **75**
Internet use 94–95, 100, 165
intervention
    evaluation of outcomes 113–115, 118–120
    justifications and problems 4–5, 120, 125–126
    ladder of government actions **126**, 126–127
    success and communication skills 79
interviewing, motivational **101**, 101–103, 104
issue framing 69

Jakarta conference (1997) 11–12, 54, 147
Johari window 85–86, **86**

knowledge
    epistemology 118

one-way transfer **82**, 82–83
    sharing and assimilation 83–84, 116, 141
Kyoto Protocol (2010) 55

Labonte's model of well-being 17, **18**, 173
Lalonde Report (Canada, 1974) 9, 147, 150
Lasswell Formula (communication) 79–80, **80**
lay people
    concepts of health 17–21, 89–90, 100, 152, 168–170
    health champions 129, **129**
    health knowledge and traditions 39–40, **40**, 145
    perspectives, as evidence 119
    self-care capacity 71
leadership
    importance for grassroots action **38**
    in organizational change **116**, 138
    in partnerships 72
    skills requirement, health promoters 140–141
learning disability 158
learning organizations 115–117, **117**
Leeds, UK
    infant mortality **15**
    Metropolitan University, health promotion
        studies 21, 136, 163
        collaboration and partnerships 65, 130, 151,
            167–168
    transport policy 65
legislation
    compared with voluntary approach **76**
    as counterproductive for change **47**, 48
    impacts on health 59–60
    influence of lobby/interest groups 70
    situations where laws needed 132, 134
leisure studies 152
liberalism **64**, 73
life expectancy, national statistics 13
lifestyle choices
    factors affecting health 5–6, 99–100
    fatalism or self-control 19–20, 125
    influence of media 90–91
    unhealthy, global spread 160
linking networks, social capital 34
literacy, health 98–101, 144–145
lobby groups 63, 65, 70, **76**
local governance
    less developed systems, community solutions 130
    participatory budgeting 45–46
    quality in healthy communities 38
    responsibility for public health, UK 150
London conference (2008) 2

malaria **97**, 163
malnutrition
    causes and effects 7
    elimination, public policy actions 11
Maori people 27–28
marginalized groups
    access to health care initiatives 42, 112–113, **114**
    community action **45**
    engagement by storytelling 49, **50**
    exclusion and oppression 22, 153–158
    lack of health data on 13–14

Marxism 36, 49, **61**, **64**, 156–157
mass media 87–89, 90–92
maternal mortality 13, 65, 93
McGuire's communication/persuasion model 80
measurement
    effectiveness of motivational interviewing 102–103
    health promotion capacity, tracking indicators 164, **164**
    indicators of health 8, 15, 16–17, 136
media *see* communication
mediation, required in health promotion **10**
medical profession
    focus on illness and pathology 8
    partnerships with lay health workers 42–43
medicine
    clinical trials, methodology 118–119
    distribution of resources 128, 162–163
    ethical framework 123–124
    see also biomedical model of health
men
    male attitude to health concerns 20, 94–95,
        145–146
    participation in education programmes **47**
mental health
    elderly people 156
    linked with happiness 171–172, 174
    policy development 59, 68
    Wye Wood project (UK) **164**, **172**
    young people 155
Mexico conference (2000) 12, 54, 147
Millennium Development Goals (MDGs) 72, 74, 138,
    165, 178
mobile phones 94, 95, **95**
models
    advocacy 69, **69**, 71
    behaviour change 102, 103–106, **105**, 174
    communication
        cyclic and reciprocal 80–81, **81**
        mass media influence 91–92
        traditional linear 79–80, **80**
    of education 82
    of health
        medical and social 7–8, **8**, 16, 28
        spiritual 173–174, **174**
    health promotion (Beattie) 134, **134**
    of participation 44, **44**, 47
    policy implementation 67
    Red Lotus model (Gregg & O'Hara) 28, 175, **178**,
        179, **180**
    settings-based problems and solutions 111, **111**
    of well-being (Labonte) 17, **18**, 173
moral codes 4, 20, 124
mortality *see* deaths, causes of
motivational interviewing 101, 101–103, 104

Nairobi conference (2009) 12, 148–149
'nanny state' 5, 56, 57, 144
nation states
    differing social policies 59
    global influences 58, 131
National Health Service, UK (NHS)
    information access strategy 95
    non-political status 7

National Health Service, UK (NHS) (continued)
    restructuring policies **62**, 62–63, 150
    workforce training 139
nationalism **64**
neo-liberalism 3, 58, **62**, **64**, 144
networks
    effects of membership on health 35, **35**
    management and leadership 141
    in policy making **61**, 66, **66**
    scope, in health promotion 116
    types within communities 34–35
New Zealand
    Maori people, health promotion relevance 27–28
    Prostitutes Collective (NZPC) **24**
NICE (National Institute for Health and Clinical
    Excellence, UK) 48, 118, 129
non-communicable diseases (NCDs) 6, 162
non-governmental organizations (NGOs) 48, 74, **75**,
    131–132, 165–166
non-verbal communication 86–87
'nudging' 65, 97–98, 123
'nutcracker effect' 2–3, 31–32
nutrition *see* diet

obesity 35, 55, 124
    in children 124, 136, 161
    and physical inactivity 60
old people
    ageism 156–157
    community involvement **45**
    grandmothers, role in maternal/child health **40**
    information technology access 95
    opinion leaders 91–92
oppression 22, 24, 83, 153–158
Organisation for Economic Co-Operation and
    Development (OECD) 171
organizations
    assets of **51**
    businesses (private sector) 112
    community-based enterprises 130, 132
    influencing global policies 74, **75**
    steps to transformation 115–117, **116**
Osgood and Schramm model (communication) 80, **81**
Ottawa Charter (1986)
    action areas suggested 9–11, 55, 68, 139, 144–145
    compared with Bangkok Charter 146
    ethos and aims 3, 9, 13, 109

parenting issues 7, 58, 136, 161, 173
participation
    by children 130–131, 155–156
    and community empowerment 25–26, **26**, 43–46, **44**
    in education 83–84, 87
    encouragement, top-down/bottom-up
        approaches 45, **47**, 47–51
    evaluation, spidergram methods **46**, 46–47
    information sharing 79, 93–94
    motivation for, in active citizens 128–131
    in policy-making process 66, 71, 73
partnerships
    health professionals and lay workers 42–43, 136

multi/trans-disciplinary studies 152, 163
    policy-making alliances 72
    universities and communities 166–168
patients, health expertise 39–40, 79
pedestrians *see* traffic/car accidents
peer education 92, 116
People in Public Health project (UK) 42, 129, **130**
People's Health Movement 3, 74
personal skills development 10–11, 99–103, **101**, 144–145
philanthropists 4, **75**, 132
photography, tool of empowerment initiatives **24**
pluralism
    in evaluation frameworks 120
    medical (biomedical and alternative therapies) 145
    in policy making **61**, 71, 73
    world philosophical outlook 170–171
policy, definitions 58–59
policy, public
    consequences and effectiveness 55–58, **57**, 73, 122
    coordination between sectors 10, 65–66, 72
    global action 55, 73–75
    ideological basis 63, **64**, 150
    national and international commitments 54
    Ottawa/Adelaide conference suggestions 10, 11,
        55, 144–145
    policy-making process
        actors/stakeholders 63, 65, 68, 144, 159
        advocacy 68–71, **69**
        citizen participation 73, 132–133
        factors influencing change **62**, 62–63, 66
        implementation 66–68
        theories, and in practice 60–62, **61**, 76
    scope of social and health policies 58–60
political action
    justifications for 4
    likelihood in communities 35
    role of third sector 131–132
political will (commitment)
    driving policy change, effectiveness 57–58
    given at conferences, and outcomes 12–13, 143
    ideological basis 63
    spending/taxation priorities 2
pollution 59, 60
Polynesians, concepts of health 18, 19
population control policies 56, 124–125
Portman Group 70
poverty
    as cause of disease/illness 13, 41
    effects of globalization on 159–160
    and healthy choices 89, 169
    poor communities, disadvantages 32–33
power
    balance
        ethical principles 123–124
        need for redistribution 2–3, 21, 23, 180–181
        between teachers and learners 83–84
    challenges, conflict and resistance 45, 50–51
    degrees of citizen control 44, **44**
    forms of oppression 22
    held by policy actors 63, 65, 72
    maintenance of status quo 51, 146, 165
    political, as policy determinant 58, **76**
    sharing and partnerships 73

powerlessness
    personal consequences 22, 23, 69
    sources of 22
    see also exclusion
prejudice *see* racism; stereotyping
prevention of illness, programmes 8, 42, 59
primary health care (PHC) 41, 72, 145, **145**, 148
prisons
    challenges for research 114–115, 163
    health promotion strategies 113, **114**
    prisoner empowerment 25–26
    as settings 109, 111, 114
    staff attitude to health promotion 67–68
private sector in health care 63, 128
professionals
    characteristics, defined 138
    communication skills and problems 39, 100
    competence and learning 139–140,
        164–165
    definitions of health 15–17
    discretion in policy implementation 67–68, 72
    relationships with clients 31, 39–40, 123–124, 152
    resistance to community involvement 46, 71
propaganda 80, 90, 91
Protection Motivation Theory 103, 104
public health
    contrasted with health promotion 3, 54–55, 138
    decision-making model 71
    effect of health literacy 100–101

quality of life 173
questions, framing (research) 121, 122–123

racism 154
randomized control trials (RCTs) 118–119, 120
rational (linear) policy development 60, **61**, 67
receivers, health messages 89–90
Red Lotus model (Gregg & O'Hara) 175, **178**,
    179, **180**
religion 4, 171, 174, **175**
reproductive health *see* women's health
responsibility (for health) 5, 7, 19–20, 63
risks
    environmental and modifiable factors 6, 13
    literacy and perceptions 99–100, 103, 153
Roseto community (USA), heart attacks **33**
Russia, post-Soviet 18, 19, 33, 147

salutogenesis concept 8–9, 16, 38–39, 175
Scandinavia, use of salutogenic approach 9
schools
    evaluation of health in 109, 113
    health issues important to children 155–156
    healthy eating promotion 55, 88–89, 136
    improvement approaches 135
    quality and access to 2, 5
    as settings 108, 109, 111, 112, 113, 115
    style of education 83, **96**, 130–131
seatbelt legislation 59–60

sectors
    public administration 65–66, 72
    society/communal life 132, **132**
self-esteem
    links with empowerment 23
    measures, in obesity prevention 124
    and mental health 104
self-harming 155
senders, health messages 85–87
Senegal
    grandmother strategy **40**
    Totsan village empowerment programme **47**
Sense of Coherence (Antonovsky) 16, 39
settings for health promotion
    effectiveness concerns 141–142
        marginalized groups 112–113
        workplaces **110**, 111, 112, **113**
    prisons 109, 111, 114
    rationale and terms 108–110, **109**
    schools 108, 109, 111, 112, 113, 115
    transfer to local context 121
    variability of practice 110–112, **111**
sex workers, community empowerment **24**
sexual orientation 124, 158
sexually transmitted infections 93, 95
Shannon–Weaver model (communication) 80, **80**
skills
    for active citizenship 128–129
    communication 79, 85, 87
    evidence-based decision making 120–122, **121**, 123
    literacy 99–101
    needed by community organizers 49, **49**, **50**
    needed by health promoters 136, 138–141, 165
sleeping sickness 162–163
smoking
    COMMIT trial programme 133
    community self-help for quitting **35**, **43**
    health warning effectiveness 89–90
    reduction policies and legislation 55, **76**, 126
social capital
    concept interpretations and understanding 35–36, **37**
    criticisms and problems of application 36–37, **38**
    empirical evidence for links with health **32**, 36, 93
    mutual support and community ties 32–34, **33**
    networks, types in communities 34–35
    trust and shared norms 35
social determinants of health
    community aspects 32–35, 38–39, 44
    component factors 1, 3, 5, 9, **12**
    discourse analysis 147
    people's awareness of 169
    WHO Commission (CSDH) report 2–3, 165
social justice
    community action 23–24
    definition 1, 174–175
    windows of opportunity 68
    see also equity
social marketing 96–97, **97**
social model of health 7–8, **8**, 151, 157–158
social movements 70–71, 128–129, 146
social policy
    definition 58–59
    impacts on health 59, 60

socialism 41, 44, 58, **64**
socio-economic groups *see* class
spiritual health 173–174, **174**, **175**
Sri Lanka
 communication problems, safe
  drinking water 39
 life expectancy 13
stakeholders, categories in policy making 63
stereotyping
 in consumer culture and marketing 97
 of stigmatized groups 22
 tools for challenge of **50**
storytelling 49, **50**, 89
structural adjustment programmes (1980s) 44, 74
Sundsvall conference (1991) 11
supportive environments
 aspects and requirements 11, 110
 global access 10
 for peer education 92, 116
sustainability, environmental 160–161
symbols 28, 80, 175

taxation
 resources in poorer countries 130
 of unhealthy products 57, 59, 67, **126**
 for wealth redistribution 2, 35, 56
television 87, 91, 93
theatre 93
Theory of Planned Behaviour 104
third sector *see* non-governmental organizations
threshold concepts 6–9, 84
tobacco
 industry and smokers' rights lobby 68, **76**
 public policies on 11
top-down processes
 characteristics **135**
 communication of health messages 78, 80,
  82, 86
 education 84
 legislation **47**, 48, 132
 policy implementation 67, 132–136, **137**
Tostan, rural women's empowerment (Senegal) 47
tracking indicators, capacity building 164, **164**
traffic/car accidents 7, **45**, 59–60, 124
training
 community health workers 41, **41**, 43, 138
 Galway consensus on skills 138–140
 sustainability, in peer education 92
transactional analysis (Berne, 1964) 86, **86**
transport policies, health benefits 59–60, **60**
Transtheoretical Model (behaviour change) 102, 104
travellers, discrimination and health 22, 158
trust, radius of 35, **38**, 168
two-step flow model, mass media 91–92

UK
 community development support 50, 51
 Health Act 2007 (smoke-free legislation) 55, **76**
 health care reorganization **62**, 62–63, 150
 introduction of happiness indicators 16–17, 171
 offenders' health delivery plan 25–26

United Nations (UN)
 Meeting on Non-Communicable Diseases 6
 role in global governance 74, **75**
Universal Declaration of Human Rights 1
universities 144, 149, 163, 167–168
'upstream' thinking analogy 6–7, **7**, 118
USA
 Data for Decision-Making (DDM) project 122
 health care access 145
 health intervention trials 133
 life expectancy 13
 power of industrial sector 70
 usefulness of lay health workers 41–42

values *see* ethics
victim blaming 13, 37, 82
village empowerment programmes (VEPs) **47**
visual literacy 100
voluntarism (free choice) 23, 97, 125
Voluntary Health Association of India **133**
voluntary sector organizations 73, 167
volunteers, displacement of paid workers 43

waste management 130, **131**, 168, **168**
water
 boiled, for diarrhoea prevention
  (Sri Lanka) 39
 clean water supply 13, 59, 72, 149, 162
 fluorination 125
wealth distribution 1–2, 35, 56, 157, 180
well-being, elements of concept 17, **17**, 170–173
'wicked problems' 62
windows of opportunity (Kingdon) 68, 74–75, **76**
women's health
 active involvement of women 40, 46, 71,
  154–155
 female genital cutting 47, 125
 public policy aims 11
 reproductive
  Fankanta initiative 93–94
  Yuannan programme 24
 risks and vulnerability 13
 support for breast feeding 122
workplaces, health promotion in 110, 111,
 112, **113**
World Bank 44–45, 56, 74, **75**, 159
World Health Organization (WHO)
 concern for health equity ('Health for All') 2, **14**,
  54–55, 154
 Copenhagen discussion paper (1984) 9, 27
 definition of health (1946) 16, 171, 173–174
 Framework Convention on Tobacco Control
  (2005) 55
 Healthy Cities programme 22, 31, 113
 healthy eating guidelines 70
 support for settings approach 109
World Trade Organization (WTO) 56, **75**

Yuannan women's health programme 24